Dyslexia Association of Singapore
1 Jurong West Central 2,
#05-01, Jurong Point
Singapore 648886
www.das.org.sg
UEN: S91SS0096B

CLEARLY DIFFERENT

Dyscovering the Differences

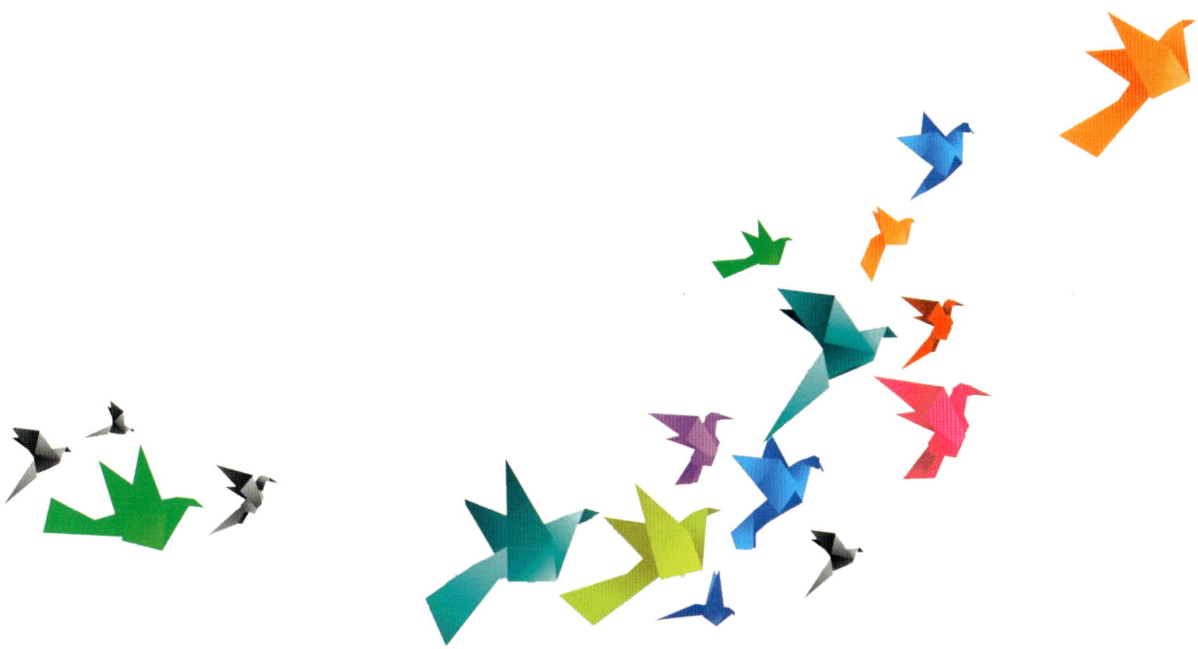

EDITORIAL NOTE

The views expressed in this book are those of the individual contributors, and do not necessarily represent the policy of the Dyslexia Association of Singapore (DAS). Whilst every effort has been made to ensure the accuracy of information provided, DAS cannot accept responsibility of the consequences of any errors or omissions in that information.

National Library Board, Singapore Cataloguing in Publication Data

Names: Wan, William, 1947- | Dyslexia Association of Singapore, issuing body.
Title: Clearly different : dyscovering the differences : 25 years of helping people with dyslexia achieve / William Wan.
Other titles: Clearly different : discovering the differences : twenty five years of helping people with dyslexia achieve
Description: Singapore : Dyslexia Association of Singapore ; World Scientific, 2017.
Identifiers: OCN 992725404 | 978-981-11-4108-9 (paperback) | 978-981-11-4107-2 (hardcover)
Subjects: Dyslexia Association of Singapore--History. | Dyslexics--Services for--Singapore--History. | Dyslexics--Singapore.
Classification: DDC 362.22095957--dc23

Published and Distributed by World Scientific, Singapore

Dyslexia Association of Singapore
1 Jurong West Central 2,
#05-01, Jurong Point
Singapore 648886
www.das.org.sg
UEN: S91SS0096B

DAS is a registered charity under the Charities Act, 1994. Registered Charity No.: 1155

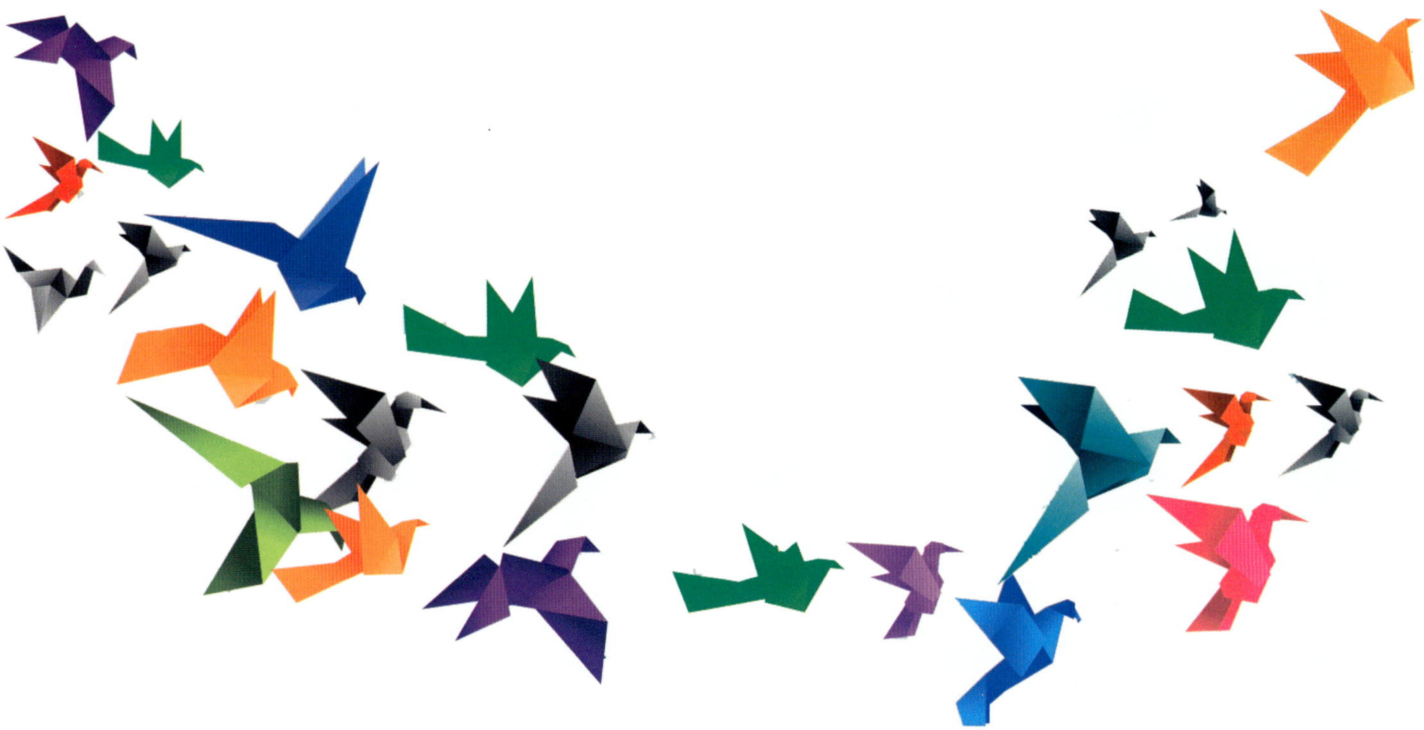

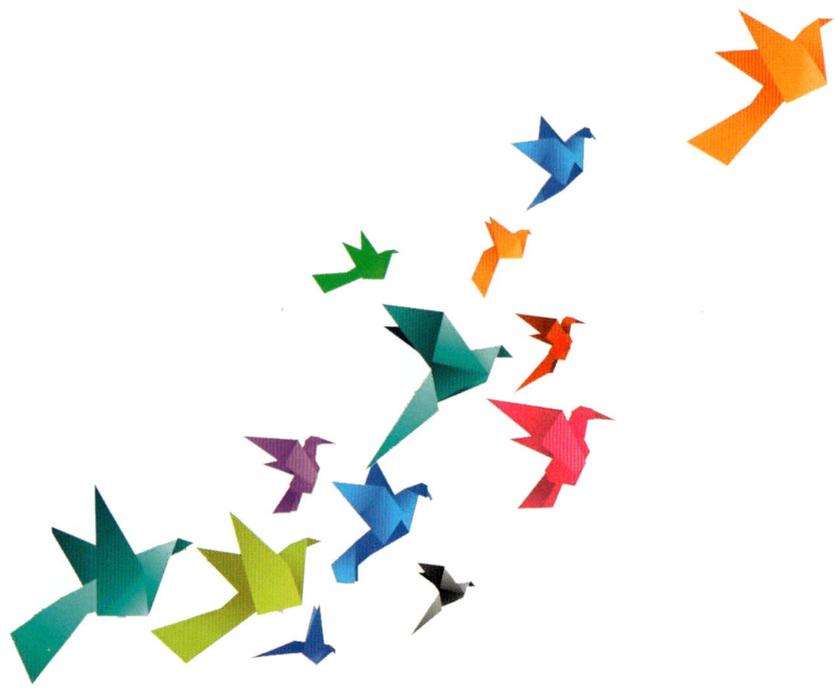

ACKNOWLEDGEMENTS

It has been a pleasure to work on this 25th Anniversary Book for the Dyslexia Association of Singapore (DAS). Not unlike any other book I have written, this work is possible only because of the collaboration of a good number of wonderful people for whom I am much indebted. My research assistant, Ms Bernice Lee, fully supported by Mrs Deborah Hewes and her Publicity and Publications team at DAS, interviewed the pioneers, the beneficiaries of DAS and their parents who co-operated enthusiastically.

I would also like to thank the staff at DAS who helped to compile the DAS history, through photographs and publications. Special mention to long-term employees, Mrs Kharyati Kamsani and Mrs Tey Ching Ching, whose institutional memory helped with the naming of individuals in the historical photos and the verification of important DAS events.

Finally, I would like to thank Mr K. Kesavapany, the Executive Committee Member of DAS, and Mr Lee Siang, DAS CEO, who supported this project in every way.

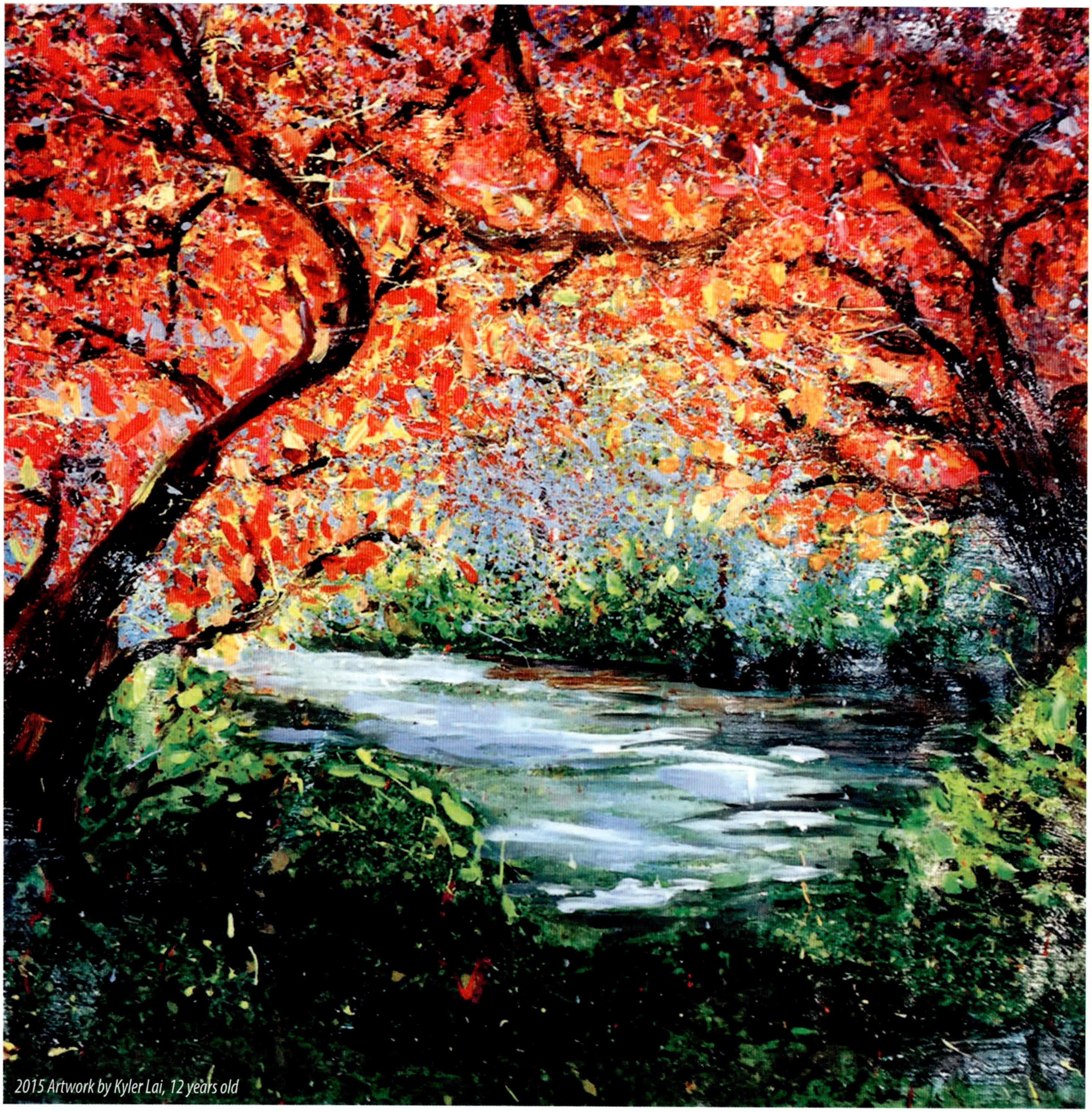

2015 Artwork by Kyler Lai, 12 years old

CLEARLY DIFFERENT

Dyscovering the Differences

William Wan

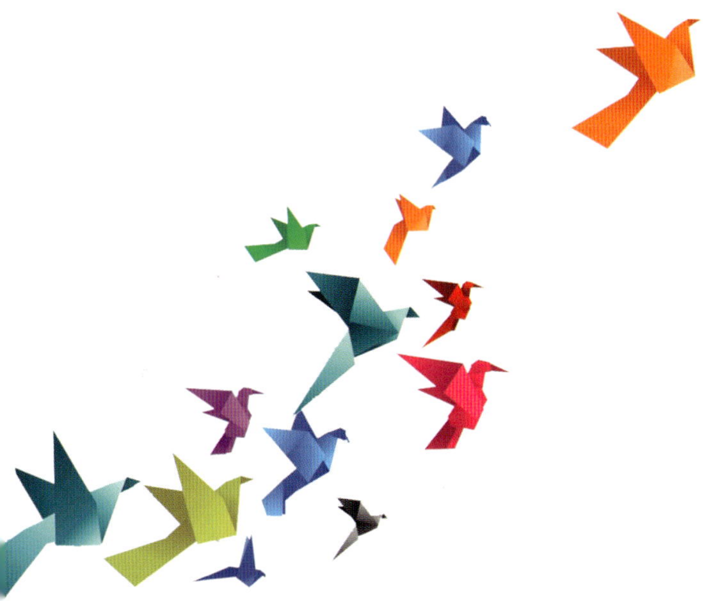

25 years of helping people with dyslexia achieve

World Scientific

DYSLEXIA ASSOCIATION DAS OF SINGAPORE

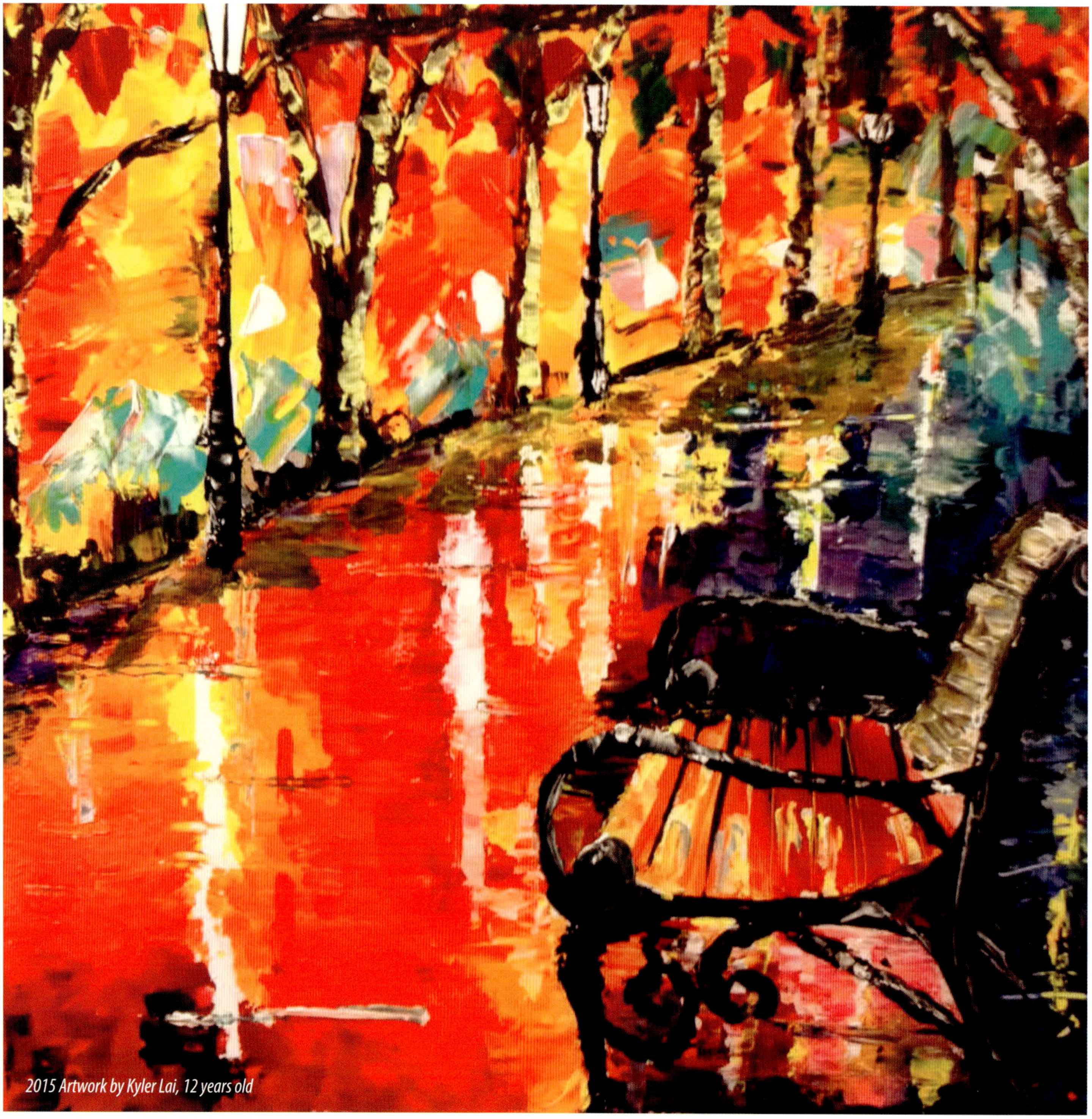
2015 Artwork by Kyler Lai, 12 years old

CLEARLY DIFFERENT

Dyscovering the Differences

CONTENTS

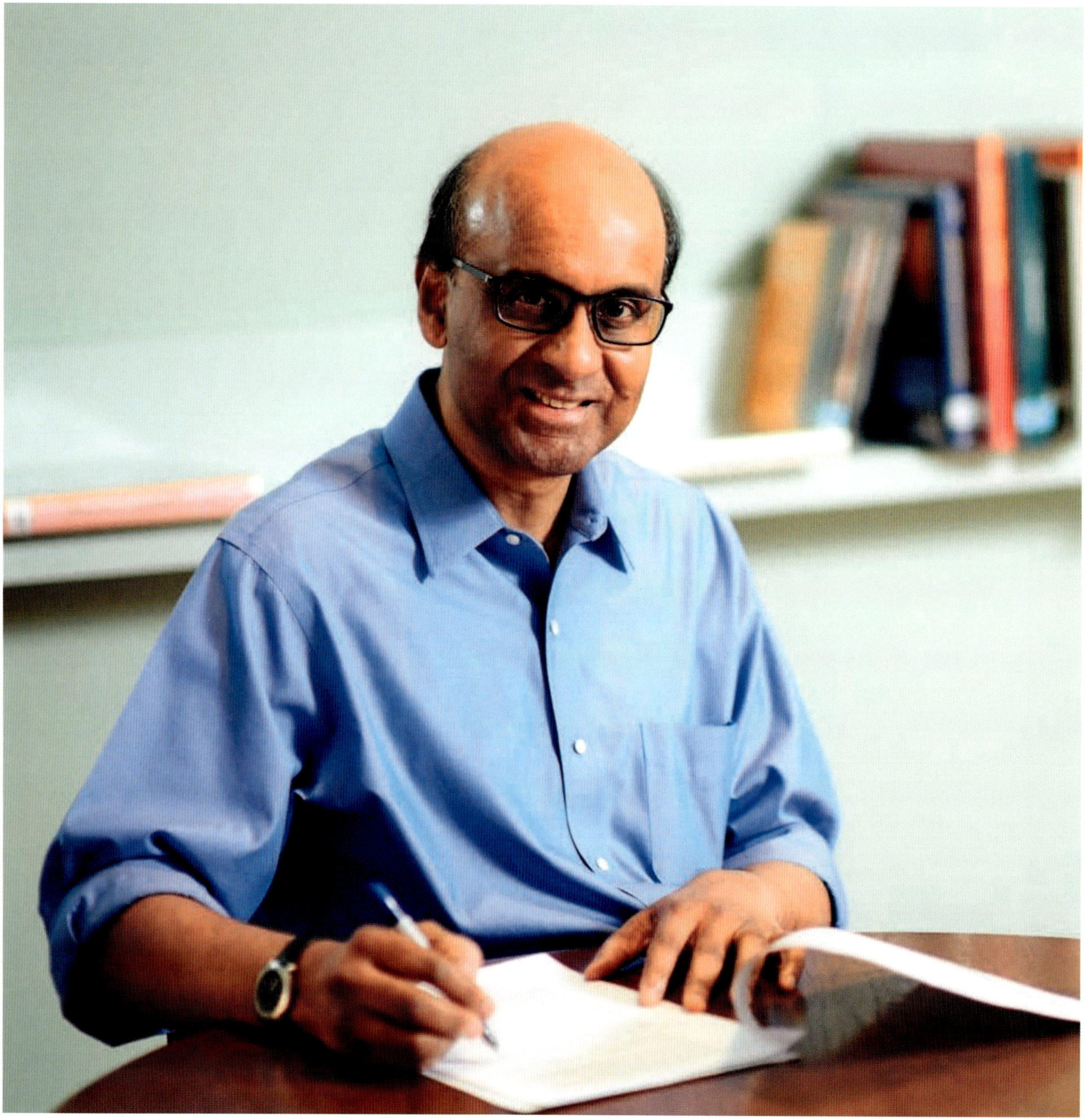

FOREWORD

Tharman Shanmugaratnam

Deputy Prime Minister and Coordinating Minister for Social and Economic Policies

My heartiest commendations to the Dyslexia Association of Singapore (DAS) for your commitment and efforts in aiding an important group of children with special needs over the last 25 years. DAS has from inception been a wonderful reflection of civic action in support of an inclusive society. Your belief that no child should be left behind because of his or her learning difficulty has led to thousands of children being helped over the years.

It has been my privilege to witness the passion and energy of the individuals behind the cause. When I visited DAS in 2004, I was impressed by your network of learning centres across Singapore offering assessment and diagnostic services, a growing team of educational therapists, speech and language therapists and specialist psychologists, and a dedicated professional training team. In 2006, I saw the strengthening of early intervention through your preschool programme, and in 2012, when I attended your 21st Anniversary celebrations, the initiation of your efforts to help children with Chinese dyslexia.

We were all saddened by the passing of the founding President of DAS, Dr Jimmy Daruwalla, in July 2016. I am confident that DAS will under its new leadership team build on all you have achieved and continue to help every individual discover their potential and realise their aspirations.

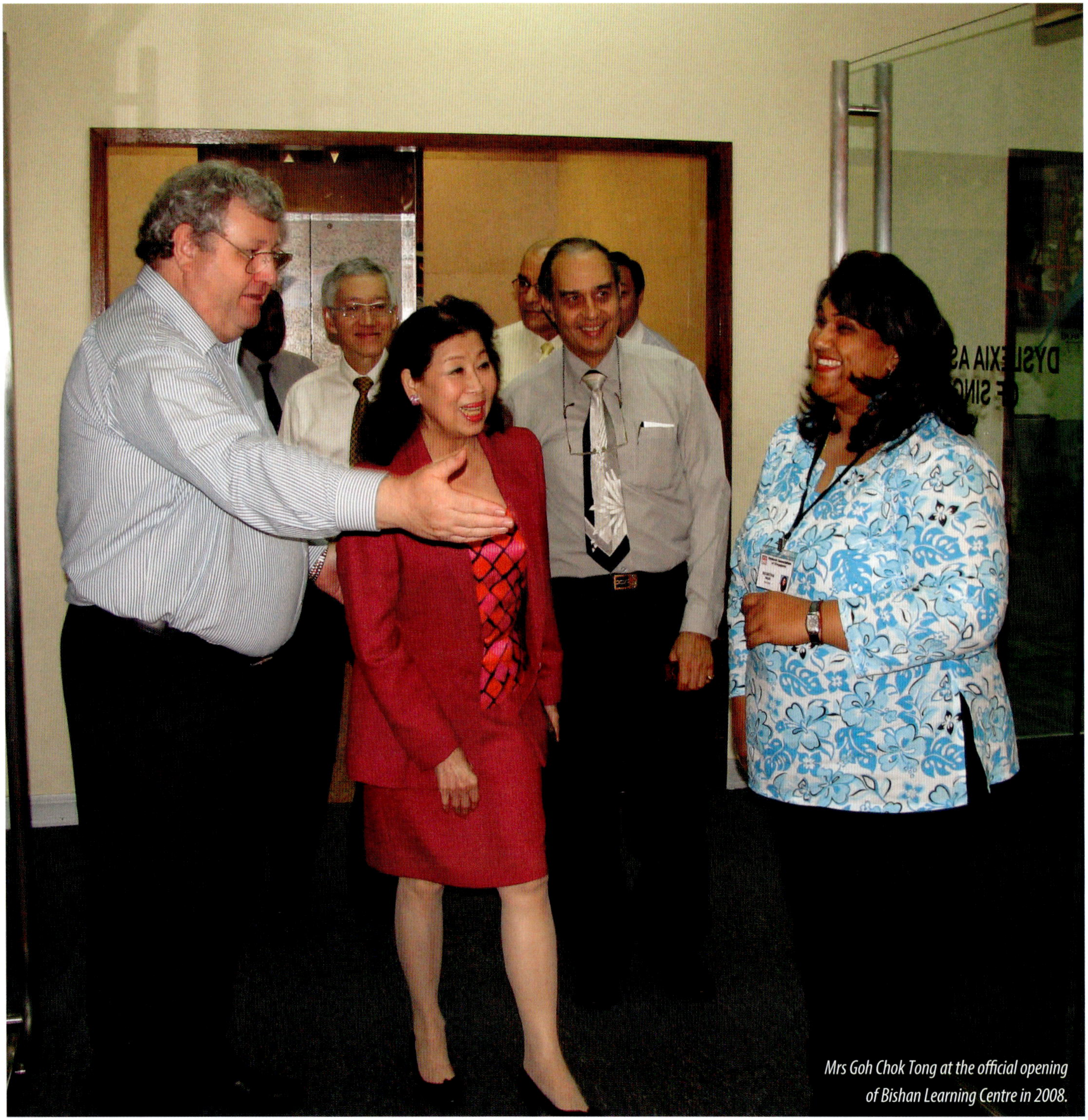

Mrs Goh Chok Tong at the official opening of Bishan Learning Centre in 2008.

MESSAGE FROM DAS PATRON
Mrs Goh Chok Tong

No one likes to stand out for reasons that they don't comprehend. One can only imagine the enormity of frustrations endured by people with dyslexia in Singapore many years back, when it was rarely talked about openly. But DAS has turned the situation around quite significantly over the past 25 years. It has been no easy task. I compliment DAS for moving from strength to strength, expanding from a humble single-service set-up to a dynamic one-stop centre offering not just educational therapy, but psychological assessments, training for parents and teachers ,and an array of other services.

In my years as the patron of DAS, I have looked forward to attending every activity – especially the annual graduation ceremonies. It is a profound joy to see DAS students beam with confidence and their parents with unbridled pride. Each cohort unleashes inspiring anecdotes characterised by courage, determination and love. Supporting people with dyslexia is an imperative endeavour. I am deeply grateful to the brilliant individuals and organisations for answering my calls to support DAS with generosity and passion. Each of you is like a beacon of light that has helped so many children with dyslexia cast their shadows behind them and march towards a brighter future. You have given them the precious opportunity to realise their full potential.

It has been a great privilege for me to be involved in an enterprise as valuable as DAS, and be part of a journey that transforms perplexity to illumination, from being awkwardly different to being clearly special. I urge everyone to embrace dyslexia and to help DAS to grow even bigger and stronger, for the benefit of those with dyslexia.

The inconceivable good that DAS has done is a collective effort of its Executive Committee, its staff and its supporters. But one man who has played an inimitable role is the late Dr Jimmy Daruwalla. His passion and vision have not only founded DAS but lifted the organisation to one great height after another. I believe that DAS will carry his baton and race forward with similar resolve and fervour.

Being clearly different is not a label for inadequacy or a passport to idleness. It is a badge of honour and an opening to making positive differences in the world. I wish DAS, its partners and all with dyslexia a rewarding journey of discovery ahead.

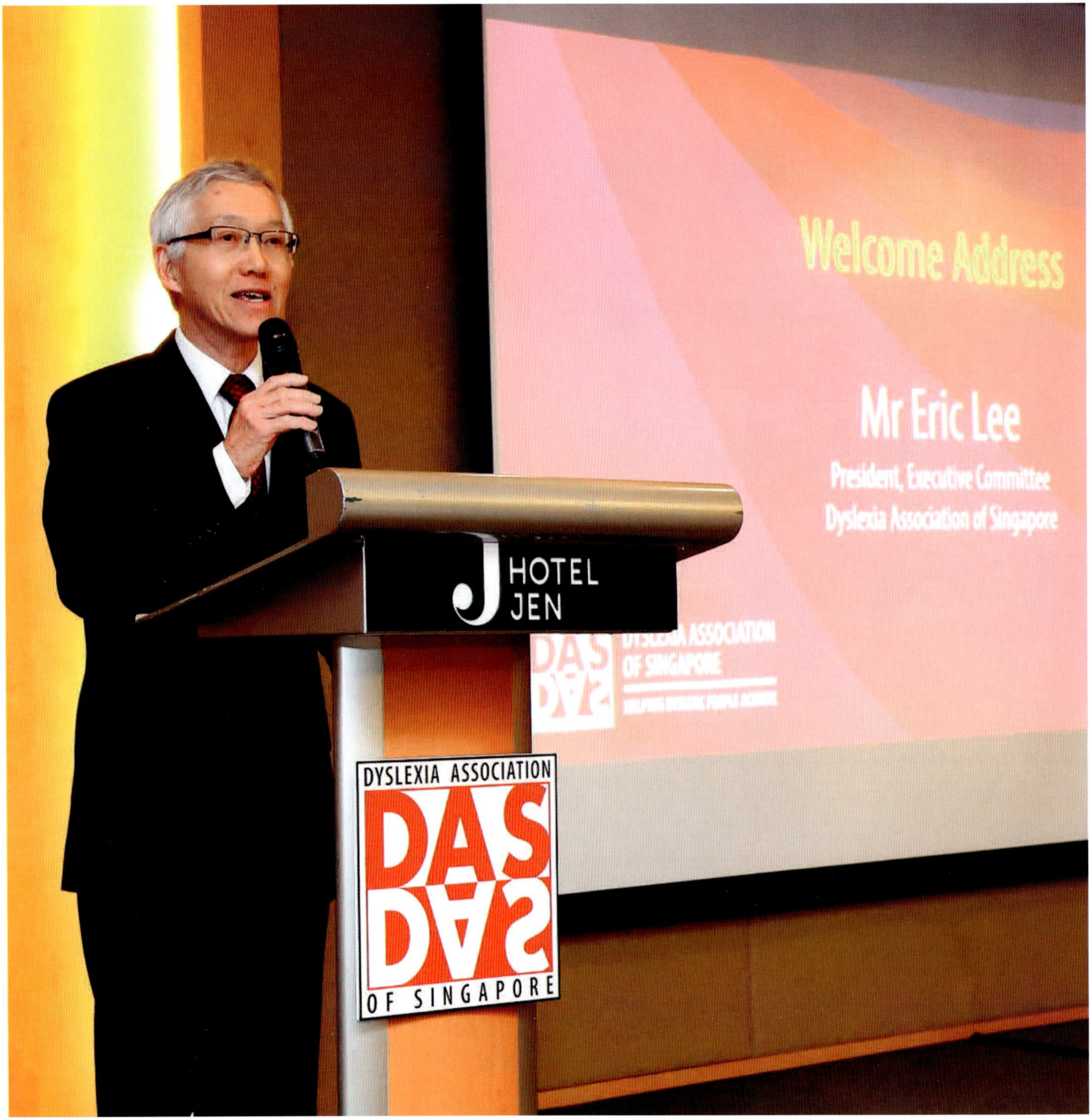

Welcome Address
Mr Eric Lee
President, Executive Committee
Dyslexia Association of Singapore
HOTEL
JEN
DYSLEXIA ASSOCIATION
OF SINGAPORE
DYSLEXIA ASSOCIATION
DAS
DAS
OF SINGAPORE

MESSAGE FROM DAS PRESIDENT
Mr Eric Lee

For an average person, facing challenges in a world that is designed for the majority is often an uphill yet manageable climb. But for people with dyslexia, dealing with these challenges can sometimes be insurmountable and overwhelming. While commonly misunderstood, countless people with dyslexia have proven to the world that it is not a disability, but a different kind of gift.

At DAS, we have spent the last 25 years attempting to unravel the world of differences that dyslexics face. From a small community service project led by our Founding President, the late Dr Jimmy Daruwalla in 1989, DAS has made great advances to become a significant charitable organisation with 13 learning centres across Singapore. It serves more than 3,500 students from preschools, primary and secondary schools, supported by a highly qualified, trained and dedicated group of 240 professional and support staff. For the thousands of students who have passed through our doors and graduated as confident individuals, we know that they will in turn become inspiring role models to others. In their own different ways, many of them have shown us the unique ways in which dyslexics think and perform. Instead of being consigned to a box that is often created for dyslexics, DAS works to unleash the varied ways in which dyslexics can contribute to Singapore and the world.

While we have come a long way in terms of providing identification and early intervention for dyslexics, the reality is that we are only scratching the surface. With many more dyslexic students in Singapore still requiring help, DAS will persevere not only to create greater awareness about dyslexia, but expanding and enhancing our efforts to provide more dyslexic individuals of all ages with greater support.

I am very grateful to Dr William Wan, ably assisted by Ms Bernice Lee, for putting together this outstanding book to celebrate the 25th anniversary of DAS. "Clearly Different: Dyscovering the Differences" reflects the paradigm shift DAS is influencing the way Singaporeans view dyslexia. We need to move ahead, not just as an inclusive society that is accepting, but one that truly acknowledges and helps each dyslexic individual achieve their full but often hidden potential. Let us continue to celebrate the successes of people with dyslexia, no matter how big or small, and just like how dyslexics try to understand the world made for the majority, perhaps the majority can attempt to view the "different" world through the eyes of dyslexics.

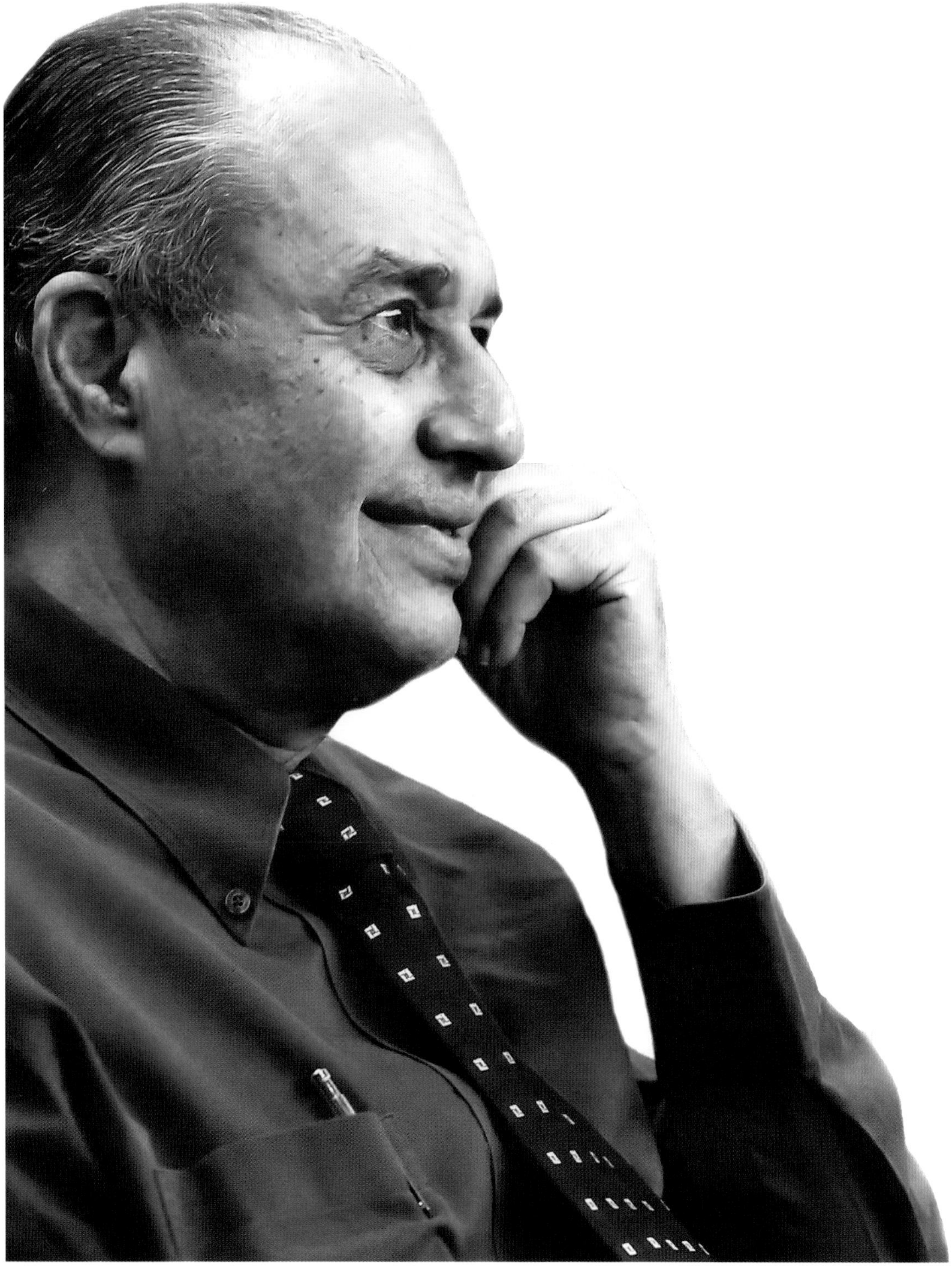

HUMILITY AND GREATNESS

Dr Jimmy S. Daruwalla

You cannot do a kindness too soon, for you never know how soon it will be too late.

Ralph Waldo Emerson

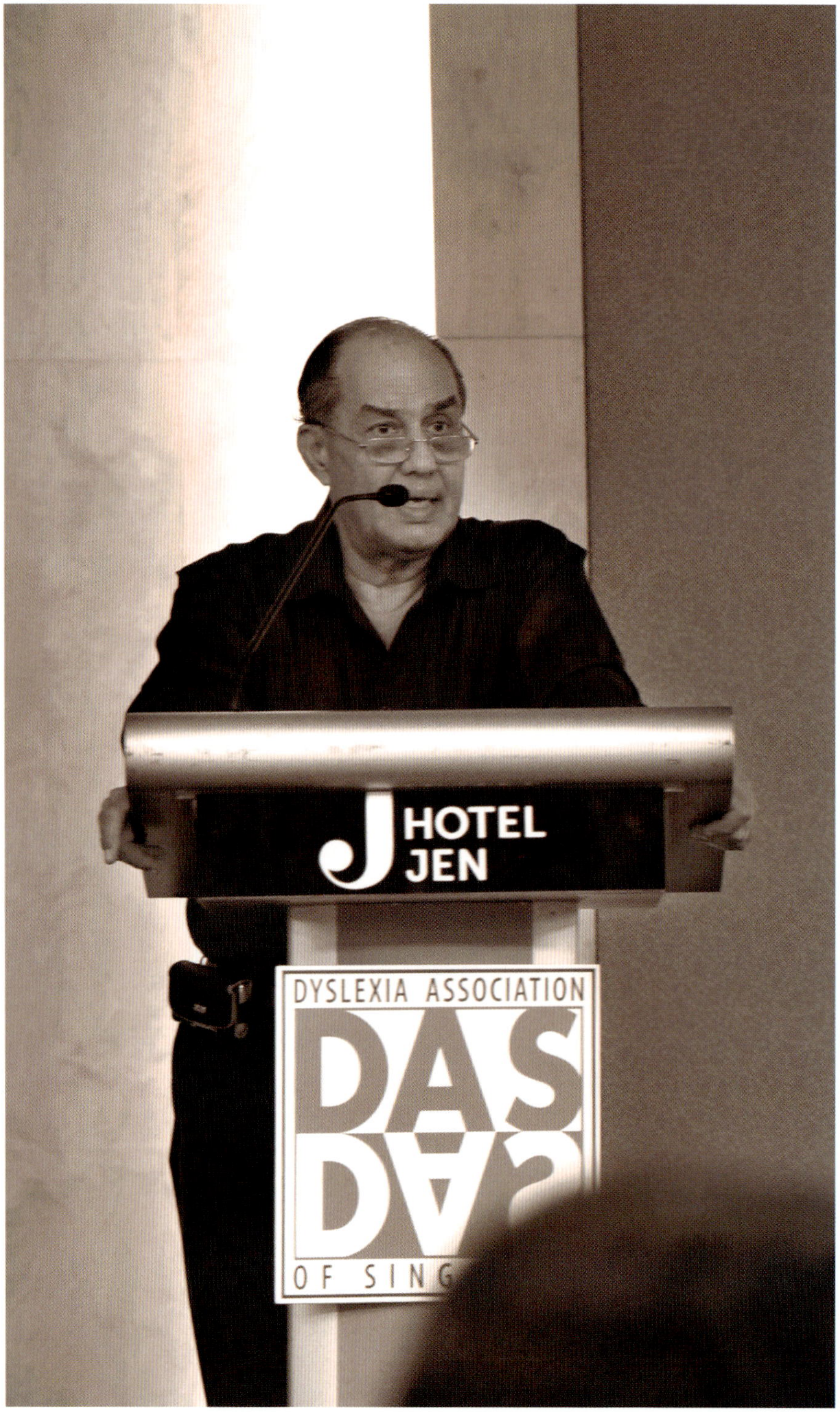

CONTINUING A LEGACY

The innate kindness of Dr Jimmy S. Daruwalla spurred him to action. And because he heeded the call, tremendous changes were effected. Generations of dyslexics have grown up finding the help they needed to overcome their challenges because Dr Daruwalla cared and championed their cause. His vision is encapsulated in his speech given at the "Embrace Dyslexia" Dinner in 2014 when he was the President.

We hope to change the way Singaporeans look at dyslexia and highlight the potential hidden and extraordinary assets of someone with a learning difference.

Dr Jimmy Daruwalla, 2014

An orthopaedic surgeon by training, Mumbai-born Dr Daruwalla learnt early on from his father's example to be compassionate and caring — to share one's success by giving back to society so that the less fortunate can be helped. This character trait has been the motivational force for all that Dr Daruwalla has achieved in his career and community service.

He found a soulmate in his first wife, Roshen, who also had a soft spot for the underprivileged and who, as a member of the Lion's Club, regularly prepared food for residents of an old folks' home. From her example, he began to volunteer at the Spastic Children's Association of Singapore and the Red Cross Home for the Disabled.

Having lived in Singapore for 35 years, he felt that it was only right to do something for society, and so he joined the Rotary Club of Raffles City. Soon after, he was asked by his Rotary Club President, Mr George Abraham, to be the Director of Community Services. More specifically, to head up a project for dyslexia. He agreed, on the understanding that it would be a one-year commitment.

It didn't take much for Dr Daruwalla to be hooked. The one year turned into two and, with a growing realisation of how great the needs were, it wasn't long before a more organised association was mooted to help address the issues. The natural choice for president was Dr Daruwalla.

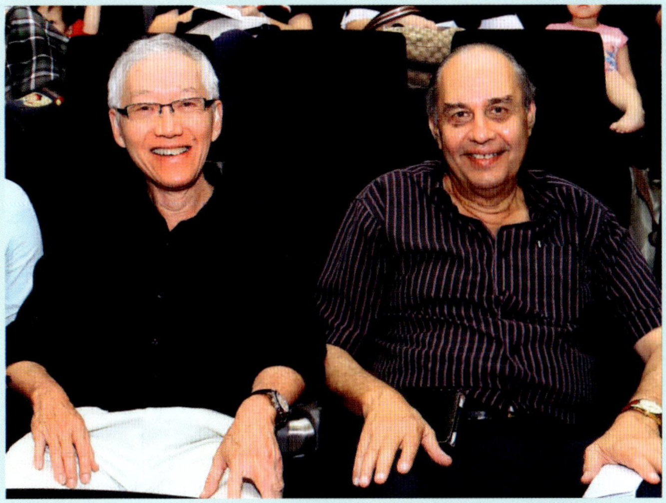

The interest and wellbeing of DAS, its goals, the management, the staff, the parents, the children, were constantly on Jimmy's mind. He took a very strong interest in every aspect of the organisation and shared with us in the Executive Committee his innermost thoughts, frustrations and visions of what the DAS could achieve.

Mr Eric Lee
DAS President
"Dr Daruwalla's Legacy"
FACETS, Apr–Jun 2016

Although he was a successful and sought-after surgeon by then, his quiet nature meant that while he willingly donated his time and effort, he was always conscious of the fact that he lacked the connections to deep pockets. His humility was to prove disarming time and again.

Financial help came from the most unexpected places, often as a result of some kind gesture on his or his wife's part. But, once the word went out among their friends and acquaintances, the funds began to come in and by 1993, the DAS was able to employ its first expat teacher.

In spite of constant frustrations over finances, staffing and bureaucratic challenges in the early days, his heart for the children and their challenges never wavered. His was a pure altruism. He had no family members grappling with dyslexia so he did not take on the responsibility for personal gain. The joy of seeing lives changed for the better was reward enough. He was unflagging in his attempts to set up a specialist school for dyslexics, and met with minister after minister to further this dream.

In 2011, the Indian community and the *Tabla!* weekly newspaper honoured him with an award to recognise his 20 years of public service as president of the Dyslexia Association of Singapore. Even then, in his acceptance speech, he was self-effacing, giving several reasons for declining the award.

Indeed, it was not a solo effort and Dr Daruwalla credited many who had played pivotal roles in the development of DAS. But he saved the best for last, and acknowledged the two women who had been serving alongside him right from the inception of the association — his first wife

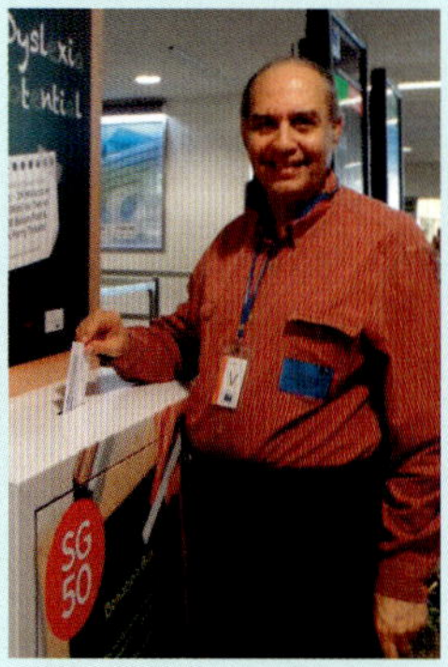

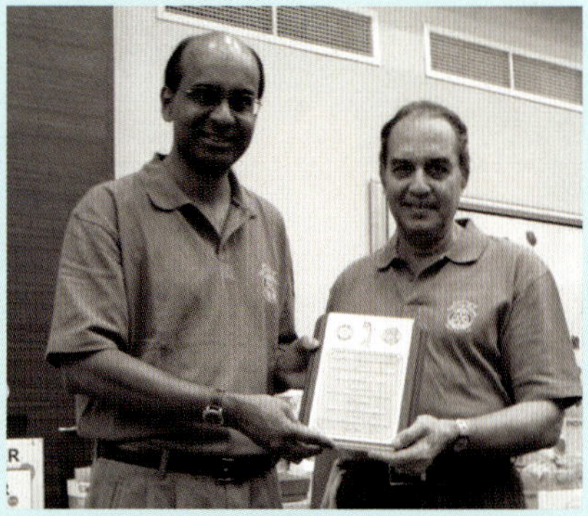

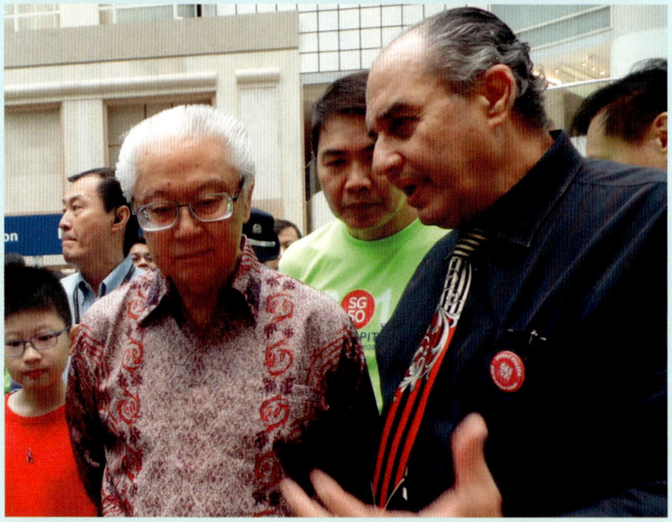

I never knew him to refuse a request for help. Jimmy's networking skills were quite incredible and I lost count of the number of times he contacted me to say he had met yet another person who could help the DAS in some way or other. Jimmy was one of a small number of people of whom it could truly be said that he left this world a better place than he found it.

Mr Robin Moseley
Retired DAS CEO (2002–2014),
"The Success of the DAS"
FACETS, Apr–Jun 2016

I am not a person who enjoys publicity. In fact, I prefer to keep a low profile... There are many more deserving candidates than myself... More importantly, there are many persons who had contributed to the success of DAS and it was not a solo effort.

Dr Jimmy Daruwalla, 2011

Roshen and, later after Roshen's passing, his second wife Jothy, who to this day continues to provide sterling support for the vision of DAS.

His original one-year commitment stretched to 25 vital years of nurturing a dedicated team of staff and volunteers who now run DAS' 13 learning centres and a training academy.

Unfortunately, his untimely death, almost exactly two weeks after my research assistant, Bernice, and I interviewed him for this book, robbed us of a fervent crusader for this cause. But his legacy will endure in the lives he has touched and will continue to touch through the memorial fund that has been started in his name to help further the cause of dyslexia he so passionately championed. He often quoted the London Cass Business School Study which found that 30% of successful entrepreneurs identified themselves as dyslexic. They developed out-of-the-box thinking and true grit from a young age because of their dyslexia. Dr Daruwalla therefore strongly believed that dyslexia can be an asset and that people with dyslexia can achieve great things in life.

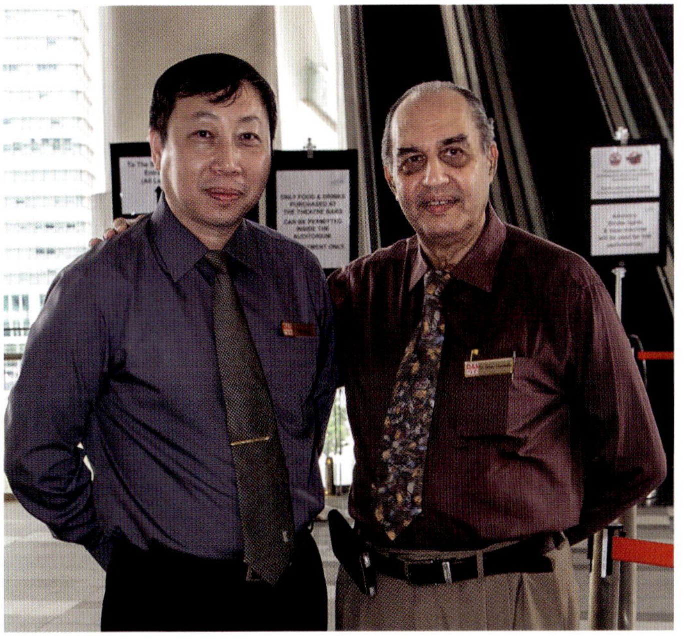

This is one of the most important things we must continue in order to carry on Dr Daruwalla's legacy. This is an area that DAS must continue to emphasise, that dyslexia is an asset, that dyslexics have great strengths, that we can help them achieve and that we must help them to embrace their dyslexia.

Mr Lee Siang
Chief Executive Officer,
"A Fatherly Figure, an Unstinting Supporter, A Unifier and a True Believer"
FACETS, Apr–Jun 2016

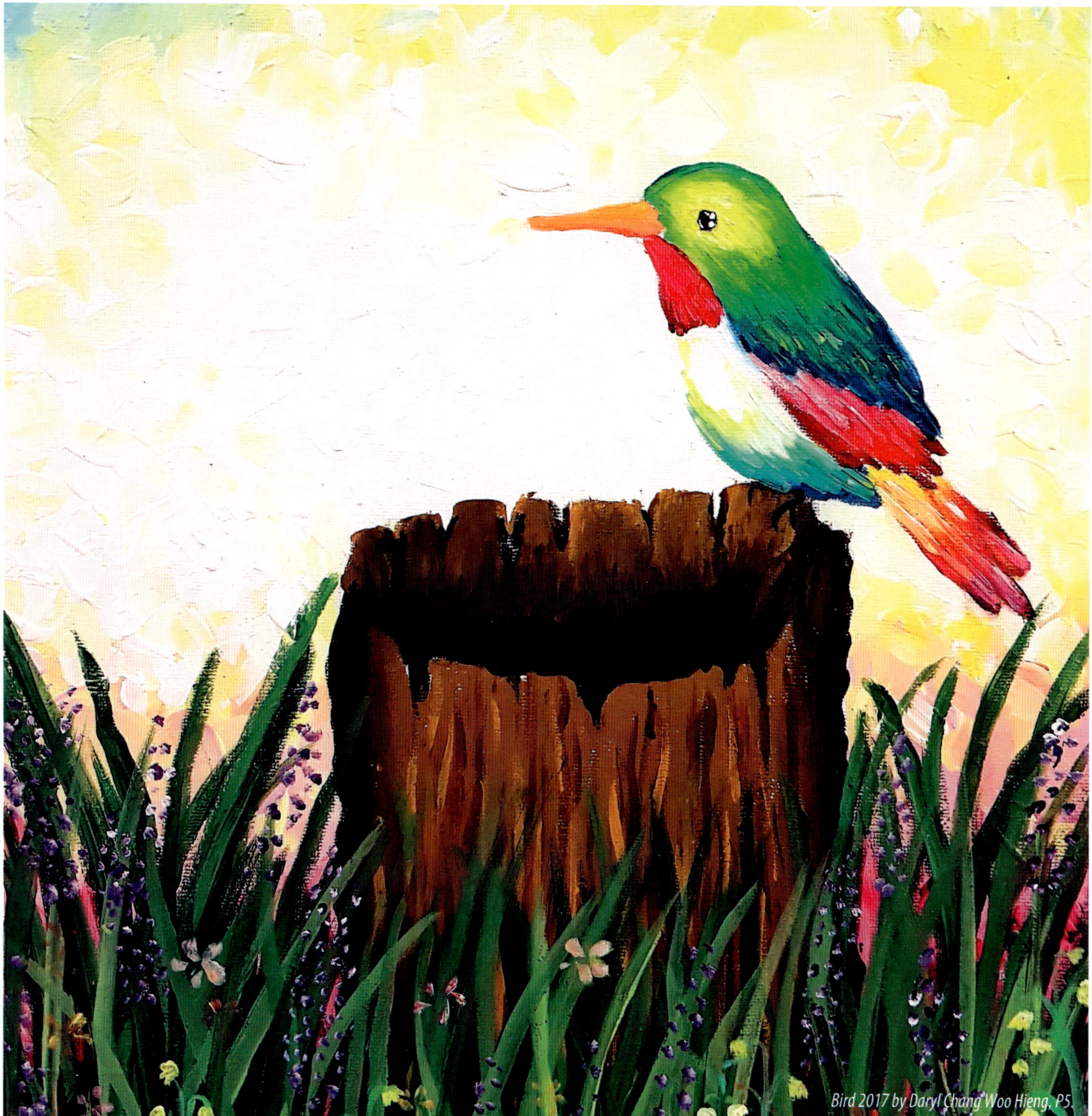

Bird 2017 by Daryl Chang Woo Hieng, P5.

INTRODUCTION

William Wan

Do what you can,
with what you have,
where you are.

Theodore Roosevelt

IN THE COMPANY OF KINDNESS AND COMPASSION

Former US President, Theodore Roosevelt, is oft-quoted to have said, "Do what you can, with what you have, where you are." This aphorism sums up the practical principles that drove the pioneers of the Dyslexia Association of Singapore (DAS). This book chronicles the inspiring journey that began 25 years ago in discovering the learning differences of the dyslexic community.

The prime movers behind this organisation chose to do what they could, with what they had, within the society that they found themselves in. Very little was known about dyslexia in Singapore in 1991, but these intrepid men saw a way to make a difference in the community.

And what a huge difference they did make!
As a fellow member of the Rotary Club of Raffles City, I count myself privileged to be in the company of these giants of kindness and compassion. As General-Secretary of the Singapore Kindness Movement, I applaud them for their generosity in contributing their time, talent and treasure, selflessly seeking only to improve the lives of dyslexics through early intervention and remediation. Their dogged commitment to increasing awareness of dyslexia has brought this learning difference into the light… in more ways than one. There is now a light at the end of the tunnel for many who struggle with dyslexia. By highlighting the many well-known personalities who have learned to cope with their challenges and even to thrive, DAS has thrown a positive spotlight on discovering and celebrating the differences that give dyslexics a creative edge.

When I was asked to write this book, I demurred, not because I don't believe in what DAS has achieved, but because I was afraid I could not do it justice. However, with the same determination that they harness to serve the dyslexic community, they were unrelenting in pursuing me to tell their story.

I am thankful for their confidence and glad for the opportunity of a ringside view to what this group of big-hearted, humble, and very giving people have done, not just for Singapore but for the wider world community of very special people as well. It is an honour to chronicle what they have done, with what they had, where they were.

I am also thankful for my own personal enlightenment in writing this book. I found to my horror that these extraordinary, kind and sensitive people are often discriminated against by many of us just because they are different from us in the way they recognise and interpret information through the senses of sight and sound more than through written words. Standard written tests and filling of forms overwhelm them as they experience high levels of stress and anxiety because their brains process information differently.

Dyslexia is much more than just having difficulty reading, writing, and using numbers. Dyslexics see the world in a completely different way, communicate differently, and have trouble organising things. It is a lifestyle challenge because it affects almost all aspects of their lives.

There is no doubt about their high intelligence. Physiologically, the left hemisphere of a dyslexic's brain is the same size as that of non-dyslexics, but the right hemisphere is about 10% larger. The left hemisphere controls the reading function but dyslexics are wired differently. The corpus callosum or the bridge of tissue between the two sides of the brain doesn't always direct information to the correct place for processing, resulting in the underutilisation of the reading side of the brain.

The right side of their brain is super active. One can even argue that dyslexia is a form of giftedness, as the right side of the brain empowers them to see things from many different angles all at once. It is a special talent but our pedagogy does not help them make sense of all those multiple perspectives.

Because they see so many different perspectives at once, they often appear incoherent and confused. The ideas they propose seem weird as they lack the

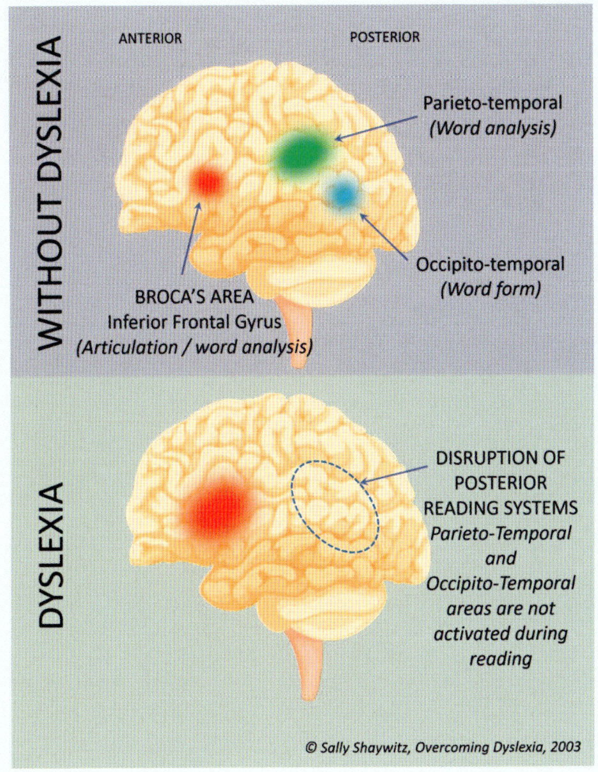

NEURAL SYSTEMS FOR READING IN THE BRAIN'S LEFT HEMISPHERE.

An anterior system in the region of the inferior frontal gyrus (Broca's area) is believed to serve articulation and word analysis. A system in the parieto-temporal region is believed to serve word analysis, and a second in the occipito-temporal region (termed the word-form area) is believed to be responsible for the rapid, automatic, fluent identification of words.

© Sally E. Shaywitz, Overcoming Dyslexia 2003

ability to check if their thoughts are suitable for conversation. Some of their ideas are wildly creative, partly because they're not constrained by the laws of physics or mathematical logic because they think in pictures. They see so many possibilities that their thoughts can become garbled and distorted. They have difficulties sorting through all that information and sifting through what's important or appropriate.

Without the ability to organise their thoughts, this special gift becomes a tragic, confusing disability especially in their social interactions. Their thoughts are often so real to them that they may fully believe that they have told you something they have not or that you have not told them something you have.

They can exhibit autism-like behaviour because they're often unaware of social rules. They do not always recognise social cues, body language or facial expressions; and tend to interrupt or ramble because their minds are flooded with so many different perspectives and ideas all at once.

Because so little was known about their special condition, many were not properly diagnosed, resulting in their suffering abuses in school for not "catching on". Inevitably, many struggled with low self-esteem and very negative feelings towards education. It is so ironic because they have brilliant minds, but they have difficulties focusing and prioritising because the mainstream educational system is not designed to cater to the way they process information.

People with dyslexia are extremely creative people. They have great strength and are often very good at reading others. They usually have fantastic memories, are often good at spoken language, and frequently spatially talented. They are highly intelligent and intuitive, with vivid imaginations and can be incredibly successful.

Some of the contemporary famous dyslexics include Sir Richard Branson, Charles Schwab, Steven Spielberg, Anderson Cooper, Whoopi Goldberg, Jay Leno, Henry Winkler, Danny Glover and Tommy Hilfiger. Famous artists Leonardo da Vinci, Andy Warhol, and Pablo Picasso; and famous authors like Hans Christian Anderson, Scott Adams, Agatha Christie, F. Scott Fitzgerald and Fannie Flagg; and iconic leaders like George Washington and Henry Ford were dyslexic.

Dyslexic Nobel prize-winning scientists include Carole Grieder and Baruj Benacerraf. Not forgetting that our own Lee Kuan Yew, the founding Prime Minister, was mildly dyslexic.

My hope is that this little book will not only help celebrate the 25th Anniversary of DAS, but that it will help its readers to see that people with dyslexia are clearly different in the way their minds function.

That they are clearly different does not make them in any way inferior. On the contrary, that they are clearly different often means that they have to strenuously swim against the tide to get to where they desire to go. And we must surely be inspired when many do get there, and achieve their potential and beyond. They are, in fact, more resilient than most of us, and to that extent, more superior.

As Sally Shaywitz, MD, the co-director of Yale Center for Dyslexia and Creativity, has summed it up so eloquently, "Dyslexics think differently. They are intuitive and excel at problem solving, seeing the big picture, and simplifying. They feast on visualising, abstract thinking, and thinking out of the box. They are poor rote reciters but inspired visionaries. Adult dyslexics are tough: Having struggled, they are used to adversity; hard work and perseverance now come naturally. Having experienced failure, they are fearless, undaunted by setbacks. Repetition and practice are a way of life. Each person I've focused on was rescued by a special person - a parent or a teacher - who saw the raw talent and nurtured it in the midst of all the naysayers. Yes, the symptoms of dyslexia persist, but they needn't interfere with success."

Dr William Wan, JP, PhD.
General Secretary,
Singapore Kindness Movement

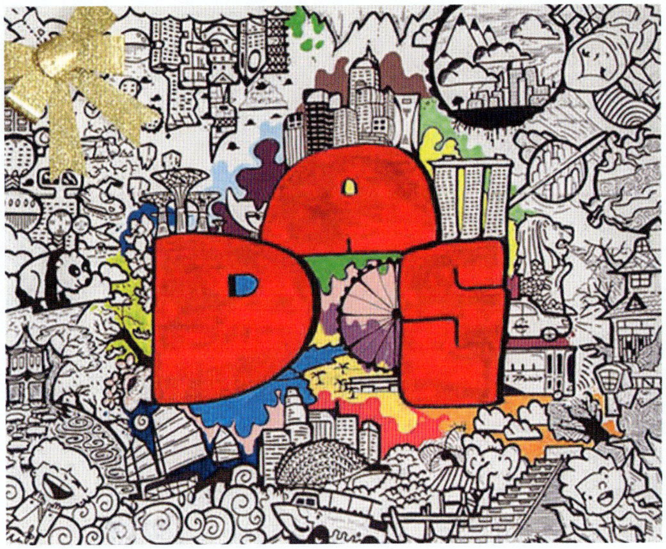

"DAS" Artwork by William Choo, 16, was created for the Student Graduation 2015. This artwork was presented to Associate Professor Muhammad Faishal Ibrahim.

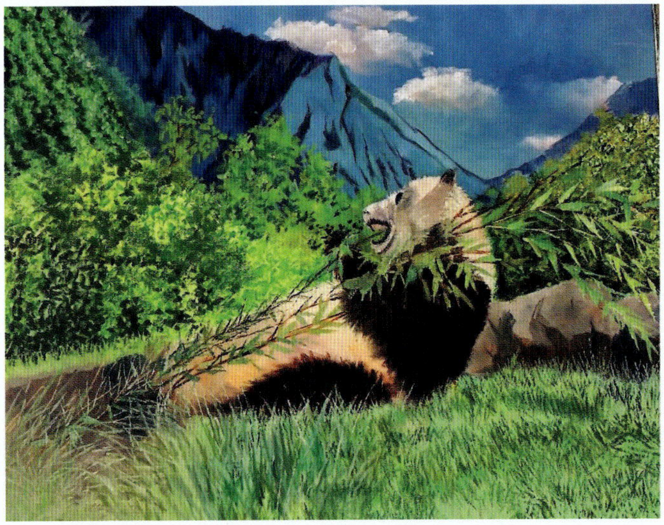

"The Spirit of the Panda" by Yue Jia Xuan, 13, was created for the Student Graduation 2015. The artwork was presented to Mrs Goh Chok Tong, DAS Patron

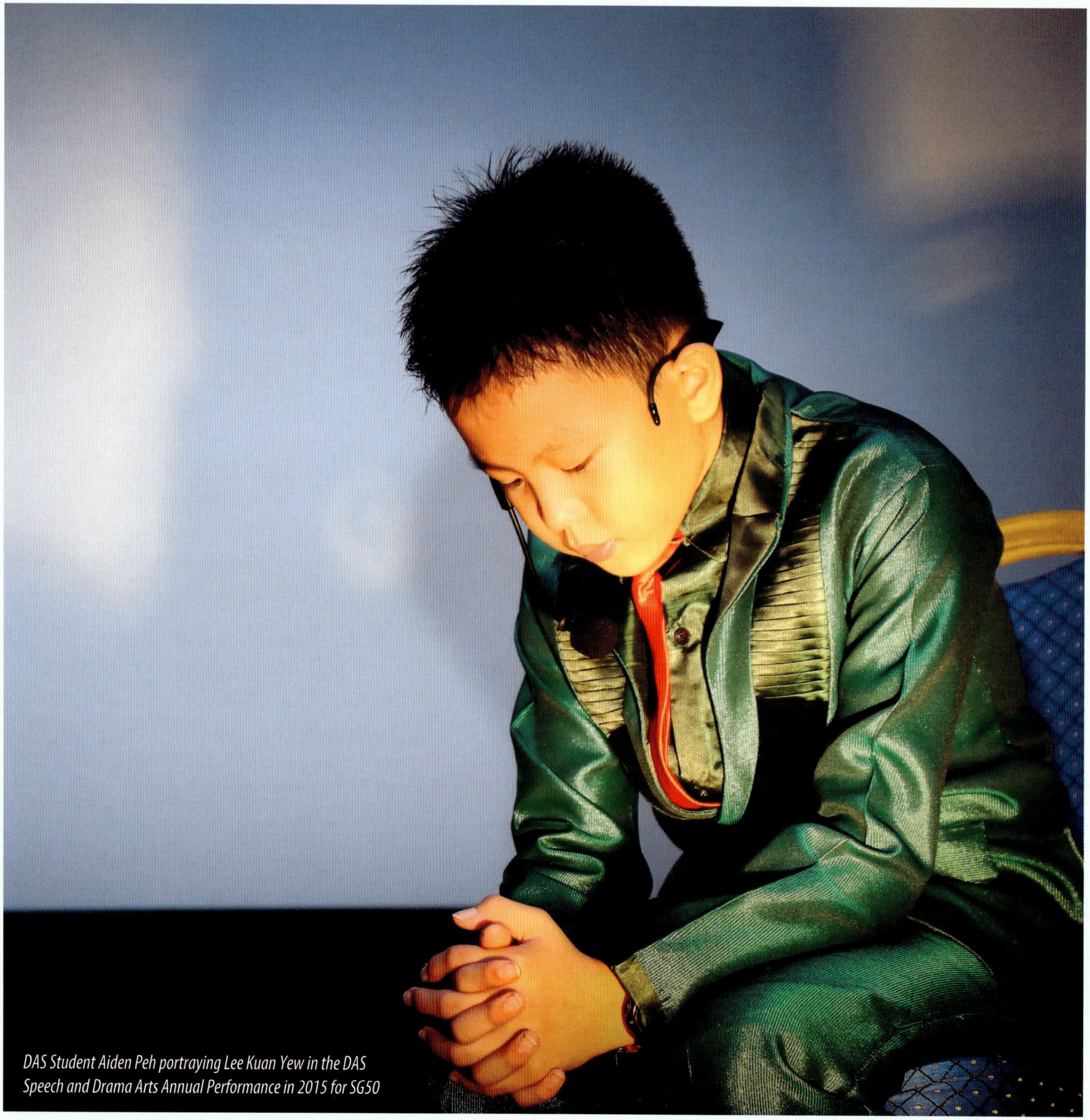

DAS Student Aiden Peh portraying Lee Kuan Yew in the DAS Speech and Drama Arts Annual Performance in 2015 for SG50

1

EMBRACING A DIFFERENT KIND OF MIND

It is more common than you can imagine. You are not alone. And while you will have this the rest of your life, you can dart between the raindrops to get where you want to go and it will not hold you back.

Steven Spielberg

THE DAS JOURNEY BEGINS

The story of the Dyslexia Association of Singapore (DAS) is one of courage and community — from the courage of those who took the first steps to address the challenges, to the courage of the ones grappling with dyslexia, to that of those who now pioneer diagnostic tools and early interventions that change the landscape of education for dyslexics.

Like the sun's rays that pierce through the mist to provide clarity, the different members of the DAS community contribute towards blazing the way forward for dyslexics and their families.

The story of the DAS begins with a vignette set in a community of friends. The "Jalan Kasau Bunch" was made up of the children of the Kwok, Khoo and Abraham families. They shared their toys, their meals and their lives. One of the young boys, Erin Khoo, was a bright little chap who found himself doing so badly in primary 1 and 2 that he developed an intense dislike for school. His difficulties with reading and the resultant inability to express himself in writing caused him great distress. His English mother, Elizabeth, who had been mildly dyslexic in her younger days but who had overcome her challenges through perseverance and support, recognised that her son was also suffering from dyslexia. Since the local school system in the late 1980s was not equipped to help him, she placed him in Dover Court Preparatory School, an international school that had teachers who could address such problems. It made the world of difference for Erin, who regained his youthful good cheer and began to enjoy school again.

Erin went on to do well enough in his studies to attain the International Baccalaureate. After serving his National Service, he promptly completed his university education and received a degree in Science.

When Mr George Abraham became the President of the Rotary Club of Raffles City (RCRC), he was looking to initiate a challenging project that would meet a need that was yet unmet, one which would leave a permanent mark on Singaporean society. Erin Khoo provided the spark of inspiration that he needed. Understanding how scarce the educational resources were at that time for providing help to dyslexics, Mr Abraham realised that a project on dyslexia would have far-reaching results. His then newly appointed RCRCs Community Services Director was Associate Professor of Orthopaedics Dr Jimmy Daruwalla.

Who better than a medical man to get this project off the ground?

Dr Daruwalla swung into action and identified Dr Lee Wei Ling, then Consultant Paediatric Neurologist and Consultant-in-Charge, Learning Disorders Clinic, School Health Services, as someone who could assist them in their endeavour. In the meantime, Mr Abraham, who travelled extensively for work, was discovering how universal the problem of dyslexia was. He was introduced by a friend to Ms Marion Welchman and Ms Jean Augur, key players in the dyslexia movement in the UK. Ms Marion Welchman was the co-founder of the British Dyslexia Association (BDA) and Ms Jean Augur the Education Director of

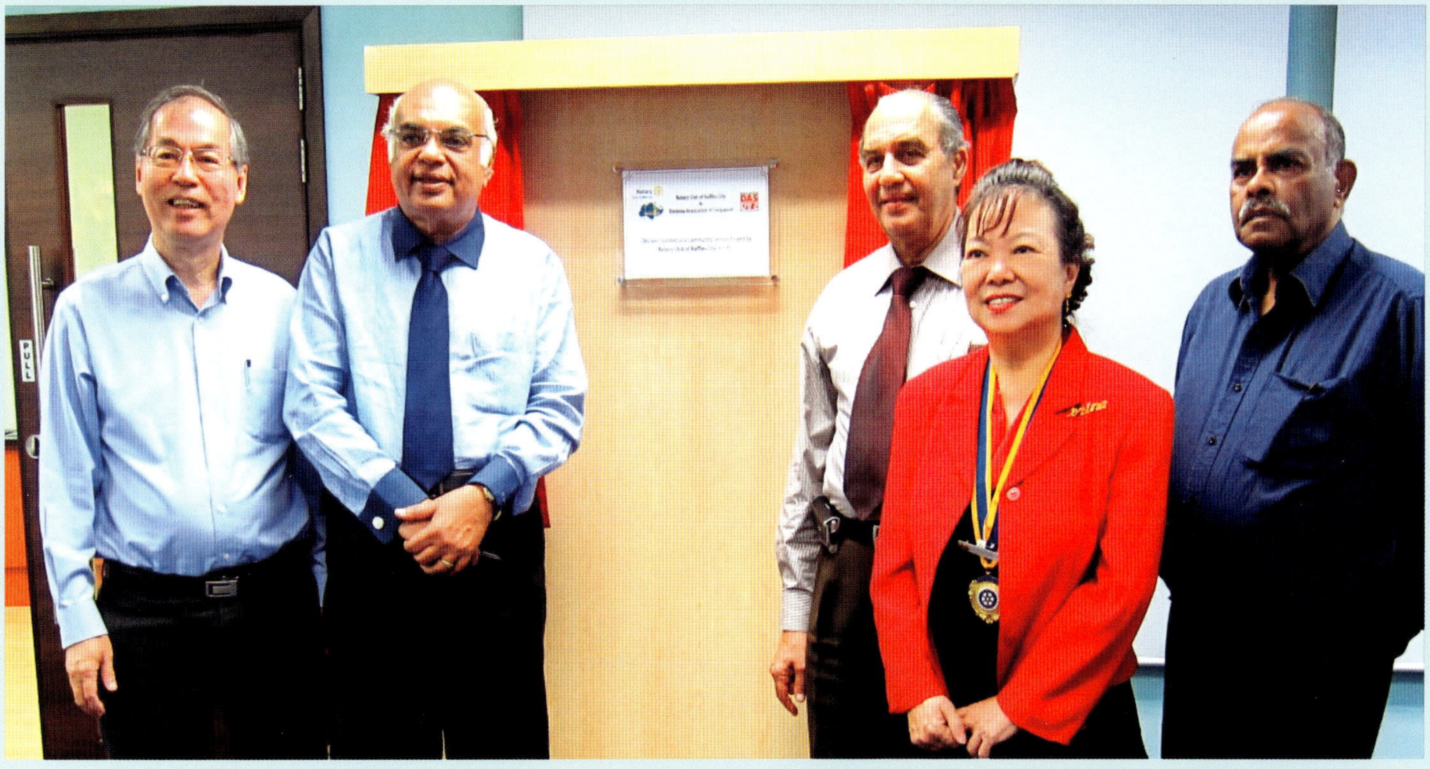

Members of the Raffles City Rotary Club (RCRC) at an event celebrating the relationship between RCRC and DAS in 2015. (L to R) Mr Vincent Chen, Mr George Abraham, Dr Jimmy Daruwalla, Mrs Corina Lai and Mr Kesavapany.

the BDA. Both agreed to support the RCRC's project and committed to coming to Singapore in April 1990 to conduct a week-long programme on understanding dyslexia.

In preparation for the launch of the dyslexia project, Dr Lee Wei Ling addressed the members of RCRC to familiarise them with the subject of dyslexia. On the 21st of April 1990, the team from the UK arrived and by the 23rd, they had swung into action with a workshop for the more than 300 teachers who had been selected by the Ministry of Education (MOE) to attend. During that week-long workshop, a public forum was also held for an unexpected 125 anxious parents who filled the hall to standing room only.

It soon became clear that there were many dyslexic children suffering in silence for want of educational assistance. As a result, an association to tackle the problem was mooted and, under the leadership of Dr Daruwalla, steps were taken to conceive a charitable organisation dedicated to helping dyslexics in Singapore. The Dyslexia Association of Singapore (DAS) was born the following year.

This book you hold in your hands is an attempt to pay tribute to and celebrate the community of countless passionate people who have contributed in ways big and small to the life-changing work of DAS under its first President, the late Dr Jimmy Daruwalla. They have brought light and clarity into lives that would have been trapped in the gloom of "un-understanding". And they continue to do so with courage, compassion, and inspiration.

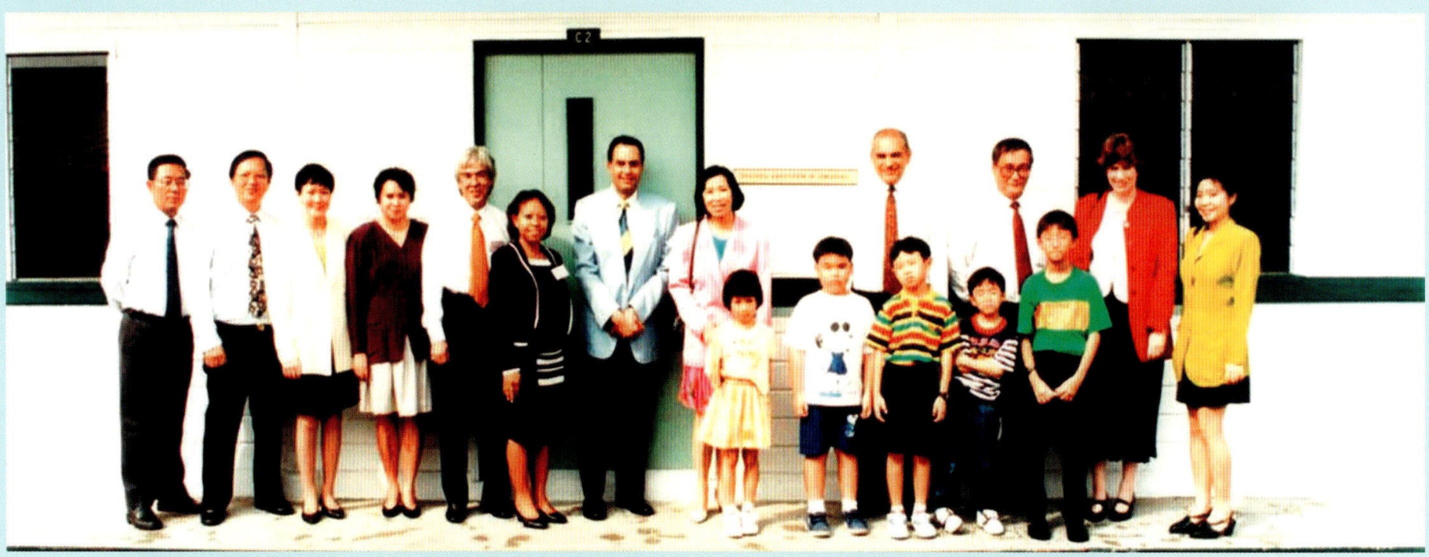

DARING TO STEP OUT

In the first year of its existence, DAS did not even have enough money to employ a secretary, much less a qualified teacher. With the help of RCRC and the Canadian Alumni, $25,000 was raised to finance the initial operations.

It was not till another two years had passed that Dr Daruwalla's many discussions with MOE finally bore fruit. Dr Aline Wong, the then Minister of State for Education, announced that MOE would give DAS a grant of $500,000 over three years.

DAS's first Learning Centre was set up at the Student Care Services Centre in Clementi, and they were able to hire their first teacher, Ms Dawn Brockett, who had a cohort of 12 students under her care. The MOE-DAS collaboration also included the establishment of another DAS Learning Centre at Ping Yi Primary School.

Things had begun to look up and there was a growing awareness of the work and its financial needs. Another growth spurt took place when Mrs Goh Chok Tong kindly agreed in 1995 to become DAS's Patron and Dr Lee Wei Ling, the Advisor.

In spite of these huge steps in the right direction, however, the social stigma associated with dyslexia remained. Public education was not far-reaching enough and many continued to suffer in silence.

Right: DAS's first Teacher, Ms Dawn Brockett, with her student and Mrs Goh Chok Tong.

Left: The official opening of the first DAS Learning Centre at Clementi Students Care Service in 1995 by Mrs Goh Chok Tong, DAS newly appointed Patron. (L to R) Four Clementi Community members, Mr Derek McCully, DAS Exco; Ms Siti Samson; Dr Jimmy Daruwalla, DAS President; Mrs Goh Chok Tong, DAS Patron; Mr Kaka Singh, DAS Exco; Community Member, Ms Dawn Brockett, DAS Teacher; and Ms Violet Kor, DAS Administration.

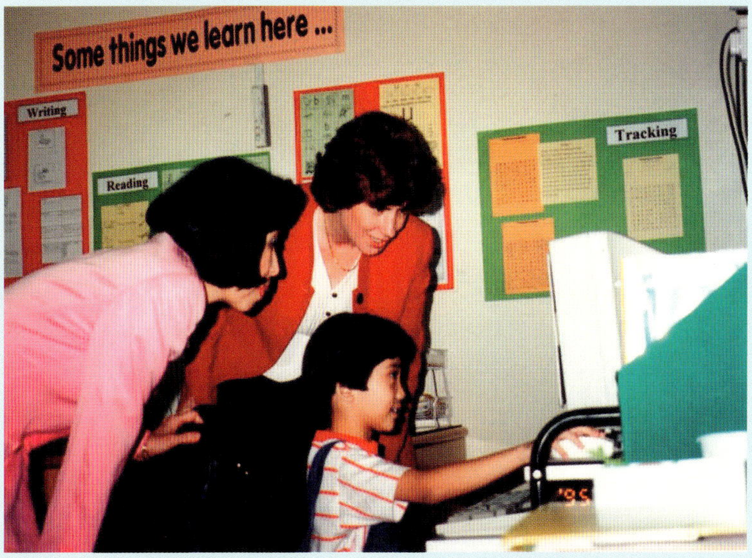

THE TURNING POINT

Back in 1991, Dr Daruwalla had already been told by Dr Lee Wei Ling that her father was dyslexic. Only in 1996 did the then Senior Minister Lee Kuan Yew announce that he was mildly dyslexic. In word and in deed, his support for DAS was unwavering. He went on to donate to DAS over $190,000 that he had received in royalties for his book Lee Kuan Yew — The Man and His Ideas.

It was the single largest individual donation to the DAS in the first decade of its existence. That generous act opened the floodgates of public interest in dyslexia.

That month alone, DAS received a thousand phone calls from parents who thought their children were dyslexic. More than the money, as Dr Daruwalla said in an interview, "The greatest thing he did for us was to remove the stigma".

With greater awareness came more opportunities to provide help where it was needed. Dyslexia Awareness Courses were organised for selected teachers from various primary schools so that the work of seeding the education system with early intervention "detectors" could begin in earnest.

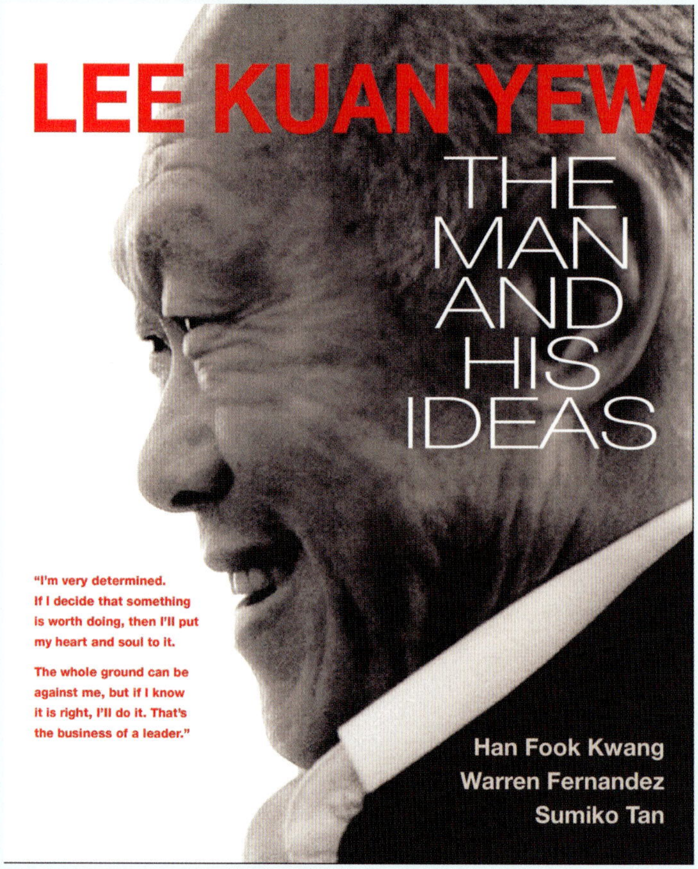

Royalties from the book, "Lee Kuan Yew—The Man and his Ideas" *were donated by Lee Kuan Yew to DAS. Mr Lee Kuan Yew was a long-term supporter of DAS and he made regular personal donations.*

Permission to print the cover image of the title, Lee Kuan Yew: The Man and His Ideas, *ISBN: 978 981 4677 62 2, © 1998 Times Editions Pte Ltd and The Strait Times Press. This paperback edition published in 2015 by Marshall Cavendish Editions. An imprint of Marshall Cavendish International and The Straits Times Press a member of Singapore Press Holdings*

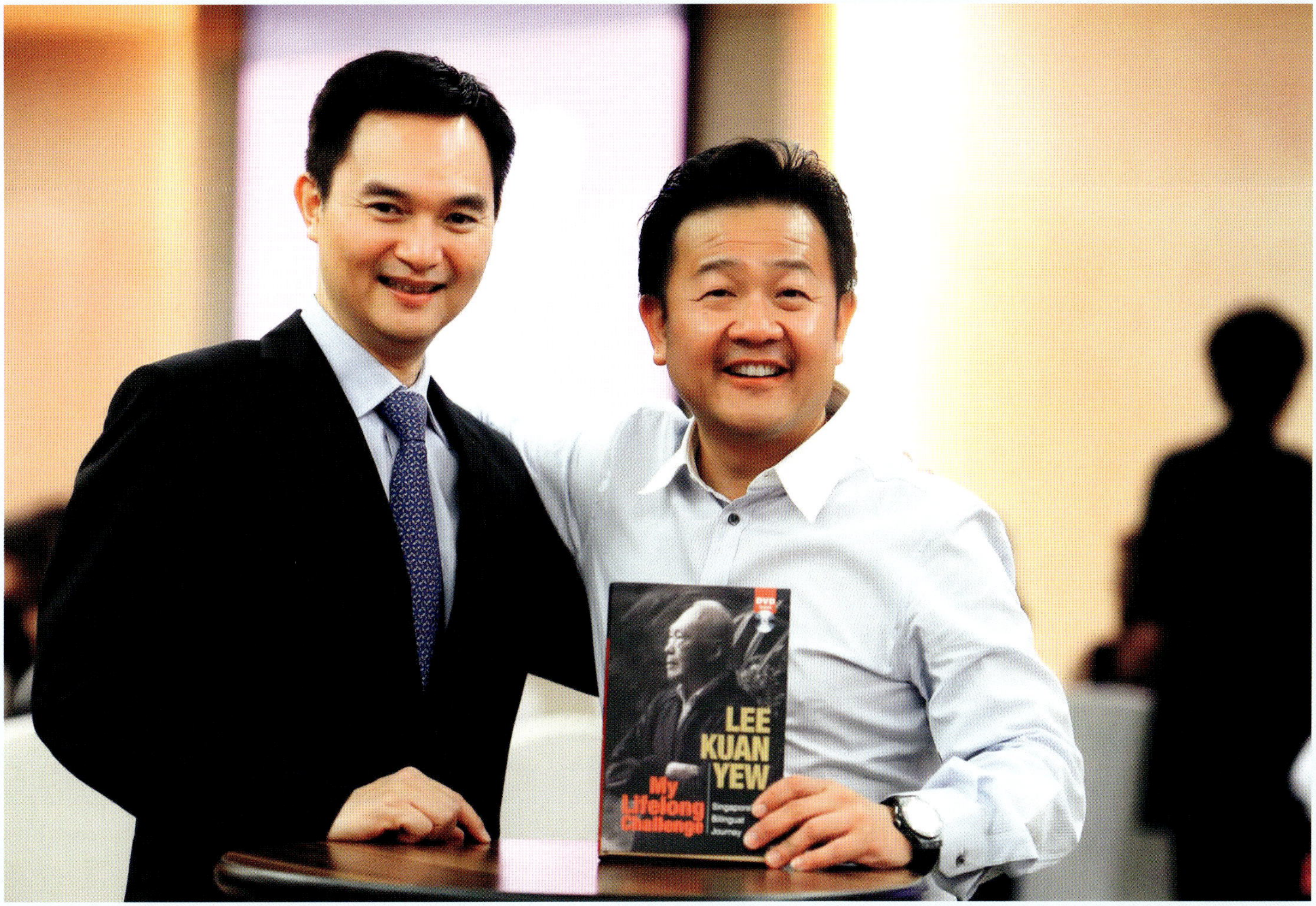

Above: Mr Kevin Kwee (R) successfully bid for Mr Lee Kuan Yew's book, My Lifelong Challenge, *at the DAS 25th Anniversary Charity Dinner in October 2016. Next to him is Mr Kevin Kwek, a DAS Executive Committee member.*

In 2012, on the occasion of DAS's 21st Anniversary, the organisation received a number of personally autographed copies of Mr Lee Kuan Yew's books. While one copy was auctioned off to Mr Kevin Kwee during the 21st Anniversary Gala Dinner, a few others were kept for future fundraising opportunities.

At the recent 25th Anniversary Charity Dinner, another of Mr Lee's books was auctioned off and, just as in 2012, Mr Kevin Kwee was again the successful bidder. He voiced his intention of passing on the two books to his daughters. While Mr Lee may no longer be with us, his legacy continues in providing much-needed funds for DAS.

YEARS OF GROWTH

The involvement and support of MOE enabled DAS to set up one new learning centre almost every year after that first one in Clementi. From the first cohort of 12 students, the numbers have steadily grown and DAS now has more than 3,500 students in its main literacy programme — the MOE-aided DAS Literacy Programme (MAP) — that is being run at its 13 learning centres.

Growth in the DAS has taken place at many levels, both quantitatively and qualitatively. Assessments by educational or specialist psychologists have grown in sophistication to enable earlier diagnosis and intervention. Aside from the main literacy programme, DAS now offers Specialised Educational Services with tailored programmes for preschool, Chinese language, mathematics, exam skills, speech and drama arts, and specialist tutoring.

From the early days of importing expertise, DAS realised that in order to forge ahead, it needed to provide training and professional development as well. When the previous CEO, Robin Moseley (himself a dyslexic), first took over the reins, he initiated significant changes that continue to undergird all that the DAS does. His oft-quoted mantra was that "dyslexic people don't need your charity, they need your professional service".

To have quality intervention, the organisation needed top-notch professionals and allied staff. At the same time, those from lower-income families can continue to access DAS services through bursaries provided.

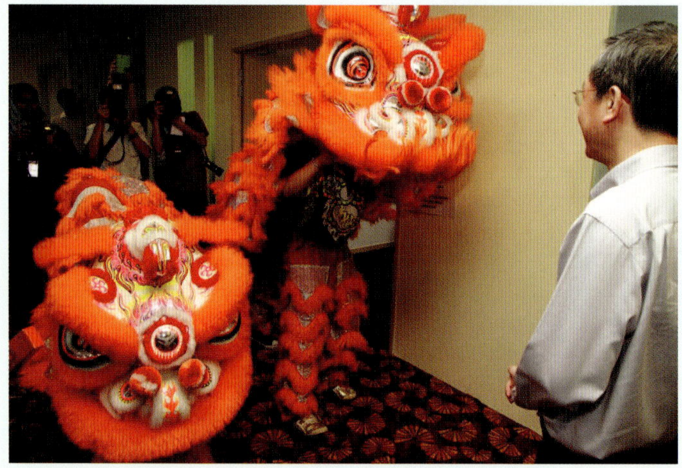

Opening of DAS 12th Learning Centre at Chinatown Point in 2013.

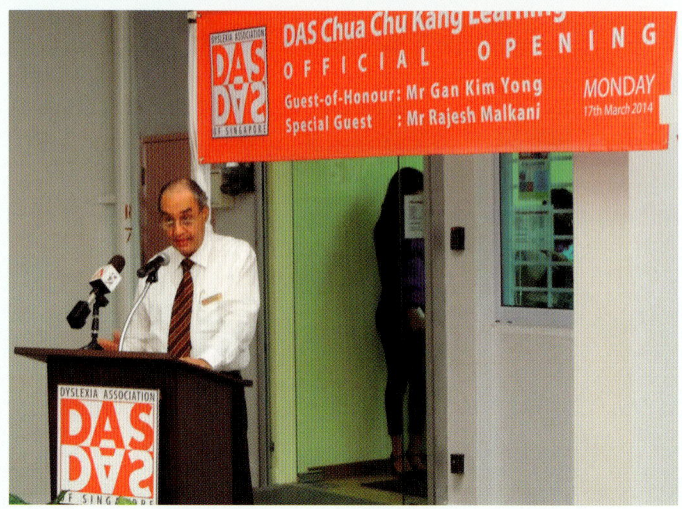
DAS Chua Chu Kang
OFFICIAL OPENING
Guest-of-Honour: Mr Gan Kim Yong
Special Guest : Mr Rajesh Malkani
MONDAY
17th March 2014
DAS
DYSLEXIA ASSOCIATION
DAS

Opening of DAS 13th Learning Centre at Chua Chu Kang in 2014.

DAS 13 LEARNING CENTRES

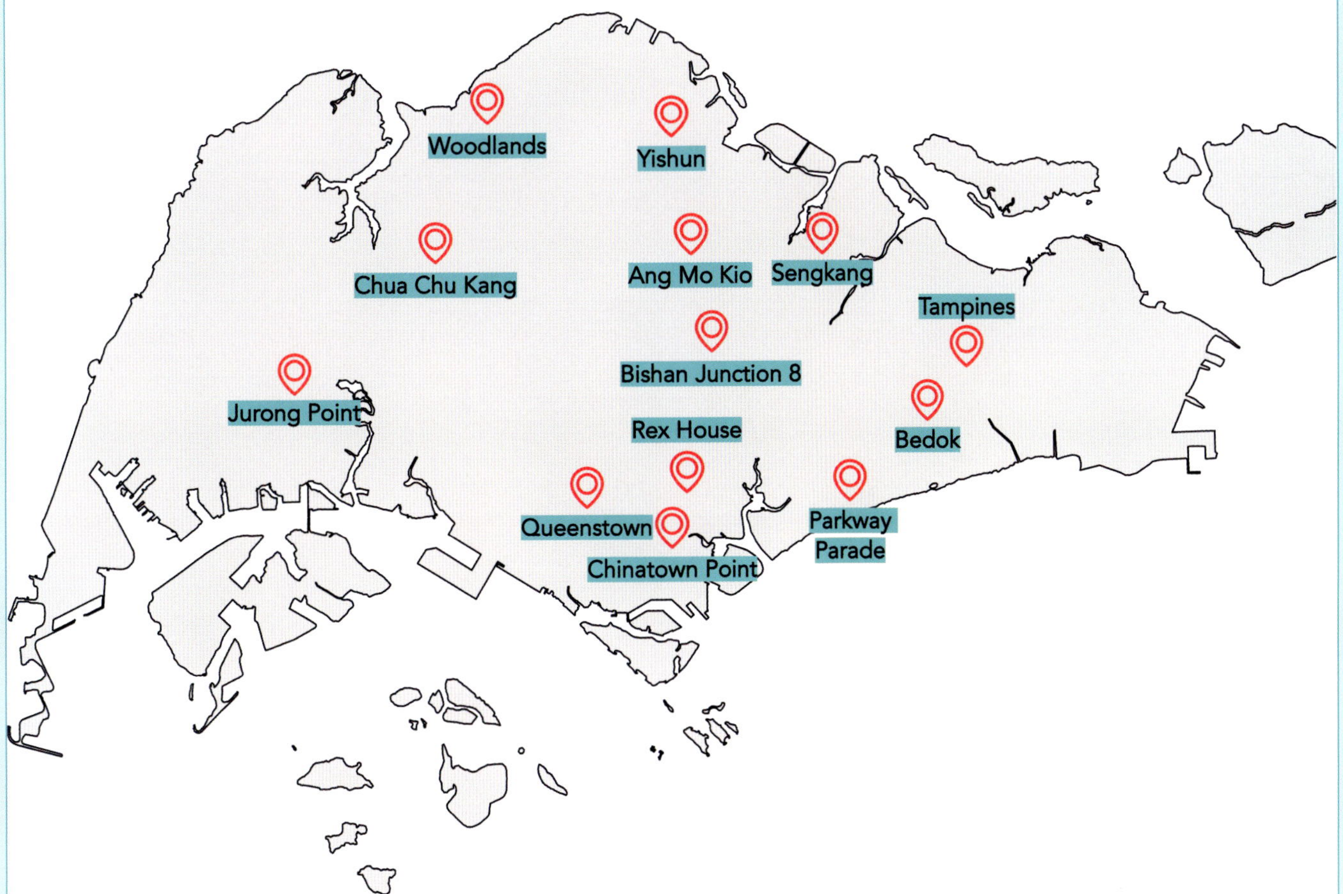
Woodlands
Yishun
Chua Chu Kang
Ang Mo Kio
Sengkang
Tampines
Jurong Point
Bishan Junction 8
Rex House
Bedok
Queenstown
Parkway Parade
Chinatown Point

OUR MISSION: Helping Dyslexic People Achieve

OUR GOAL: To build a world class organisation dedicated to helping dyslexic people, those with specific learning differences and reaching out to the region.

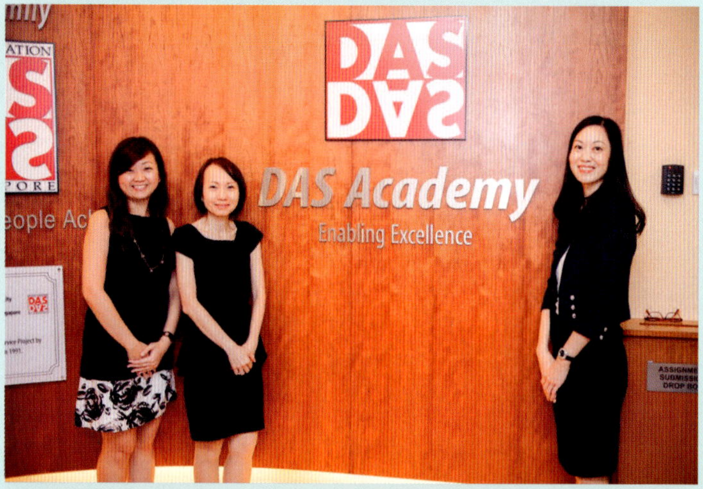
DAS
DAS Academy
Enabling Excellence

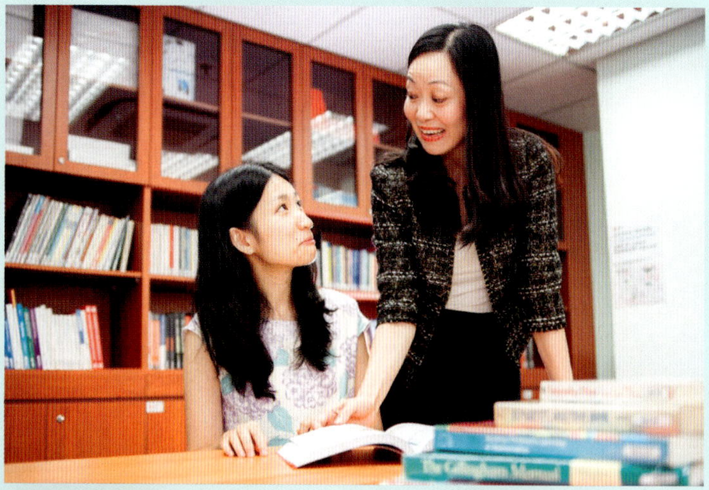

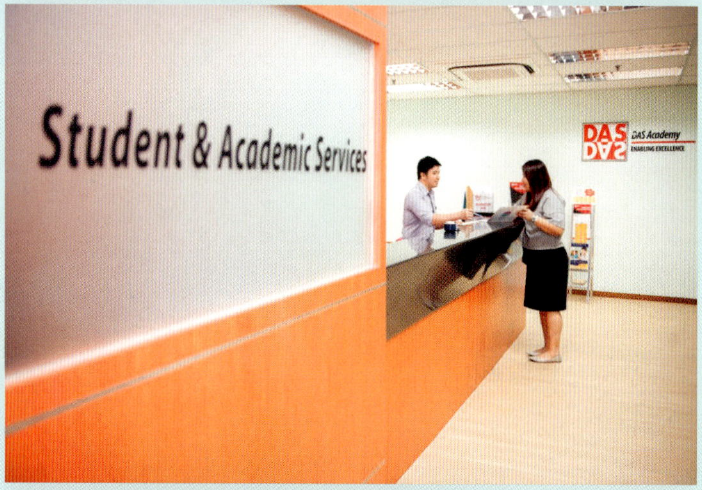
Student & Academic Services
DAS Academy

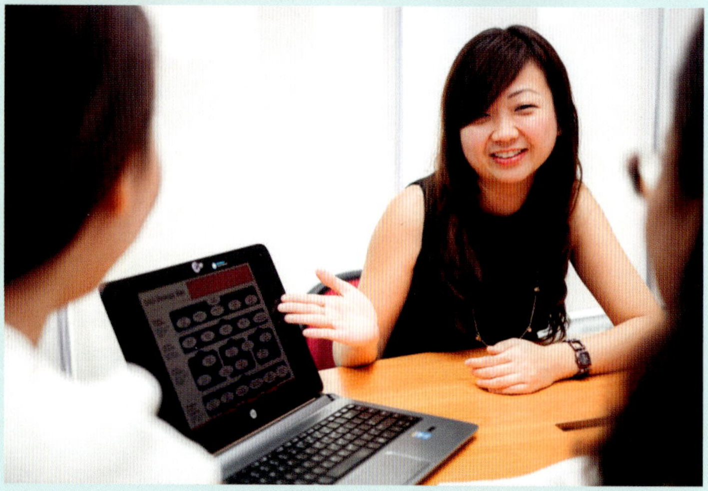

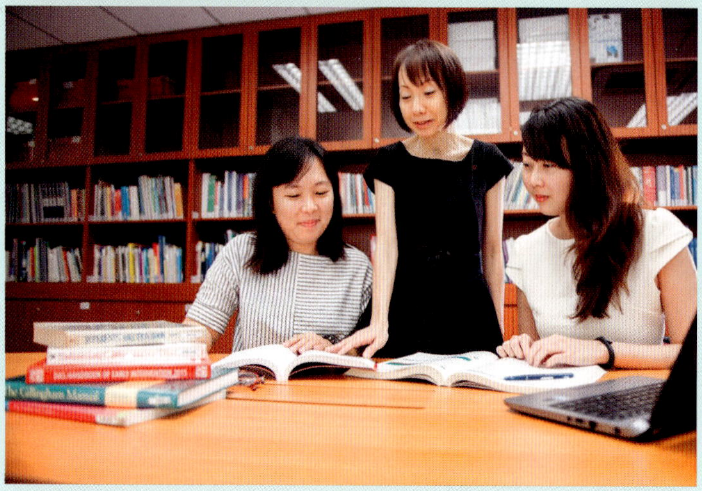

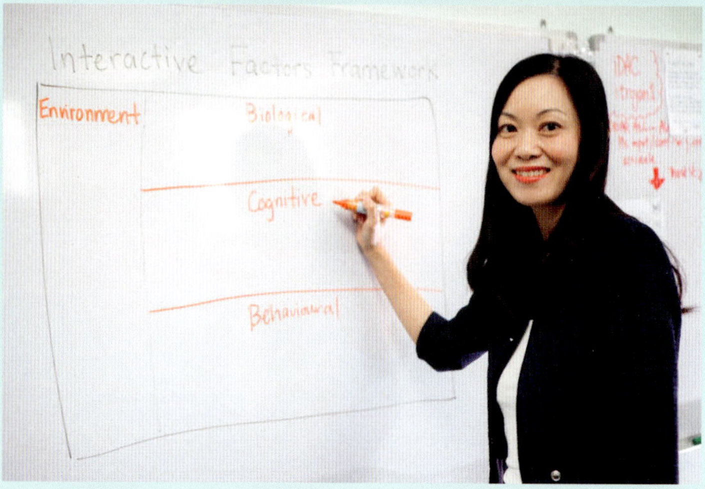
Interactive Factors Framework
Environment
Biological
Cognitive
Behavioural

Under Robin's watch, the Training Division was set up to groom local trainers and lecturers. This meant that DAS could increase its teaching capacity in response to growing demand for assessments and therapy. The Training Division eventually evolved into the DAS Academy, a private educational institution registered with the Council of Private Education, offering training courses specialising in dyslexia and other specific learning differences (SpLD). Led by a multi-disciplinary team that has extensive experience in providing direct support to people with SpLD, the DAS Academy's programmes provide an academic pathway in the field of SpLD from foundation to postgraduate levels.

In 2013, the DAS Academy partnered with the University of South Wales, UK, to launch the Master of Arts degree in Special Educational Needs (MA SEN). Accredited by the University of South Wales and jointly delivered by the DAS Academy, this programme has been well received by both educators and caregivers of people with special educational needs since its launch.

Working with professional and educational bodies in Singapore and the region (Brunei, Hong Kong), the DAS Academy also caters to the specific training needs of schools — mainstream, international, and special — to equip their teachers and Allied Educators with the skills and strategies required to help learners with SpLD reach their true potential.

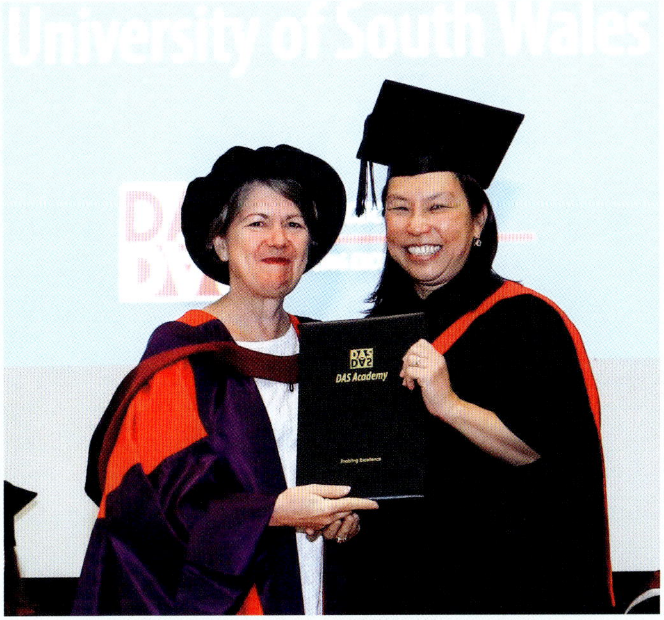

Ms Christina Chia at the 2016 MA SEN Graduation Ceremony with Dr Shirley Egley of the University of South Wales

Professionally, it renewed my zeal and confidence as an educator. It allowed me to apply a lot of what I studied to my practice, bringing theory to life.

This experience has made me more understanding as a teacher and also given me more empathy in my teaching. But more than that, it has also made me a better person. In wanting to make a difference, we learnt resilience, tenacity, courage and resourcefulness.

Ms Christina Chia
Valedictorian, MA SEN, DAS Academy Graduation Ceremony,
19 October 2016

THE KEY TO SUCCESS

DAS was started by people who genuinely care for other people. This continues to be the driving force and a hallmark of DAS's work. It comes as no surprise therefore that people are their key resource. In the DAS family, everyone is valued and has a vital role to play.

It was their first President's dedication and unrelenting commitment that enabled them to build their network of supporters and volunteers at the speed they did. Their vision-led CEOs have helped flesh out and execute the mission set before them and successfully led the organisation to progressively higher levels.

Without the professional expertise of the educational and specialist psychologists, DAS would not be able to diagnose and refer the dyslexic clients who come to them for help. The innovativeness and creativity of their teachers have been instrumental in enabling DAS's students to be fully functioning and contributing members of society. Their communications and publications department has been at the forefront of getting their message out to the wider society and increasing public awareness. Without their efficient and caring administrative staff, operations would grind to a halt. And the janitorial crew are the ones

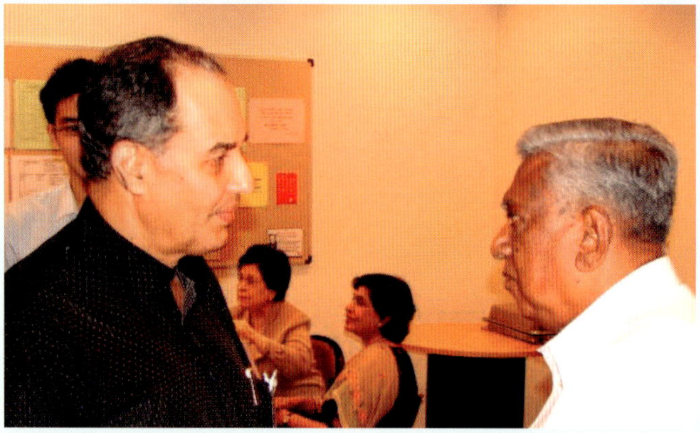

Dr Jimmy Daruwalla pictured with the former President of Singapore, Mr S. R. Nathan when he visited DAS in 2005

My aim is to enable dyslexic children to learn happily and effectively at school and my vision is that DAS is recognised both here and internationally as a world-class organisation and as a leader in specialist education. ... DAS has also evolved over the years from being simply a charity organisation to a professional one dedicated to providing the essential services that are necessary to enable a dyslexic to achieve.

Yet, we still maintain our charitable work by providing bursaries and subsidies for children who come from needy families. As a psychologist, I am especially pleased that we have been able to develop our Assessment Service from an initial team of four graduate psychologists.

Mr Robin Moseley
Former DAS CEO (2002–2014), "My Journey in the DAS" in *FACETS*, Oct–Dec 2008

who maintain cleanliness and help promote a clean and conducive environment for all who use their centres. In line with Robin Moseley's constant exhortation for DAS to achieve credible professional standards, excellence and self-improvement have remained high on the DAS's priority list. At the heart of it all is the desire to give their students the best care and teaching possible. DAS epitomises the truth that it takes a whole village to ensure that no dyslexic child is left behind.

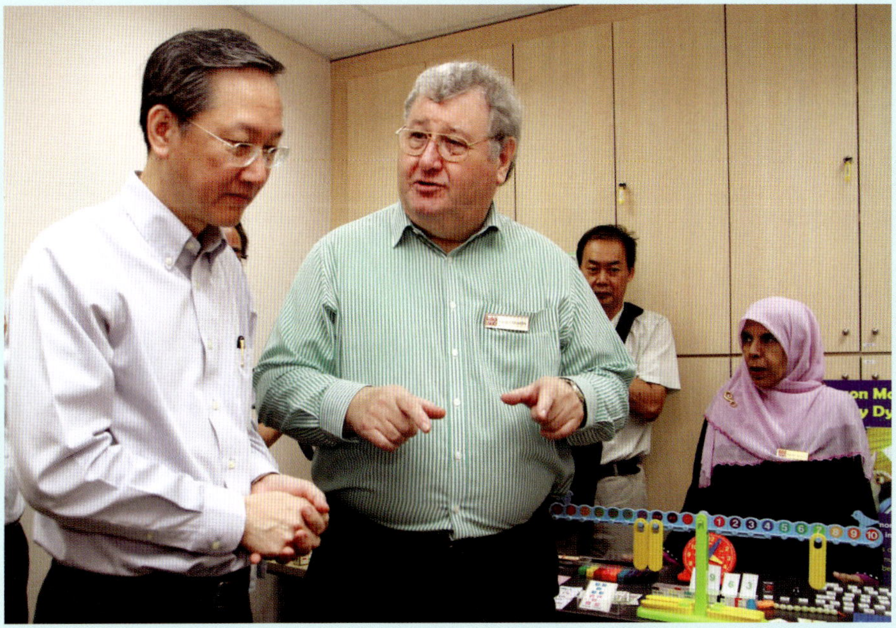

Mr Sam Tan, at the time the Senior Parliamentary Secretary, Ministry of Foreign Affairs and Ministry of Culture, Community and Youth, and Mayor, Central Singapore District, was the Guest of Honour at the DAS Chinatown Point Learning Centre's Official Opening in March 2013. Mr Tan is pictured above with DAS CEO Robin Moseley

If you speak to any of our educational therapists or psychologists or speech and language therapists, the one thing they're very happy about DAS is the professional development that is given... In the past decades there has been a great focus on basic training. In the last 2 years, we have started providing a lot of specialist diplomas to various people. For example, we have over 30 people attending a math certificate course right now because we want to move even bigger into mathematics. All our Chinese teachers are also taking Chinese-teaching diplomas. And of course, for our main literacy programme, we are encouraging more to take on the Masters programme, so that they can also help to do curriculum development, research work, and so on.

DAS Academy provides the bulk of the training, but we don't have expertise in Chinese teaching, for example. So we have sent them to another training institute to receive their training, locally. We've also brought in consultants to ensure the organisation continues to learn from others. One of the main objectives of DAS is to build a pool of expertise in dyslexia and specific learning differences here in Singapore.

Mr Lee Siang
DAS Chief Executive Officer

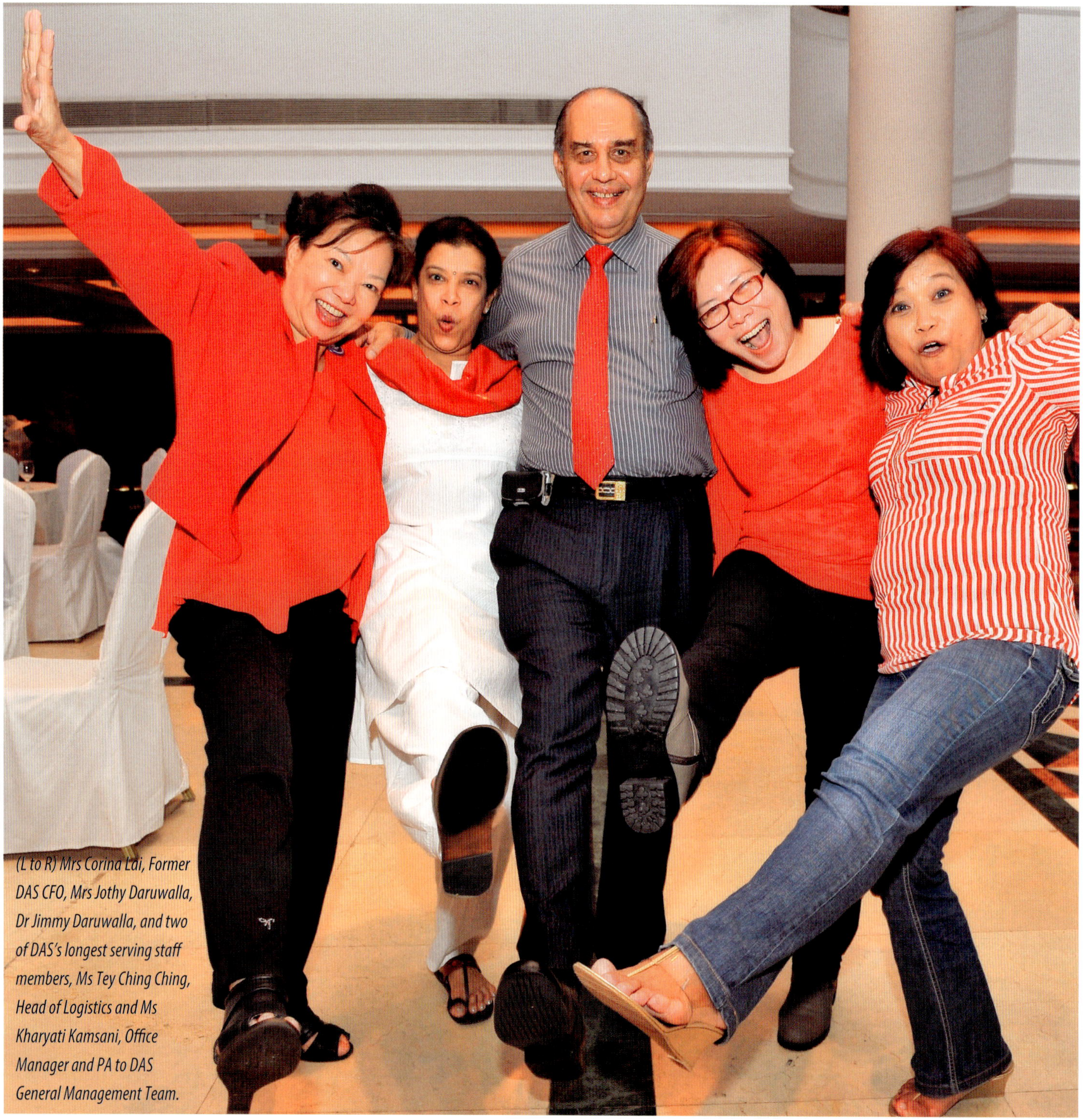

(L to R) Mrs Corina Lai, Former DAS CFO, Mrs Jothy Daruwalla, Dr Jimmy Daruwalla, and two of DAS's longest serving staff members, Ms Tey Ching Ching, Head of Logistics and Ms Kharyati Kamsani, Office Manager and PA to DAS General Management Team.

2

MILESTONES IN THE PAST 25 YEARS

A business has to be involving, it has to be fun and it has to exercise your creative instincts.

Richard Branson

A REWARDING JOURNEY

The Dyslexia Association Singapore has come a long way since 1991. DAS founding President Dr Jimmy Daruwalla compiled the first milestones from 1989 before it was converted into the history of DAS on the DAS website by then Head of Corporate Services Mr Lee Siang from 2004. The DAS Publicity and Publications Team led by Ms Deborah Hewes continued the compilation of the history and milestones. The rich and colourful history of DAS has been captured in this chapter.

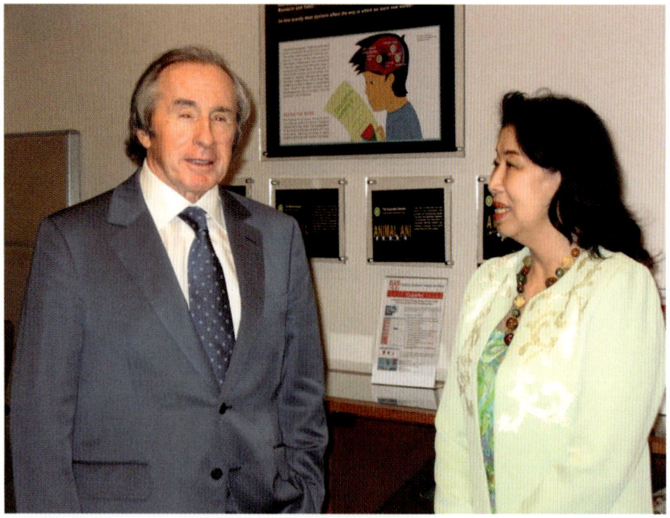

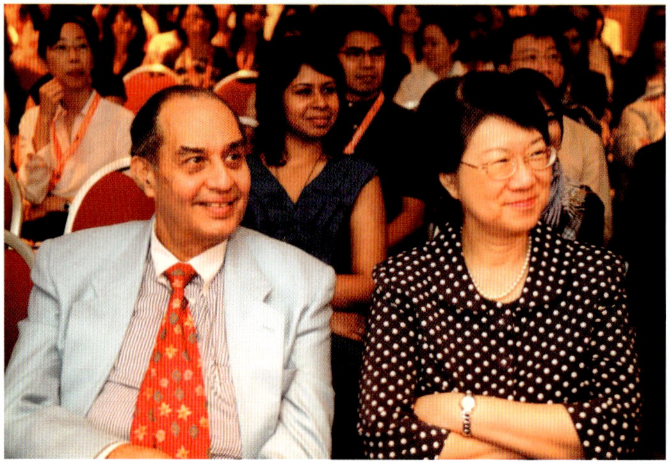

Above right: Visiting DAS in 2007, Sir Jackie Stewart is pictured with DAS Patron Mrs Goh Chok Tong. Right: Dr Jimmy Daruwalla is seated next to Ms Ho Peng from the Ministry of Education at the DAS Seminar Week held in 2010.

1989

JUL The Rotary Club of Raffles City initiated a community service project to raise awareness of dyslexia in Singapore, driven and led by Mr George Abraham and Dr Jimmy Daruwalla.

1990

APR The Rotary Club of Raffles City organised the first public forum on dyslexia. Ms Marion Welchman, Secretary of the British Dyslexia Association and Founder of the first dyslexia association in the United Kingdom at Bath, Ms Jean Augur, Educational Officer, British Dyslexia Association and Dr Lee Wei Ling, Consultant Paediatric Neurologist and Head of the Learning Disorders Clinic at School Health Services, were invited to speak at the forum. A workshop was also held for 200 teachers from the Ministry of Education (MOE).

OCT A second public forum was organised by the Rotary Club of Raffles City and the need for establishing a Dyslexia Association in Singapore was put forward.

1991

APR A committee was formed to lay the groundwork for setting up the Dyslexia Association of Singapore (DAS).

OCT Dyslexia Association of Singapore was registered with the Registrar of Societies. The People's Association provided DAS with office space at its Kallang premises free-of-charge. This was as a result of Ambassador Kesavapany's effort in speaking to Mr Lee Chong Giam.

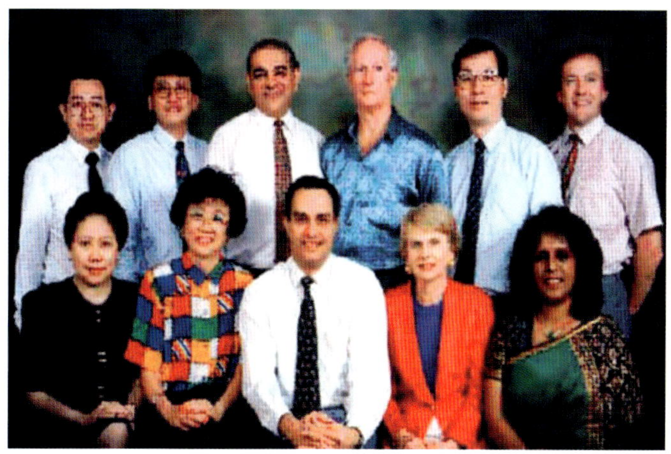

The first Executive Committee was formed. Front row (L to R) Dr Loke Loo-Pin; Ms Jenny Tang; Dr Jimmy Daruwalla; Ms Lorna Whiston; Ms Shanta Emmanuel. Back row (L to R) Mr Joseph Chew; Mr Paul Lim; Mr Kaka Singh; Mr David Smith; Mr Vincent Chen; and Mr Tony Gash.

1992

JUL DAS Committee members held an informal meeting with Mrs Barbara Bush, First Lady and wife of President George Bush, of the United States during her visit to Singapore.

At her request, the Texas Scottish Rite Hospital in Dallas presented the DAS with a set of 500 video tapes for remedial teaching.

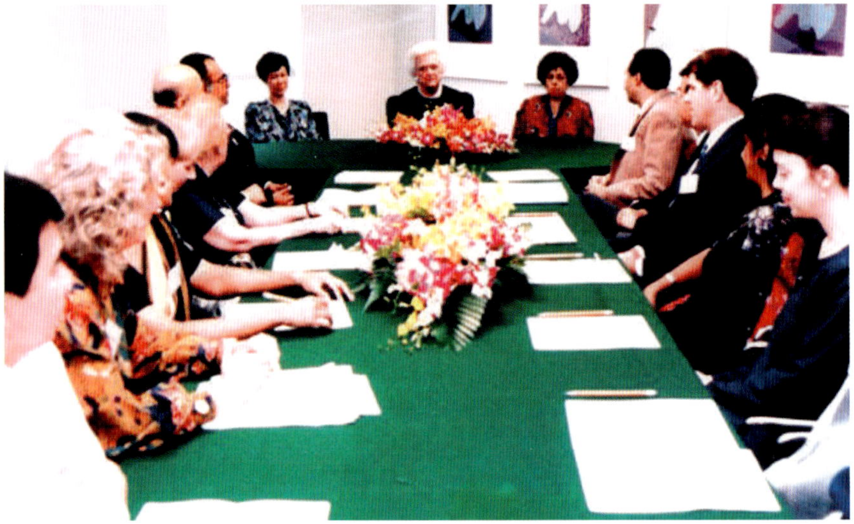

Mrs Bush wrote to Dr Daruwalla after her visit, "So many thanks for such an interesting briefing on the Singapore Dyslexia Society. I truly enjoyed learning more about your fine work. You all are doing a terrific job and should be very proud of your efforts. With all best wishes, Warmly, Barbara Bush."

MAR The Rotary Club of Raffles City and the Canadian Alumni raised $25,000 to finance the initial operations of DAS.

1993

FEB An MOU was signed with Mr Eric Low, Chairman of Students Care Service, to use their facilities at Clementi.

OCT A golf tournament organised by the Lions Clubs of Singapore Metropolitan, New Central, City and Ladyhill raised a total of $127,000 for the DAS to set up its first learning centre for dyslexic children at the Students Care Service in Clementi. DAS then hired its first teacher, Ms Dawn Brockett, to teach the first group of dyslexic students, a class of 12.

DEC DAS became the 200th affiliated member of NCSS but it is not under ComChest.

1994

FEB Dr Loke Loo Pin organised the charity concert "A Musical Affair" in aid of DAS at the Jubilee Hall in Raffles Hotel, which raised a total of $16,700.

MAR The official opening of the first DAS Learning Centre at the Students Care Service Centre in Clementi, by Mr Bernard Chen, MP for Brickworks GRC. DAS also published its first newsletter.

JUL DAS was invited by MOE for discussions.

1995

APR Mrs Goh Chok Tong became the Patron of DAS.

MAY DAS held its first Charity Dinner and Dance at the ballroom of Shangri-La Hotel. Mrs Goh Chok Tong was the Guest of Honour. A total of $250,000 was raised.

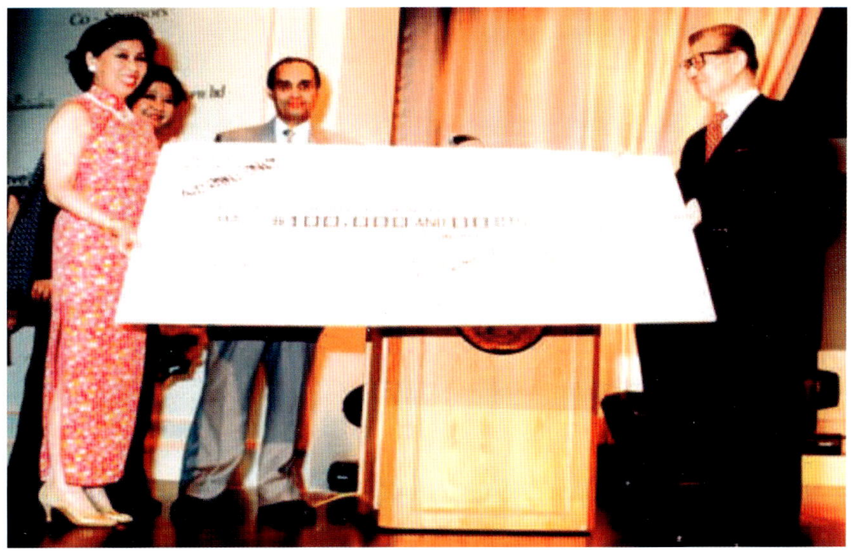

At the Charity Dinner, Mrs Goh Chok Tong, DAS Patron; Mrs Dora Chan, DAS Fundraising Chair; and Dr Jimmy Daruwalla, DAS President; received a donation from Mr Lee Seng Gee, Chairman of the Lee Foundation.

JUN Dr Lee Wei Ling, Consultant Paediatric Neurologist and Head of the Learning Disorders Clinic at School Health Services, became Advisor to DAS.

1995

JUL Dr Aline Wong, Senior Minister of State (Education & Health), announced an MOE-DAS joint project and a starting grant of $500,000 which included $95,000 for the renovation of another DAS Learning Centre at Ping Yi Primary School. The balance was a subsidy paid over the following three years.

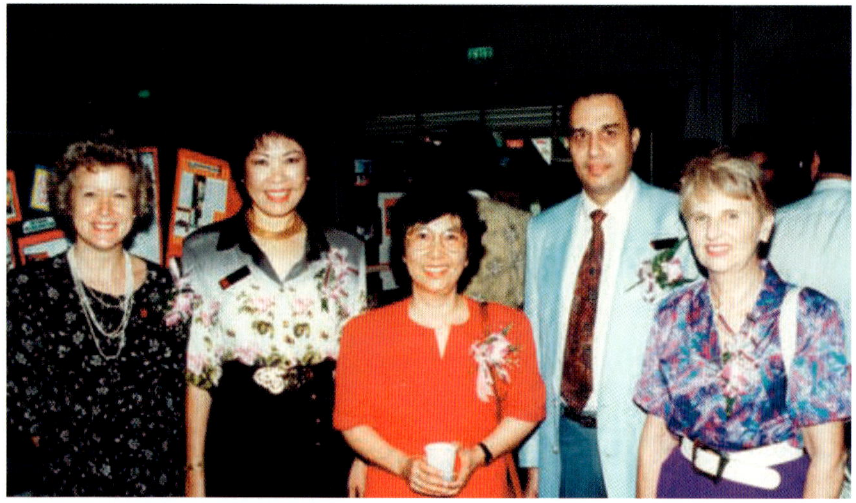

At the DAS Learning Centre at Ping Yi Primary School (L to R) Ms Janette Skeath, Ms Linda Low, Dr Aline Wong, Dr Jimmy Daruwalla, Mrs Lorna Whiston.

SEP DAS Learning Centre at Clementi Community Centre was officially opened by Mrs Goh Chok Tong, DAS Patron.

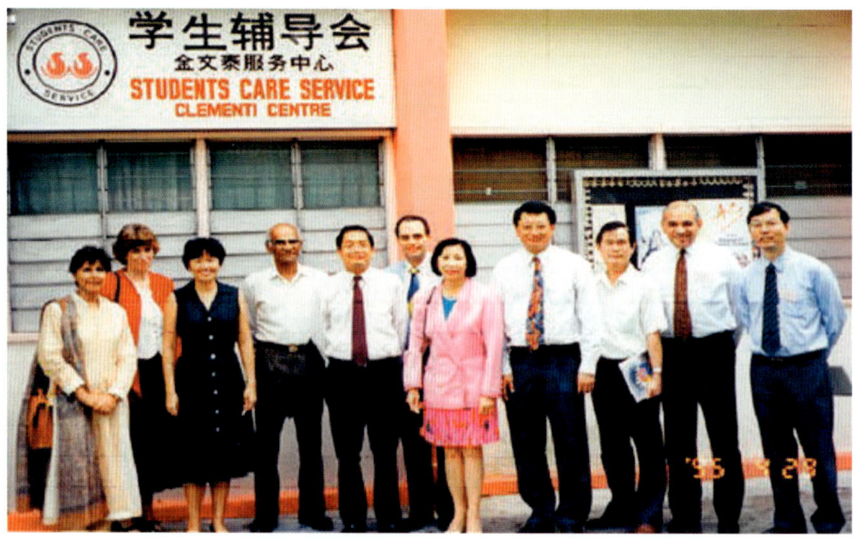

(L to R) Clementi Community Member; Ms Dawn Brockett, DAS Teacher; three Clementi Community members; Dr Jimmy Daruwalla, DAS President; Mrs Goh Chok Tong, DAS Patron; two Clementi Community members; Mr Kaka Singh, DAS Exco; and Mr Vincent Chen, DAS Exco.

1996

MAR DAS appointed its first Executive Director, Mrs Linda Low.

APR The stigma of having a learning difficulty was considerably lessened when Mr Lee Kuan Yew, former Prime Minister of Singapore, announced that he had mild dyslexia and donated a large sum of money to DAS. This created more public awareness, and there was a flood of enquiries. A symposium on dyslexia, sponsored by the British Association of Singapore, was held to increase public awareness of this learning difficulty.

DAS Patron, Mrs Goh Chok Tong, was the Guest of Honour at the opening ceremony of DAS Learning Centre in Ping Yi Primary School.

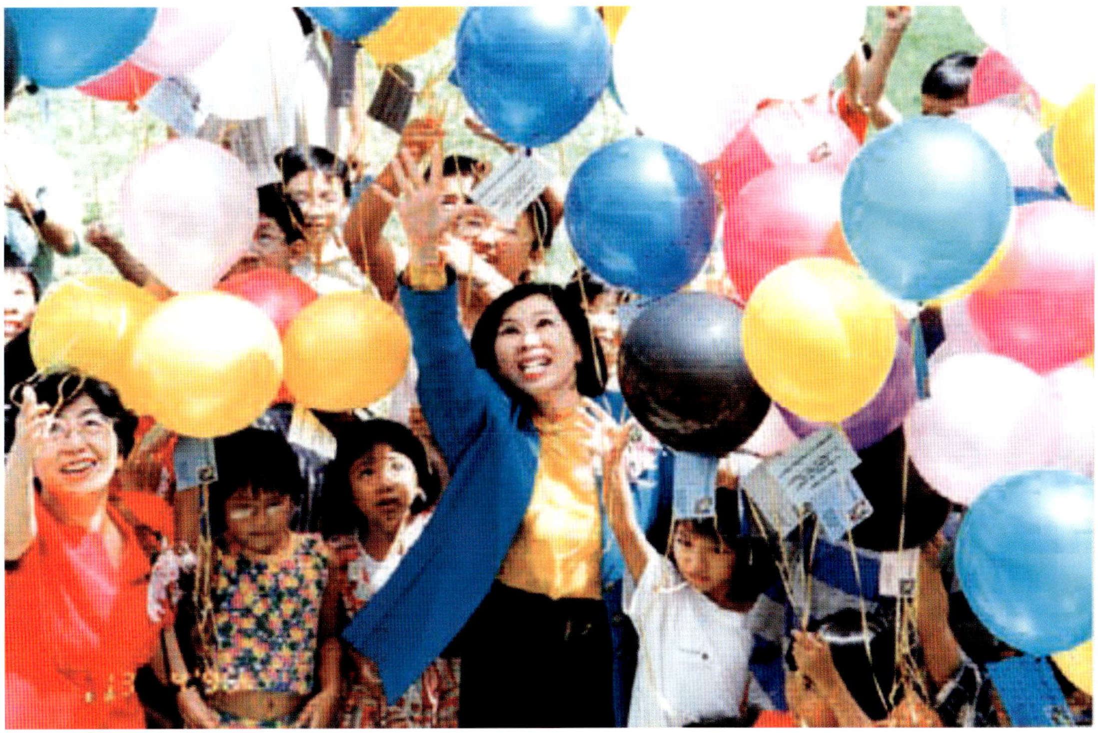

JUL 60 teachers from various primary schools attended a Dyslexia Awareness Course jointly organised by the MOE and DAS.

OCT DAS organised a Gala Dinner to celebrate its 5th Anniversary on 27 October 1996.

1997

JUN A Dyslexia Awareness Course was jointly organised by DAS and the Specialised Pupil Programmes Branch for teachers in Singapore.

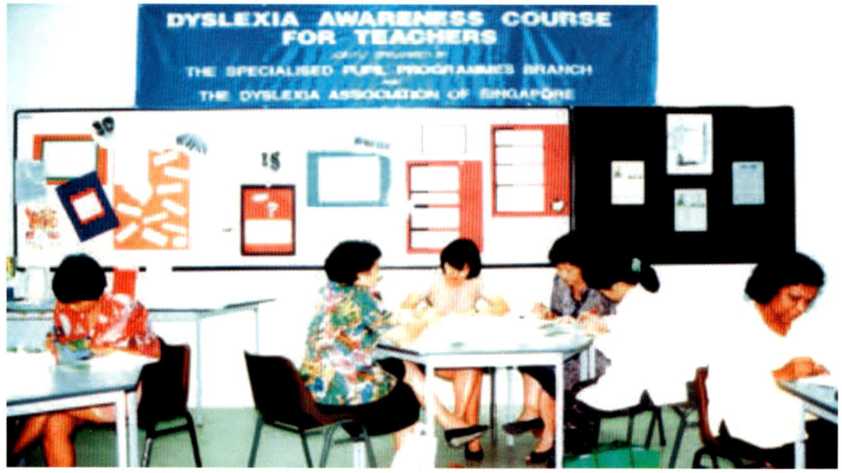

OCT DAS appointed its second Executive Director, Ms Zunaidah Shahul Hamid.

DEC Student enrolment at DAS jumped to 188. Of these students, 128 were in the Primary 1 to Primary 4 age range.

1998

JUN DAS invited Mr Ron Yoshimoto and Ms Jane Raissle to conduct the first Orton-Gillingham (OG) Course.

Mr Ron Yoshimoto, with Ms Wendy Sweeney, another Fellow of the Academy of Orton-Gillingham Practitioners and Educators (New York), conducted a total of six Orton-Gillingham Courses from 1998 to 2003, which trained about 200 DAS, MOE and private teachers.

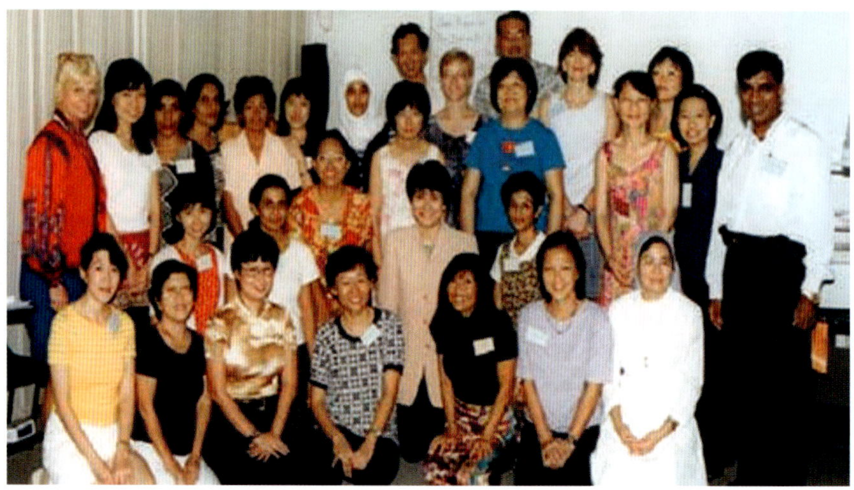

1998

FEB The Clementi Learning Centre was moved to Alexandra Primary School and renamed as Redhill Learning Centre.

OCT The Redhill Learning Centre at Alexandra Hill Primary School was officially opened by Dr Aline Wong, Minister of State (Education and Health).

JUL Enrolment of DAS grew to 223 students under the guidance of 10 teachers.

2001

JAN DAS appointed its third Executive Director, Madam Ong Phiak Kim.

MAR DAS became a Lifetime Member of the International Dyslexia Association.

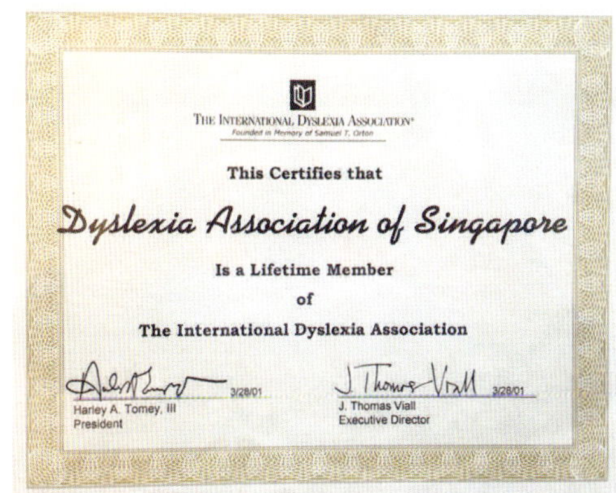
The International Dyslexia Association
This Certifies that
Dyslexia Association of Singapore
Is a Lifetime Member
of
The International Dyslexia Association
3/28/01
Harley A. Tomey, III
President
3/28/01
J. Thomas Viall
Executive Director

AUG The Roshen Daruwalla Trust Fund was set up to provide support for needy dyslexic children.

Educational Therapists from DAS conducted a Dyslexia Awareness Course for MOE teachers in August 2001.

OCT The Official Opening Ceremony of the DAS Ang Mo Kio Learning Centre at Anderson Primary School was held with Mrs Goh Chok Tong as the Guest of Honour. Enrolment stood at 341 students.

This meant that at the end of 2001, DAS had three learning centres — Ang Mo Kio Learning Centre in Anderson Primary School serving students in the North Zone, Bedok Learning Centre in Ping Yi Primary School serving students in the East, and Redhill Learning Centre in New Town Primary School serving students in the South and West Zones.

2002

FEB Mr Hawazi Daipi, Parliamentary Secretary, Ministry of Education, officially opened the Bedok Learning Centre in Fengshan Primary School.

SEP Mr Robin Moseley took over as the fourth Executive Director at DAS.

DEC Redhill Learning Centre moved to Queenstown Primary School and was renamed the Queenstown Learning Centre.

DAS Training Department commenced training with a double diploma for teachers and trainers.

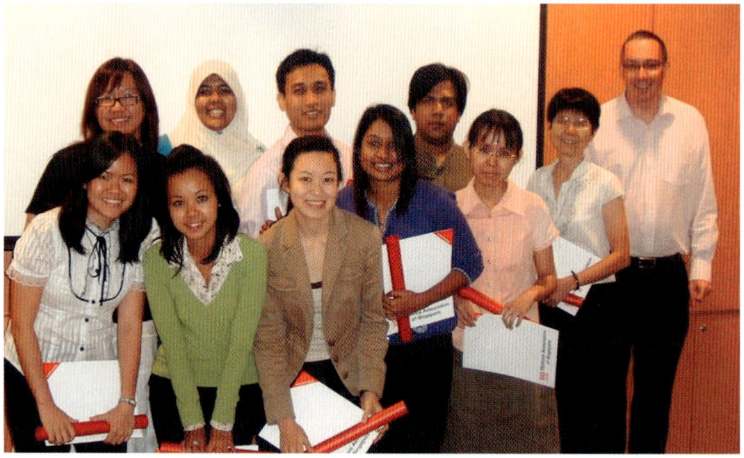

Pictured here are the first graduates of the Cambridge International Diploma for Teachers and Trainers (University of Cambridge International Examinations) at DAS. In the centre are three members of the current DAS General Management Team, Ms June Siew, Ms Geetha Shantha Ram, and Mr Nor Ashraf Samsudin. The training was delivered by Mr Kevin Smith (far right).

2003

JUN DAS began its Assessment Services with a team of seven psychologists. Dyslexic children could now be assessed by one of our DAS specialist psychologists within a month of application. Enrolment stood at 528 students.

Representatives from DAS attended the Orton-Gillingham International Conference in Vancouver, Canada. This marked the start of regular DAS participation in major conferences overseas.

DAS held a press conference to announce the findings of a dyslexia awareness survey involving more than 720 parents. There was extensive media coverage on dyslexia and DAS was featured in all major newspapers and television channels.

2004

JAN The Lee Foundation Dyslexia Centre was set up in SPRING Singapore, Bukit Merah. This centre was established to provide assessment and training services under one roof. The Lee Foundation donated $300,000 towards the renovation of this centre.

FEB DAS Training Service was launched with its first Dyslexia Support Course for parents and teachers. An ongoing series of workshops including Dyslexia and Mathematics, Exam Study Skills for Dyslexic students, etc., was conducted.

JUN DAS took over responsibility for the training of DAS and MOE teachers when the Orton-Gillingham Course was conducted by three local DAS trainers for the first time.

JUL Student enrolment at DAS exceeded 600 for the first time. DAS launched its first Diploma in Dyslexia Studies Course in a tie-up with the University of Cambridge International Examinations.

AUG Education Minister, Mr Tharman Shanmugaratnam, opened the Lee Foundation Dyslexia Centre and the Roshen Daruwalla Resource Centre in the presence of our patron, Mrs Goh Chok Tong.

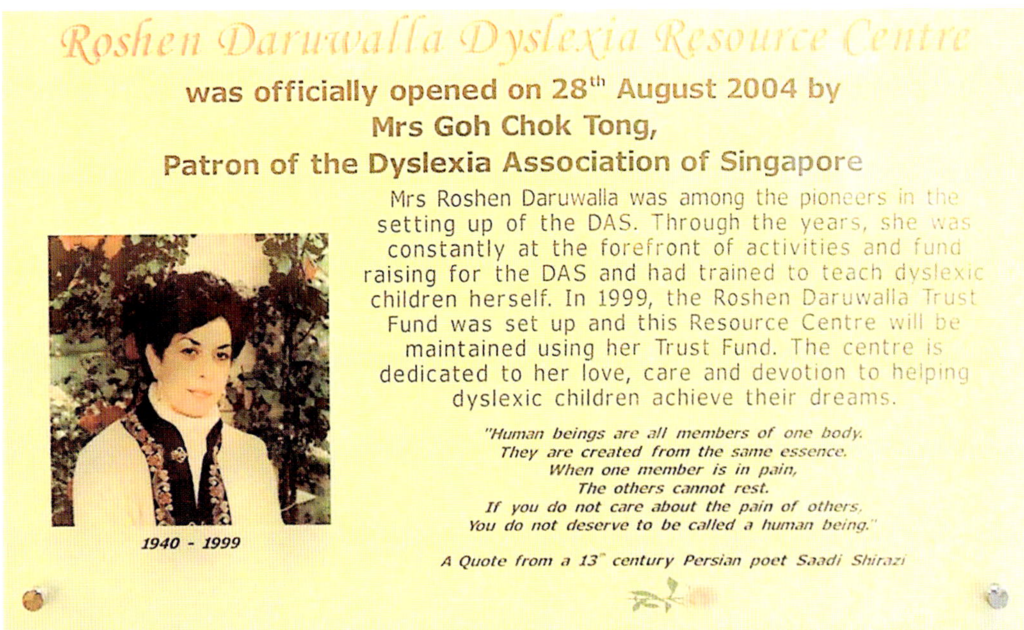

2004

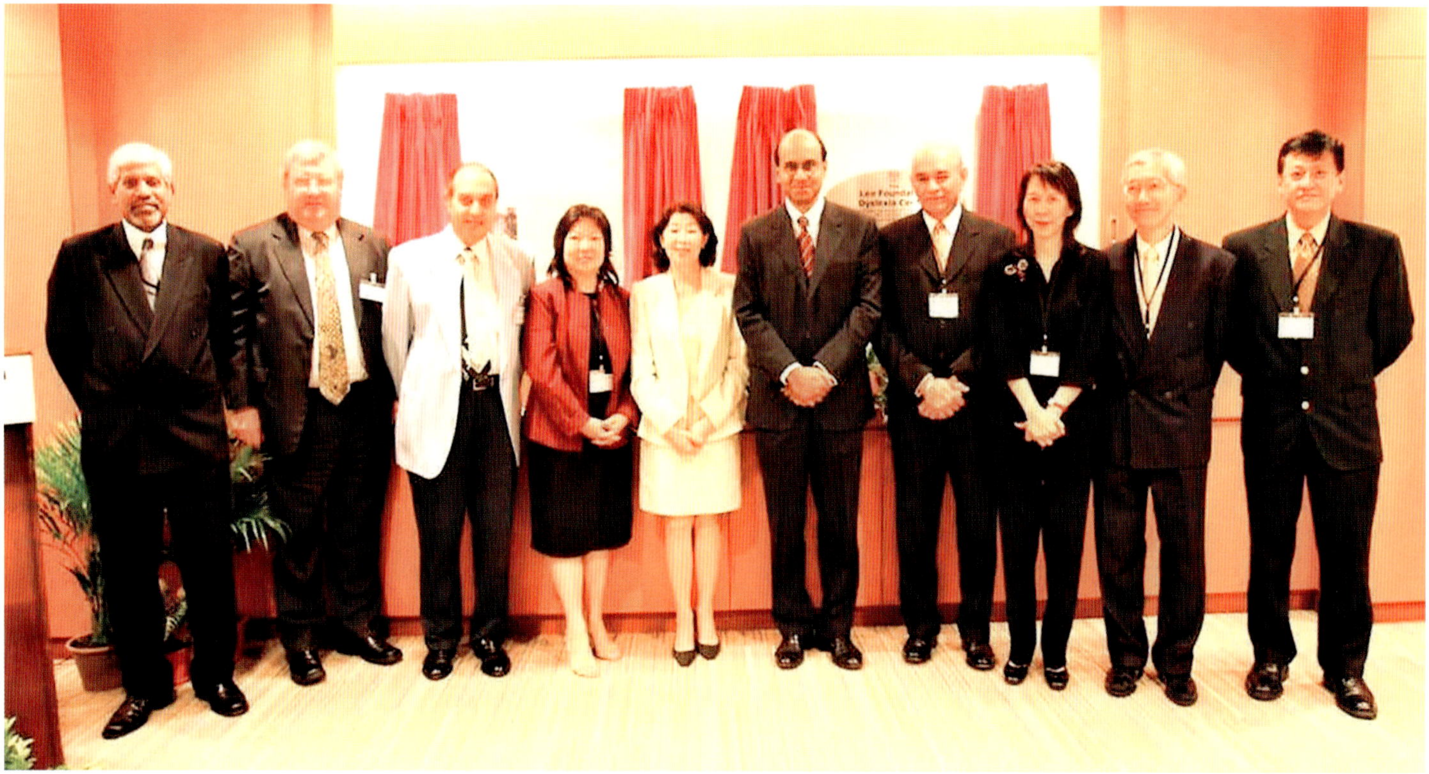

Opening of Roshen Daruwalla Resource Centre. (L to R) Mr Rajaram, DAS Exco; Mr Robin Moseley, DAS CEO; Dr Jimmy Daruwalla, DAS President; Mrs Corina Lai, DAS CFO; Mrs Goh Chok Tong, DAS Patron; Mr Tharman Shanmugaratnam, Minister for Education; Mr Kaka Singh, DAS Exco; Ms Cynthia Tan, DAS Exco; Mr Eric Lee, DAS Vice President; and Mr Paul Lim, DAS Exco.

2005

JAN Speech and Language Service was established with three Speech and Language Therapists. Enrolment stood at 778 students.

MAR The Rotary Club of Raffles City held a charity golf event in aid of DAS.

JUN DAS signed a five-year contract with MOE to provide training for MOE Special Needs Officers.

JUL DAS presented a paper at the 3rd International Multilingualism & Dyslexia Conference in Cyprus.

2005

JAN President S. R. Nathan and Mrs Nathan visited the Dyslexia Centre at SPRING Singapore.

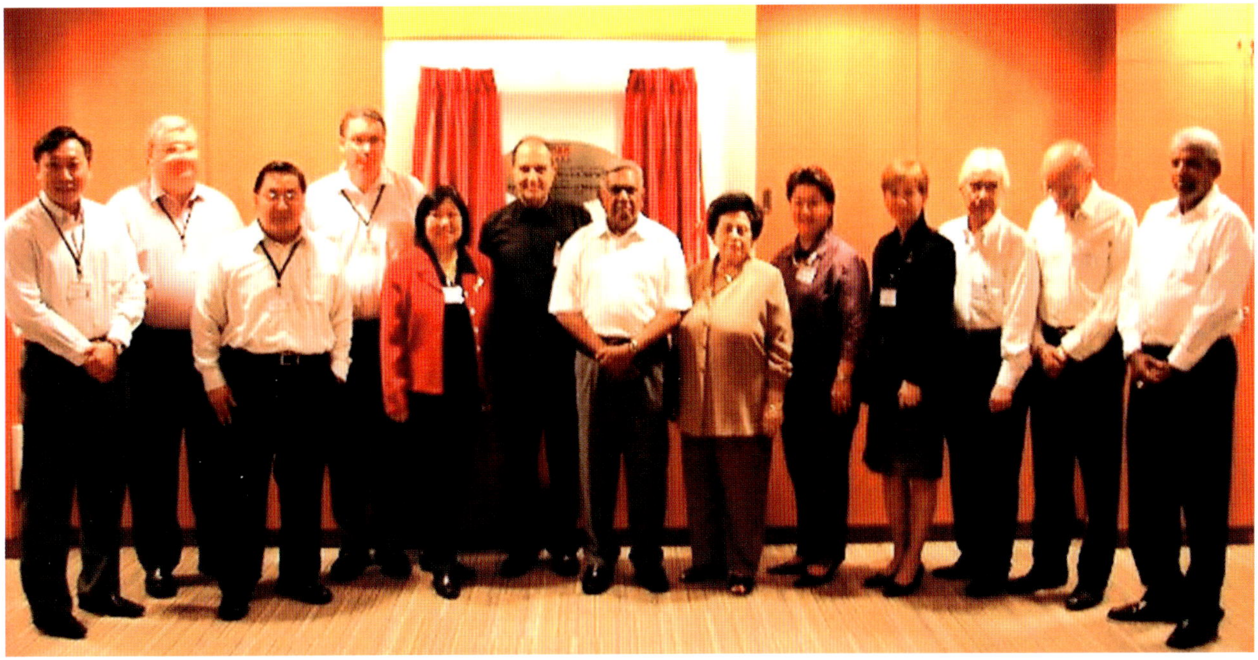

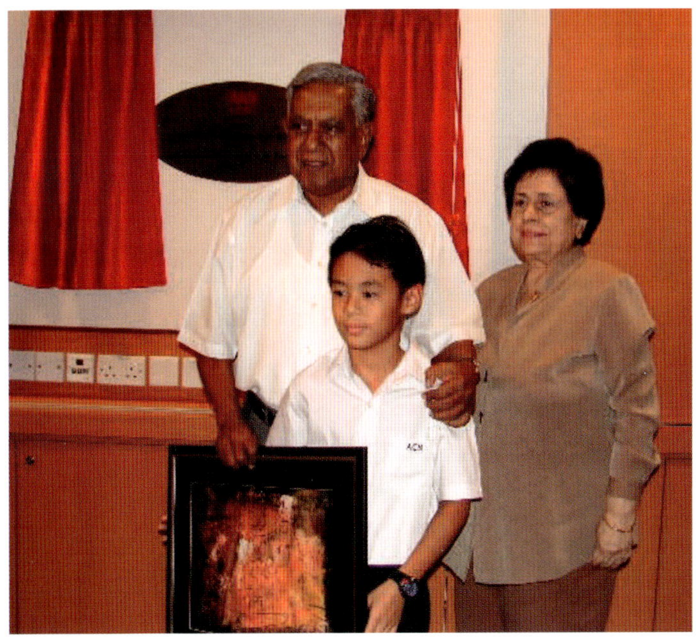

President S. R. Nathan and Mrs Nathan visit DAS. (L to R) Mr Lee Siang, DAS CCO; Mr Robin Moseley, DAS CEO; Mr Roslan Sa'ad, DAS Education Director; Mr Kevin Smith, DAS Training Director; Mrs Corina Lai, DAS CFO; Dr Jimmy Daruwalla, DAS President; Singapore President S. R. Nathan and Mrs Nathan; Ms Yat Swee Eng, DAS Exco and Chair of the DAS Parents Support Group; Ms June Tham, DAS Exco; Mr Derek McCully, DAS Exco; Mr Kaka Singh, DAS Exco; and Mr Rajaram, DAS Exco.

2006

JAN First Lady, Mrs Nathan, visited the Queenstown Learning Centre at Anderson Primary School.

DAS opened the first learning centre in a shopping mall at Bishan Junction 8.

JUN DAS launched the Preschool Service. Education Minister, Mr Tharman Shanmugaratnam, was the Guest of Honour at this event.

The National Council of Social Services provided $300,000 over two years to help the project get started.

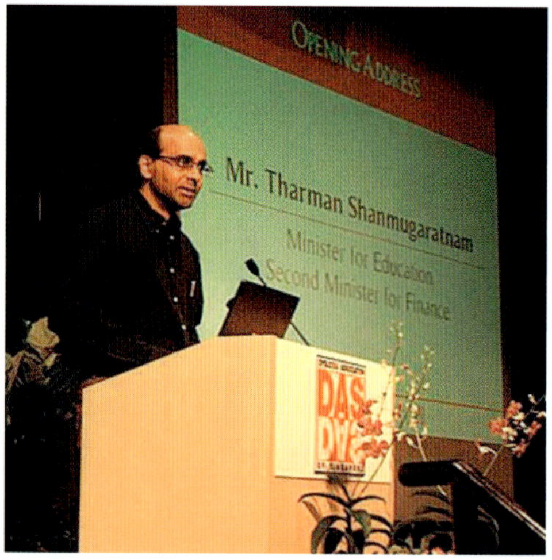

Mr Tharman Shanmugaratnam, Education Minister, was the Guest of Honour at the DAS Preschool Service launch .

JUN The Rotary Club of Raffles City, together with Lions Club of Singapore New Central, held a charity golf event in aid of DAS.

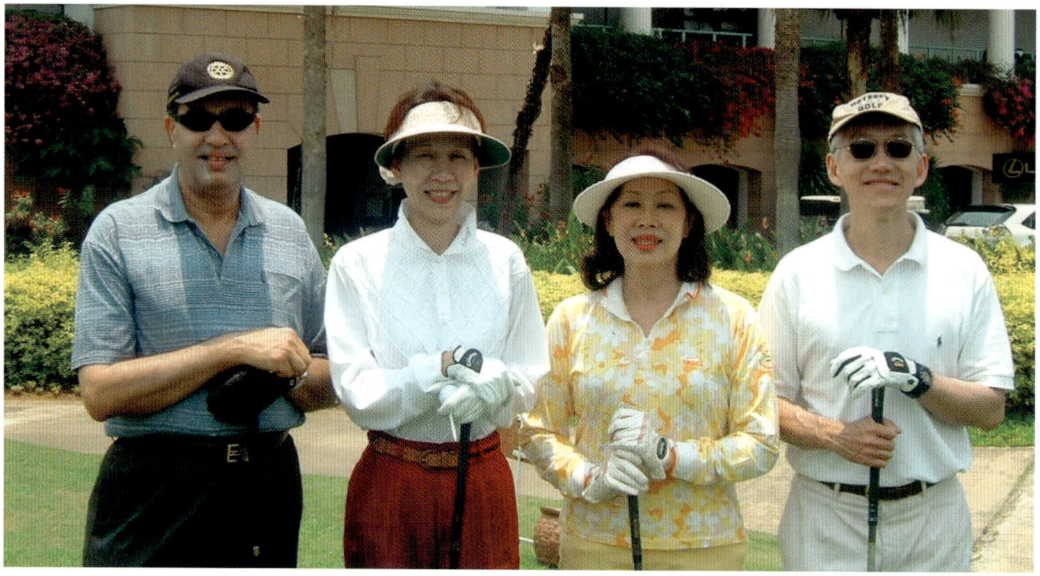

Golf Flight, Dr Jimmy Daruwalla, Ms Cynthia Tan, Mrs Goh Chok Tong and Mr Eric Lee.

2006

NOV The Rotary Club of Raffles City organised an Art Competition for DAS students at the National Library next to Bugis Junction. Volunteers from Deutsche Bank helped at the event.

DEC DAS staff spoke on the identification of dyslexic children at the "Helping Children with Dyslexia" Seminar in Jakarta organised by the Universitas Kristen Krida Wacana. DAS conducted a dyslexia workshop for special education teachers in Kota Tinggi, Malaysia, organised by the Alpha & Omega Distance Learning Centre, a non-profit organisation.

2007

MAR DAS gave a presentation on the assessment and diagnosis of dyslexia in Singapore for the Taiwan Academy of Learning Disabilities during their 2007 Annual Conference on 3 March at the National Kaohsiung Normal University.

APR F1 Champion Sir Jackie Stewart visited the Dyslexia Centre at Spring Singapore where he announced that DAS ***"could lead the world in this".***

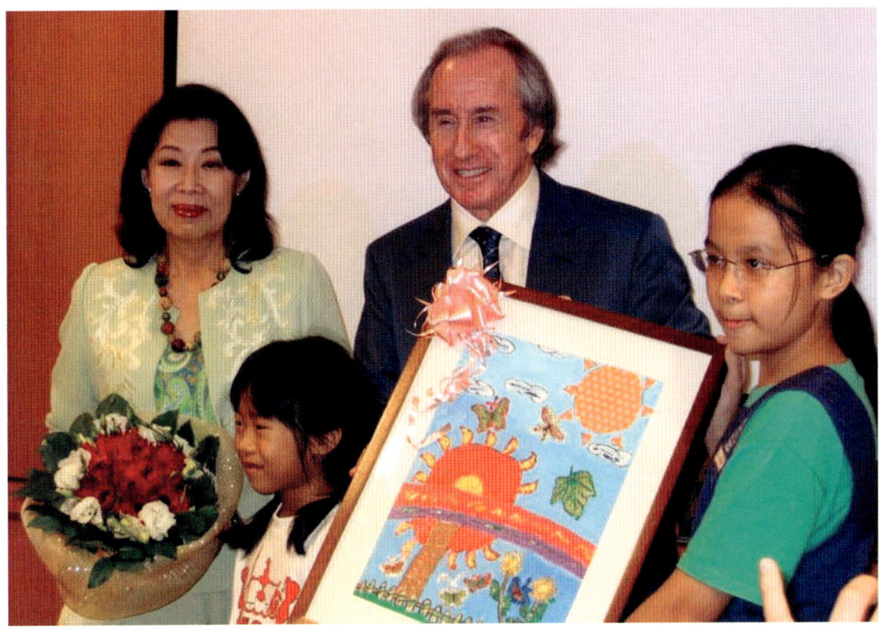

Sir Jackie Stewart with Mrs Goh Chok Tong receiving tokens of appreciation from DAS students.

JUN A two-day workshop was held at Perling Specialist Hospital, Johor Bahru for medical staff, school principals, kindergarten teachers and parents.

2007

JUL DAS reached out internationally to Hong Kong. The Orton-Gillingham course was conducted for the first batch of teachers of Tung Wah Group. This course was conducted for an additional four years.

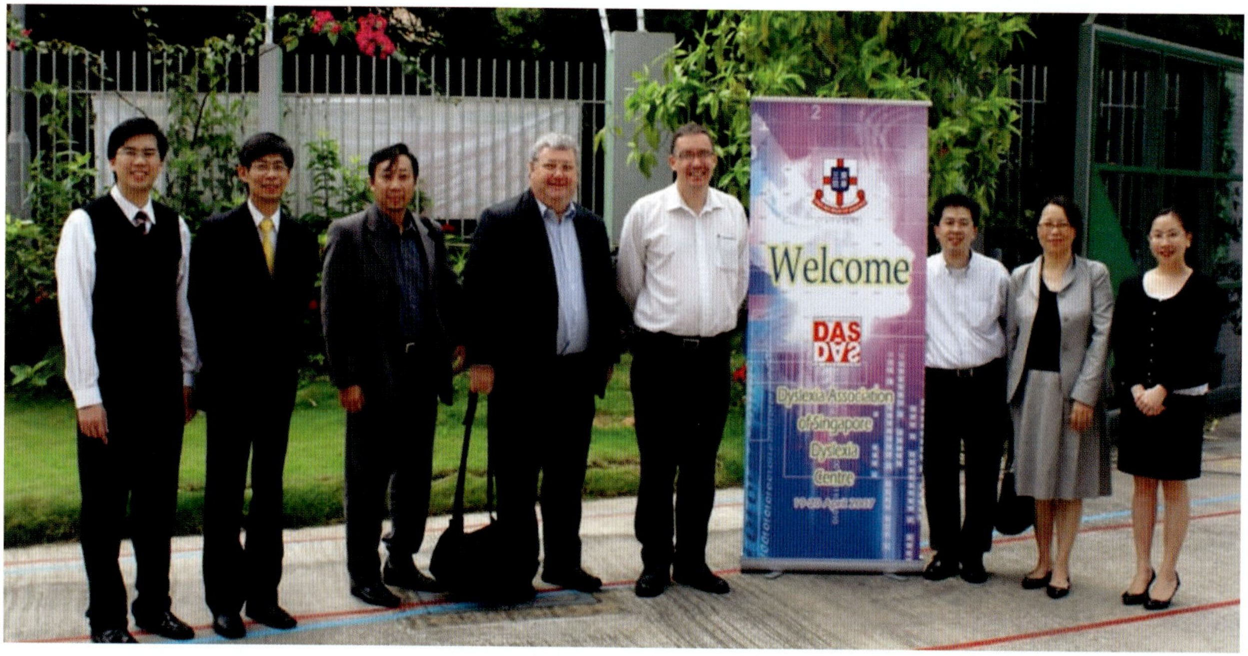

At Hong Kong Tung Wah Group – Pictured above with Tung Wah Staff, (standing to the left of the banner from R to L) Mr Kevin Smith, DAS Training Director; Mr Robin Moseley, DAS CEO; and Mr Lee Siang, DAS COO.

JUN MOE signed a five-year contract with DAS to train Special Needs Officers as part of the National Institute of Education's Diploma in Special Education in 2005.

The first two batches of Special Needs Officers who had completed their training with the NIE and DAS in August 2007 received their graduation certificates from the Minister of State for Education Mr Gan Kim Yong.

Enrolment in our main literacy programme stood at 1,032 students.

2008

MAR Official Opening of the Bishan Learning Centre, at Bishan Junction 8, officiated by Mrs Goh Chok Tong, DAS Patron.

.

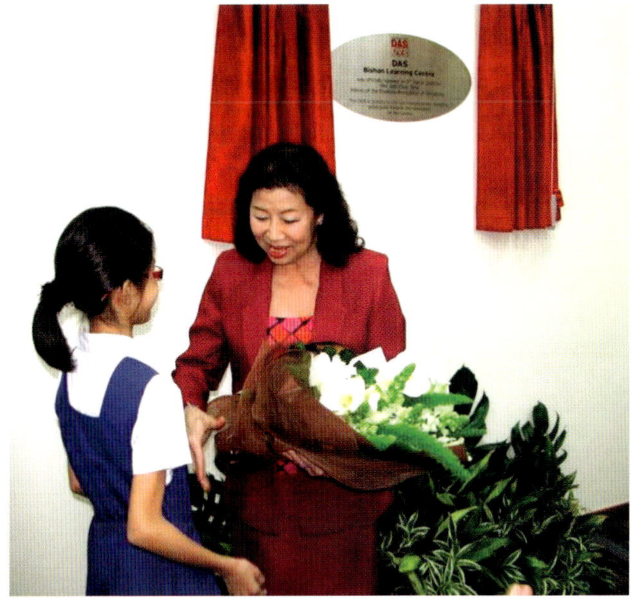

Mrs Goh Chok Tong receiving a token of appreciation from a DAS student.

DEC DAS launched its first Advertising Campaign. It was sponsored by Credit Suisse Singapore.

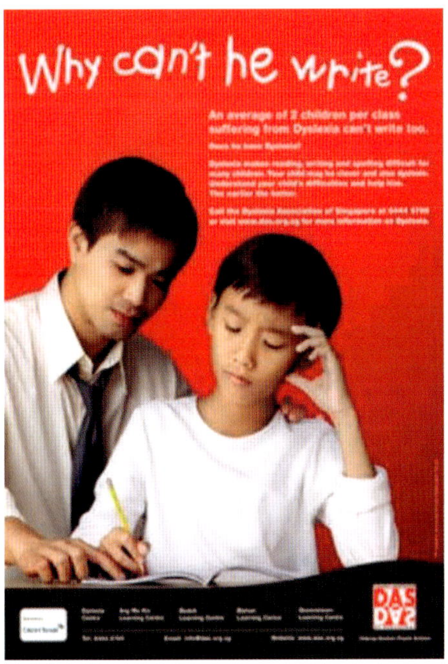
Why can't he write?

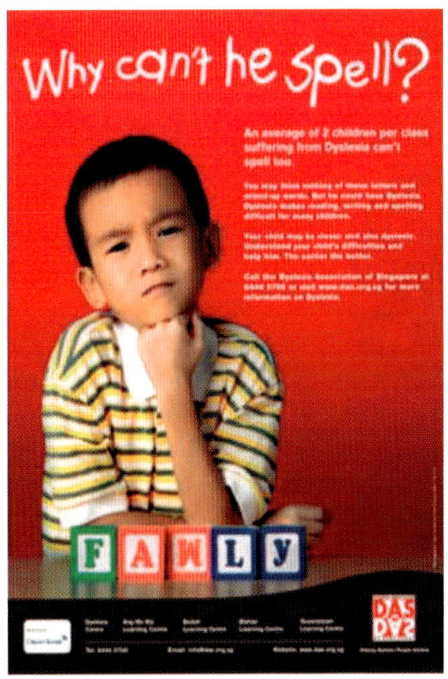
Why can't he spell?
FAWLY

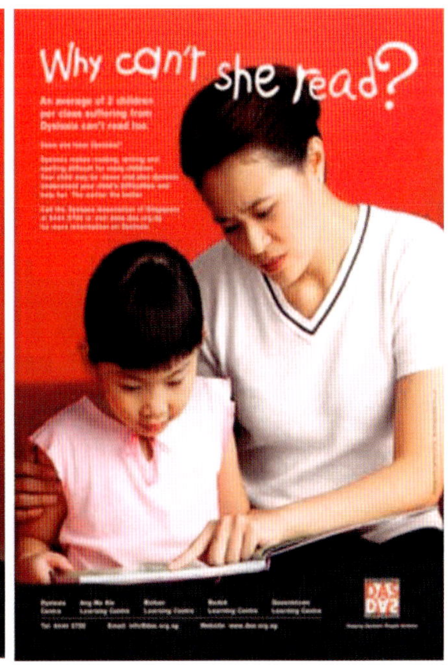
Why can't she read?

2008

AUG Raffles City Rotary Club raised $200,000 for DAS through its charity Dinner. It was held on 2 August at the Meritus Mandarin in conjunction with their Presidential Installation Ceremony. His Excellency President S. R. Nathan was the Guest of Honour. Attended by 300 guests, there was also a performance by veteran artiste Usha Uthup from Calcutta.

DAS won the Best Poster award at the British Dyslexia Association Conference for the poster titled "Dyslexia Friendly Survey in Singapore—Students' views on factors critical for learning" presented by DAS Psychologists.

JUN Graduation of the 2nd Batch of MOE Special Needs Officers trained by DAS on supporting students with learning differences was held with Guest of Honour, Ms Grace Fu, Senior Minister of State, Ministry of Education.

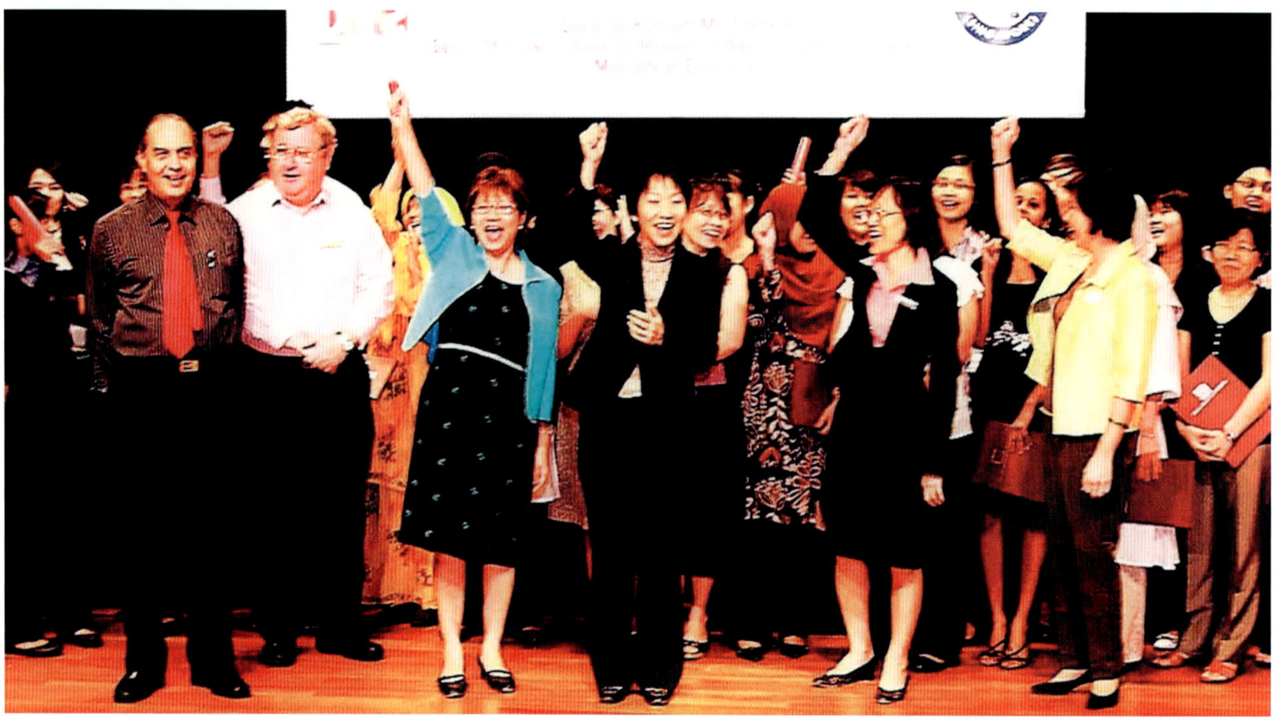

Present at the graduation of the Special Needs Officers (SNO) were (L to R) Dr Jimmy Daruwalla, DAS President; Mr Robin Moseley, DAS CEO; Ms Grace Fu, Senior Ministry of State, Minister of Education; Mrs Linda Low; and the graduating SNO's.

2009

FEB Dyslexia Centre moved to Jurong Point under the NCSS Civic and Community Institution Space Scheme. This centre, for the first time, provided assessment, training and education services under one roof. DAS also opened new learning centres in Woodlands and Tampines. This marked the first time that DAS had centres located in HDB void decks.

MAY DAS presented at a conference organised by the Tung Wah Group of Hospitals and the University of Hong Kong.

DAS launched the first Dyslexia Raise Awareness Week (DRAW).

The DAS Woodlands Learning Centre, our first HDB void deck centre, was officially opened by Mr Hawazi Daipi, MP for Sembawang GRC.

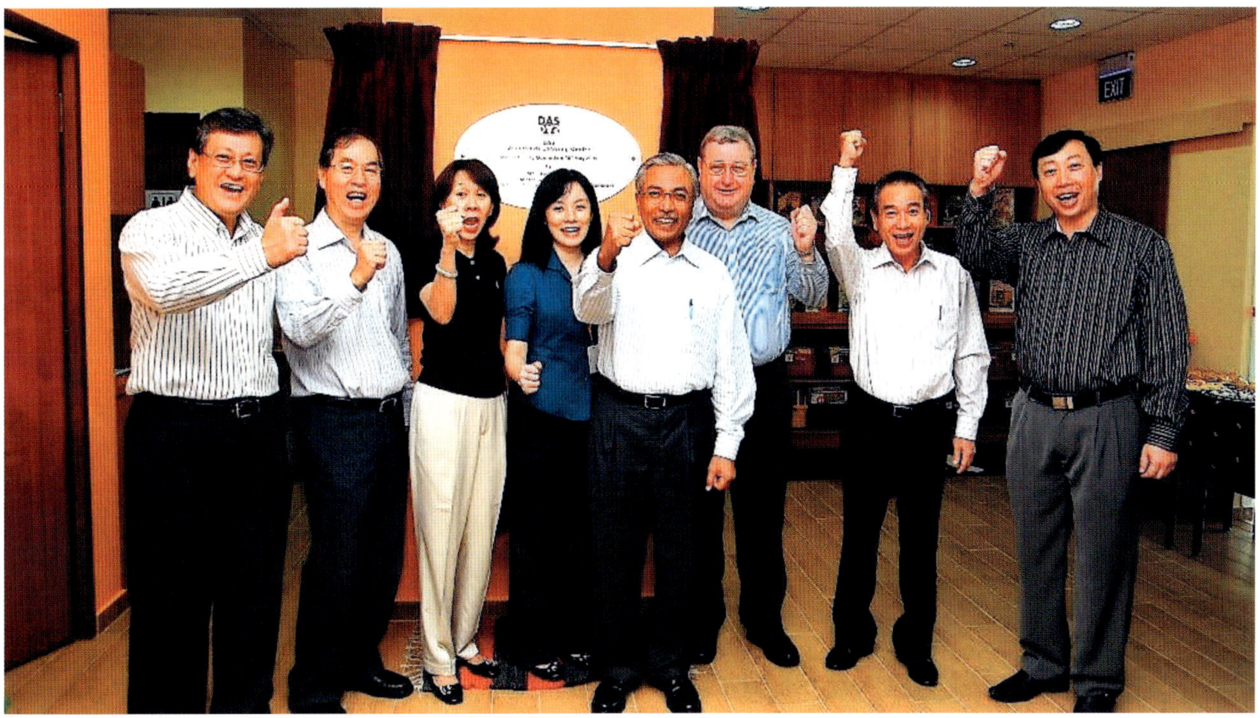

Opening of DAS Woodlands Learning Centre, (L to R) Mr Paul Lim, DAS Exco; Mr Vincent Chen, DAS Exco; Ms Cynthia Tan, DAS Exco; Ms Jane Ho, DAS Educational Therapist; Mr Hawazi Daipi, MP for Sembawang GRC; Mr Robin Moseley, DAS CEO; a Woodlands Community member; and Mr Lee Siang, DAS COO.

2009

JUL At the request of the Ministry of Education, Brunei, the DAS conducted a one-day seminar on dyslexia for 500 senior officers and teachers of the ministry. DAS lecturers subsequently delivered a two-week Certificate Course in Dyslexia Studies for 24 Special Education Officers. The course was very well received and MOE Brunei requested that DAS conduct similar courses in 2011, 2012 and 2013.

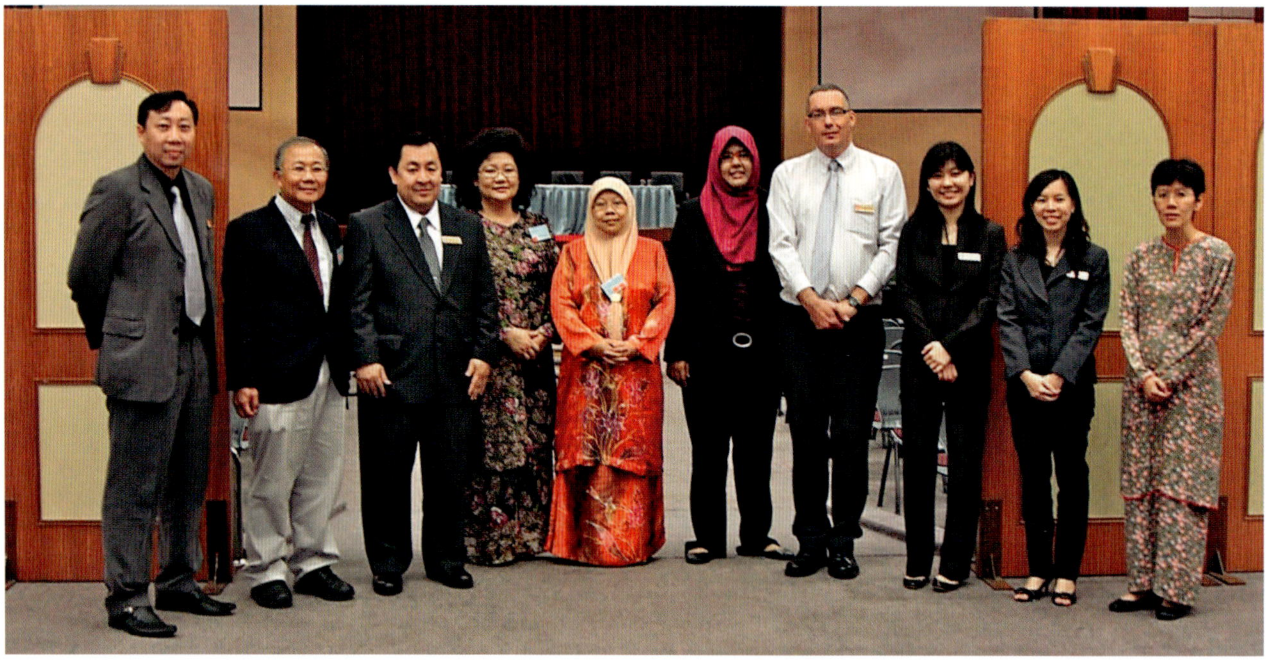

DAS Staff members with Brunei MOE Staff (BMS). (L to R) Mr Lee Siang, DAS COO; BMS staff member; Roslan Sa'ad, DAS Education Director; two Brunei MOE staff; Aishah Said, DAS Educational Therapist; Kevin Smith, DAS Director of Training; Danielle Seah, DAS Specialist Psychologist; Choo Ling Fong, DAS Specialist Psychologist; and a BMS staff member.

SEP DAS launched the Master of Arts in Specific Learning Differences course, accredited by London Metropolitan University in Singapore.

DAS opened its 8th learning centre in the Parkway Parade shopping mall.

2009

NOV DAS organised the first Dyslexia Conference in Asia which was graced by Guest of Honour, Dr Ng Eng Hen, Minister for Education and Second Minister of Defence. The Conference was attended by over 500 teachers, therapists and parents along with a number of foreign delegates from Brunei, Hong Kong, India, Indonesia, Malaysia, the Philippines and Thailand.

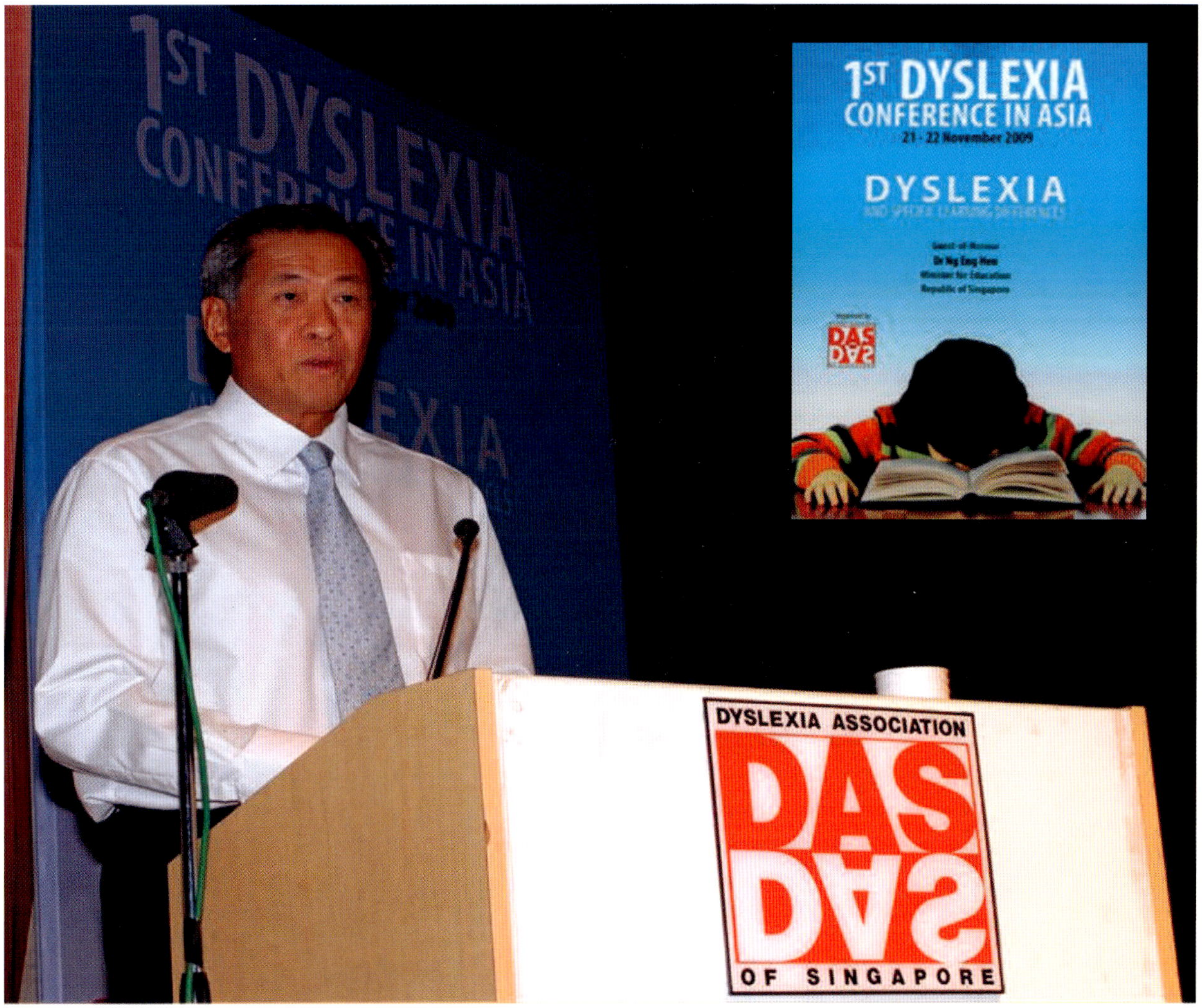

Guest of Honour, Dr Ng Eng Hen, Minister for Education and Second Minister of Defence.

DEC Enrolment for DAS Preschool Service increased to 82 students. Enrolment for the DAS Main Literacy Programme stood at 1,321 students.

2010

APR DAS launched "DAS at the Libraries" to raise awareness about dyslexia. Several awareness talks in English, Malay, Tamil and Mandarin were conducted at various public libraries.

AUG The Rotary Club of Raffles City held its 31st Installation Ceremony and the event at Hilton Hotel was graced by Guest of Honour, Mr S. Dhanabalan, Chairman of Temasek Holdings. A total of $100,000 was raised for DAS at the event.

AUG DAS Academy evolved from a need to localise professional training and development of specialist teachers in dyslexia and SpLD in Singapore. The DAS Training Service was first initiated in 2003 and when government regulations required the registration of Diploma and Masters level programmes under the Council for Private Education, DAS Academy was incorporated as a Private Educational Institution and a subsidiary of DAS.

Led by a multi-disciplinary team that has extensive experience in providing direct support to people with specific learning differences (SpLD), the lecturers are able to use their skills and expertise in the design and delivery of the programmes offered by the DAS Academy.

DAS Academy
ENABLING EXCELLENCE

These programmes provide an academic pathway in the field of SpLD from foundation to postgraduate levels.

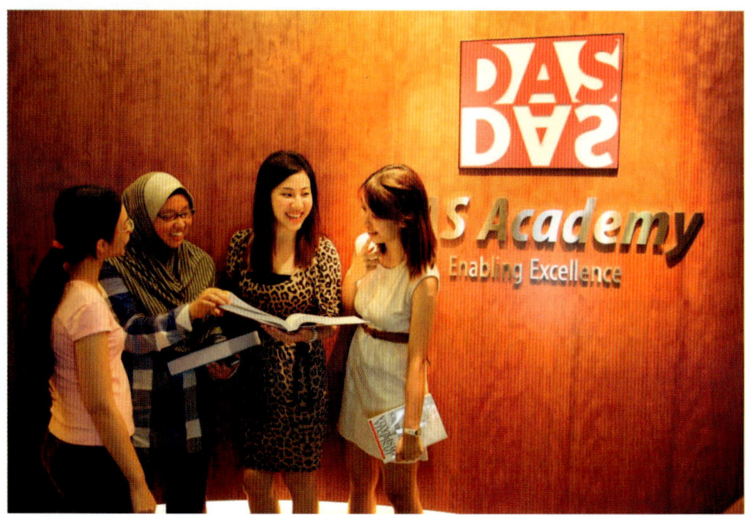

2010

NOV The annual conference adopted a Seminar Week model as well as expanded coverage to related Specific Learning Differences. The DAS Seminar Week was held over five days at the Suntec Singapore Convention Centre. The event was made possible by the Lee Foundation which contributed $50,000 to support the event. Other sponsors included SPH Foundation and the Kwan Im Thong Hood Cho Temple.

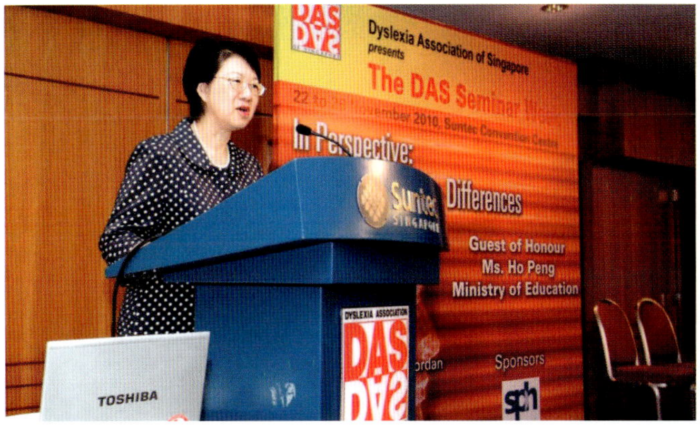

The DAS Seminar Week was graced by Guest of Honour, Ms Ho Peng, Ministry of Education

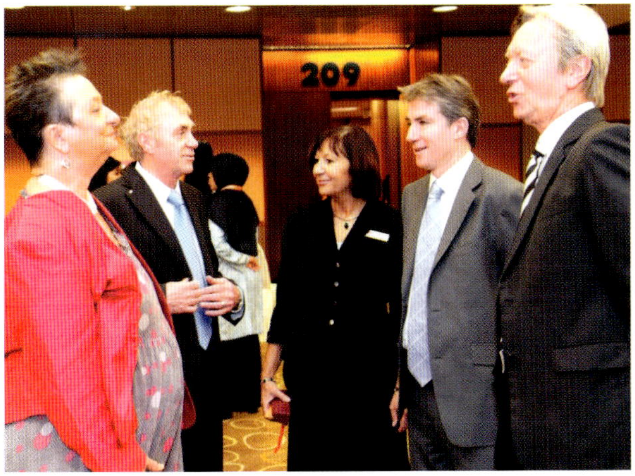

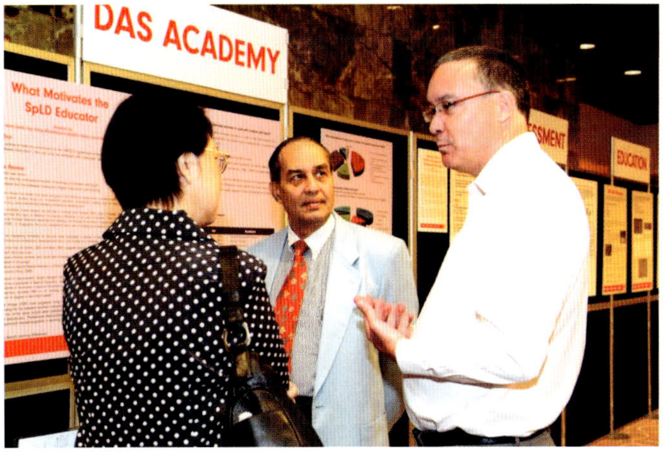

Above: (L to R) International presenters at the DAS Seminar Week, Professor Rita Jordan; Dr Gavin Reid; Ms Gaynor Brooks, DAS Consulting Educational Psychologist; Mr Fintan O'Regan; and Dr Steve Chinn.

Above right: (L to R) Ms Ho Peng; Dr Jimmy Daruwalla, DAS President; and Mr Kevin Smith, Director of DAS Academy.

Right: Robin Moseley, DAS CEO presenting at the DAS Seminar week.

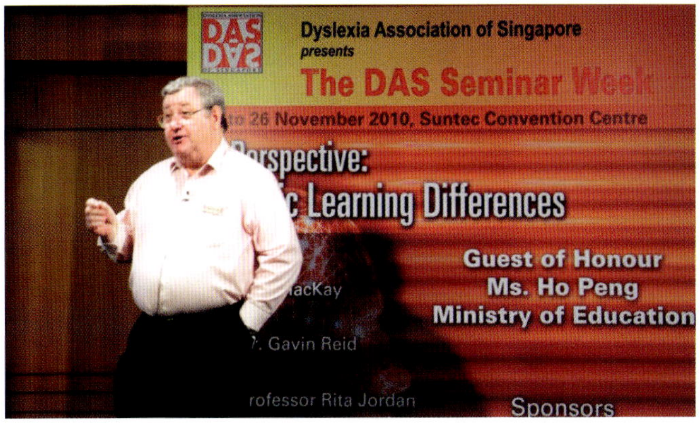

2011

MAY Dyslexia Raise Awareness Week featured week-long interactive activities such as "Building Self-Esteem" at the Singapore Management University.

DAS International was launched as a wholly-owned subsidiary of DAS. It supported Singaporeans and expatriate students on a one-to-one basis and focused on a wider range of learning differences.

JUN The Royal Bank of Scotland selected DAS as one of four beneficiaries of its Community Investment Programme.

SEP Mediacorp Radio Yes 93.3 adopted DAS.

DAS Sengkang Learning Centre was opened by Mr Teo Ser Luck, Minister of State, Ministry of Trade and Industry, and Mayor of North East district.

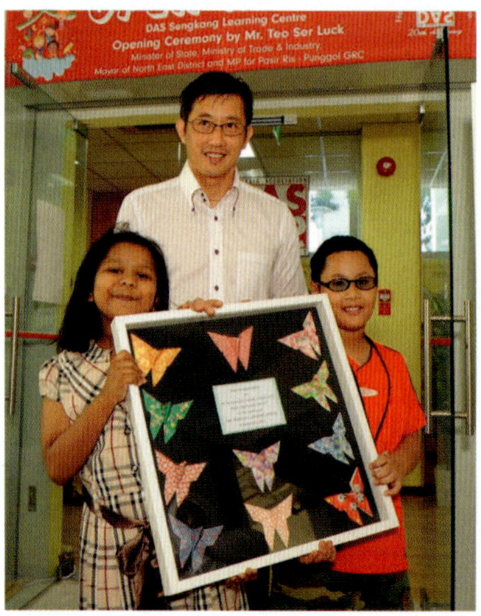
DAS Sengkang Learning Centre
Opening Ceremony by Mr. Teo Ser Luck
Minister of State, Ministry of Trade & Industry,
Mayor of North East District and MP for Pasir Ris - Punggol GRC

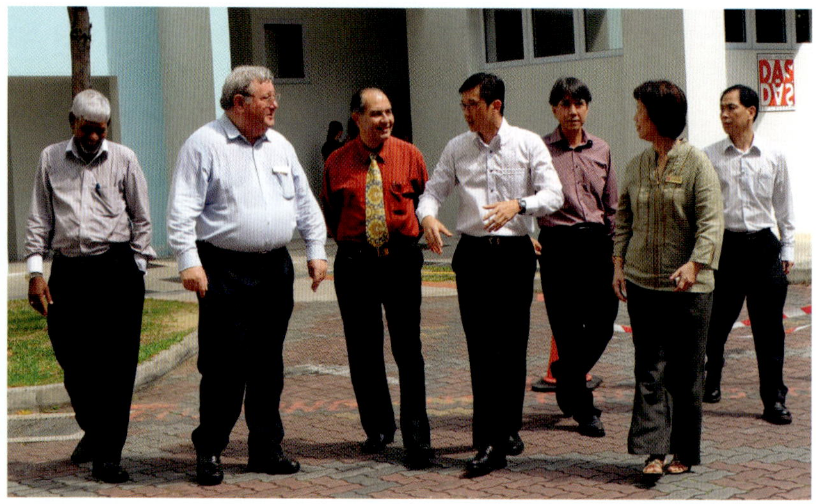

Official Opening of DAS Sengkang Learning Centre by Mr Teo Ser Luck, Minister of State, Ministry of Trade and Industry and Mayor of North East District, pictured on the left with DAS students receiving his token of appreciation and right walking with (L to R) Mr Rajaram, DAS Exco; Mr Robin Moseley, DS CEO; Dr Jimmy Daruwalla, DAS President; Mr Teo Ser Luck; two ministry staff and Mrs Carine Wong, DAS Centre Manager.

NOV DAS held its third annual conference themed "Success with Technology". The focus was on Assistive Technology and how it can benefit and facilitate children's learning.
Enrolment on the main literacy programme has reached 1794 students.

2012

APR DAS opened its Tampines Learning Centre and the event was graced by Mr Masagos Zulkifli Bin Masagos Mohamad, Minister of State, Ministry of Home Affairs and Ministry of Foreign Affairs, and MP for Tampines GRC.

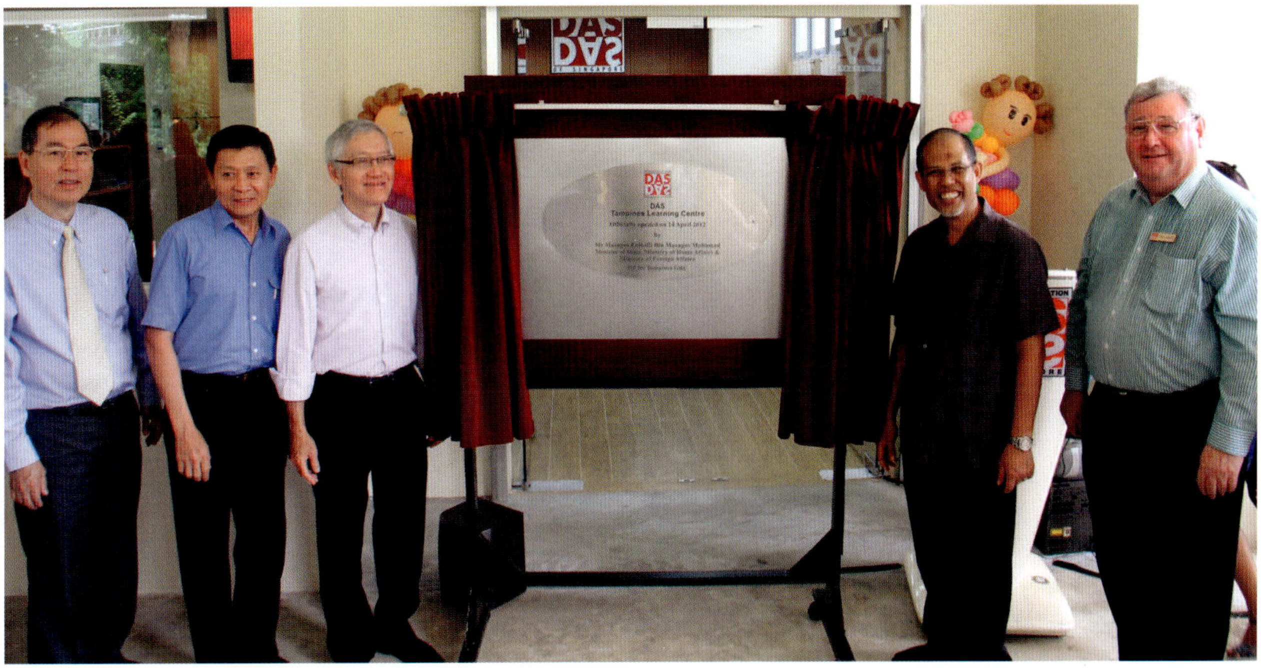

(L to R) Mr Vincent Chen, DAS Exco; Tampines Community Leader; Mr Eric Lee, DAS Vice President; Mr Masagos Zulkifli Bin Masagos Mohamad, Minister of State, Ministry of Home Affairs and Ministry of Foreign Affairs, and MP for Tampines GRC; and Mr Robin Moseley, DAS CEO.

SEP DAS published "*My Inner World: A Celebration of Dyslexic Minds*". This 70-page collection of creativity, wit and brilliance by the children we work with was a special 21st anniversary publication. It celebrates what dyslexics are capable of and invites the reader to journey into their world. Four chapters in the book feature a myriad of artwork, writing, expressions plus activities to keep the reader constantly engaged.

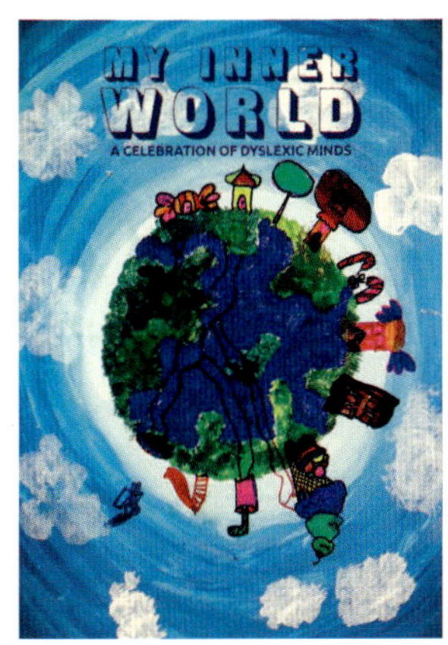

2012

SEP DAS celebrated 21 years of helping individuals with learning differences with a Charity Gala Dinner which raised a total of $1.3 million. The event was graced by Guest of Honour DPM Tharman Shanmugaratnam, DAS Patron Mrs Goh Chok Tong, DAS Executive Committee members and major donors. There was a performance by DAS students as well as a charity auction.

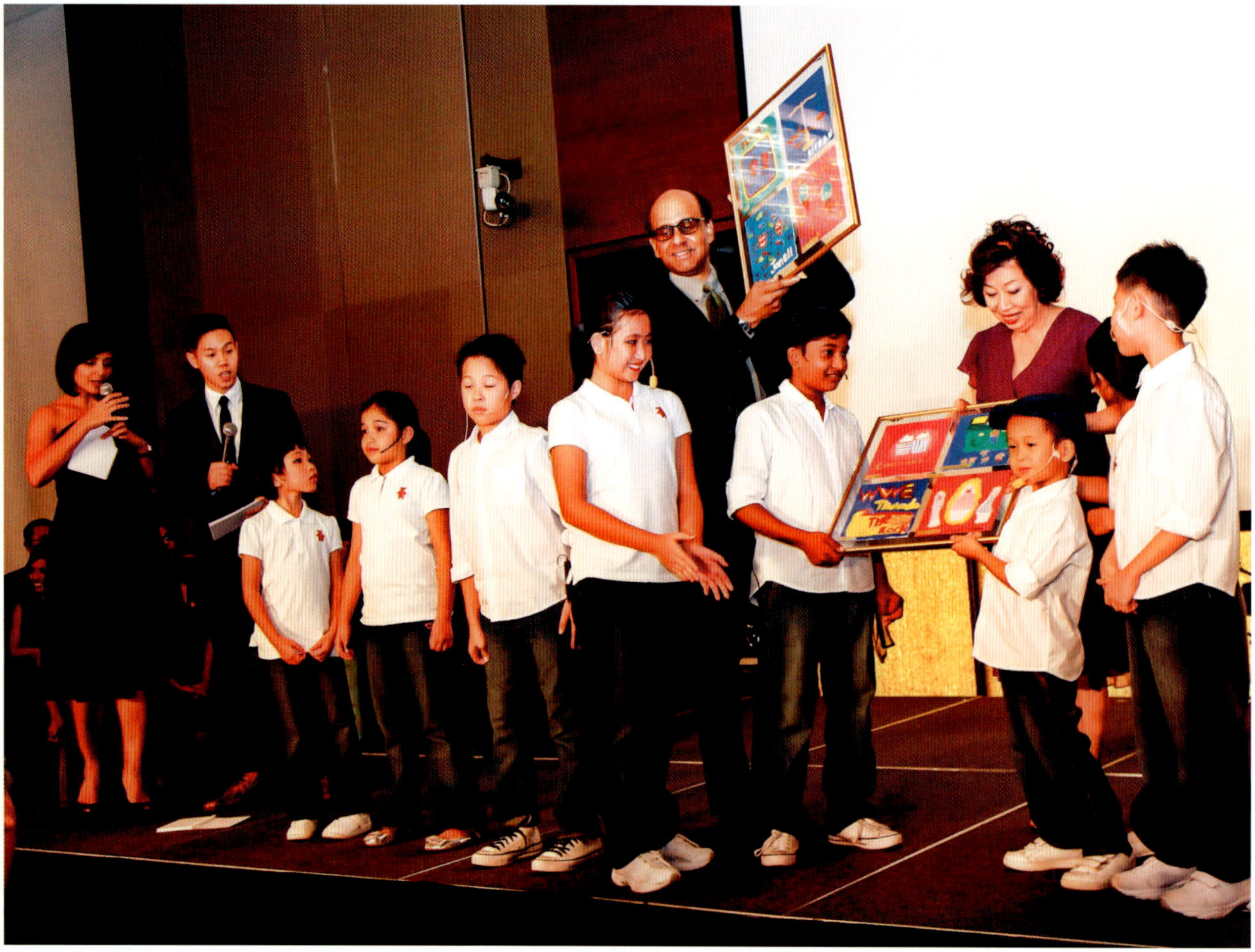

Artwork created by young DAS student performers were given as a token of appreciation to our DAS Patron, Mrs Goh Chok Tong and Guest of Honour, Mr Tharman Shanmugaratnam.

2012

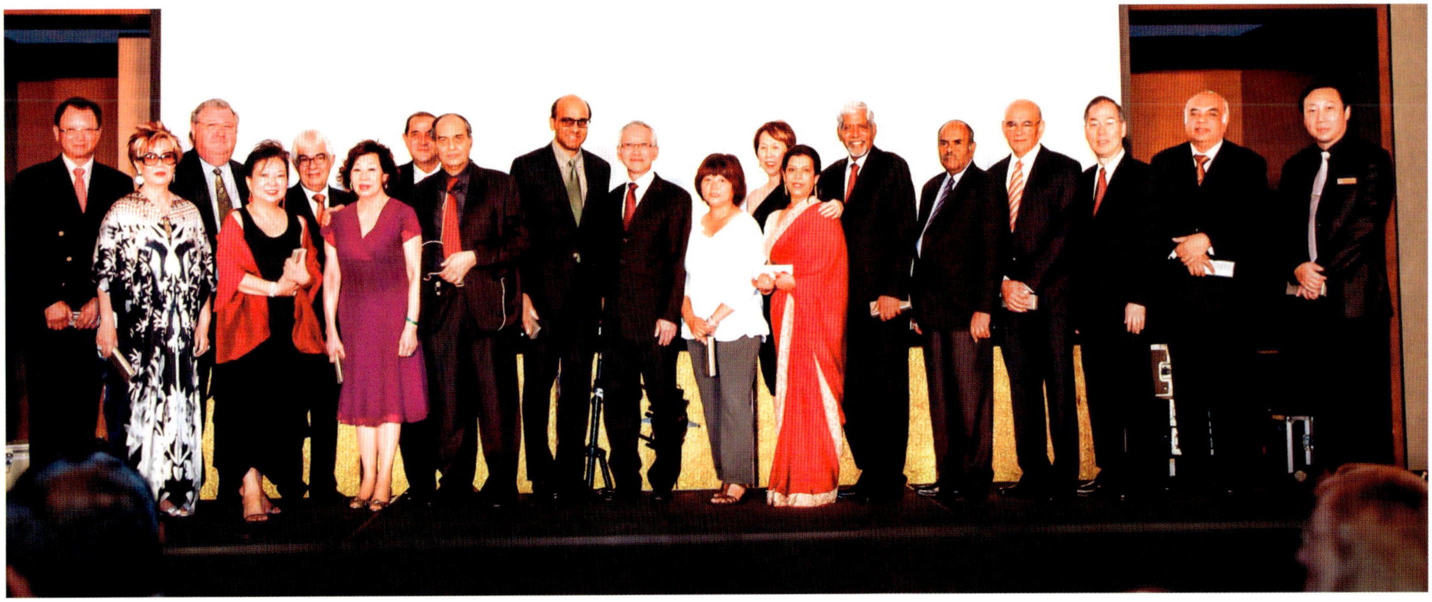

Members of the Rotary Club of Raffles City and supporters of DAS were recognised for their long-term support at the 21st Anniversary Dinner.

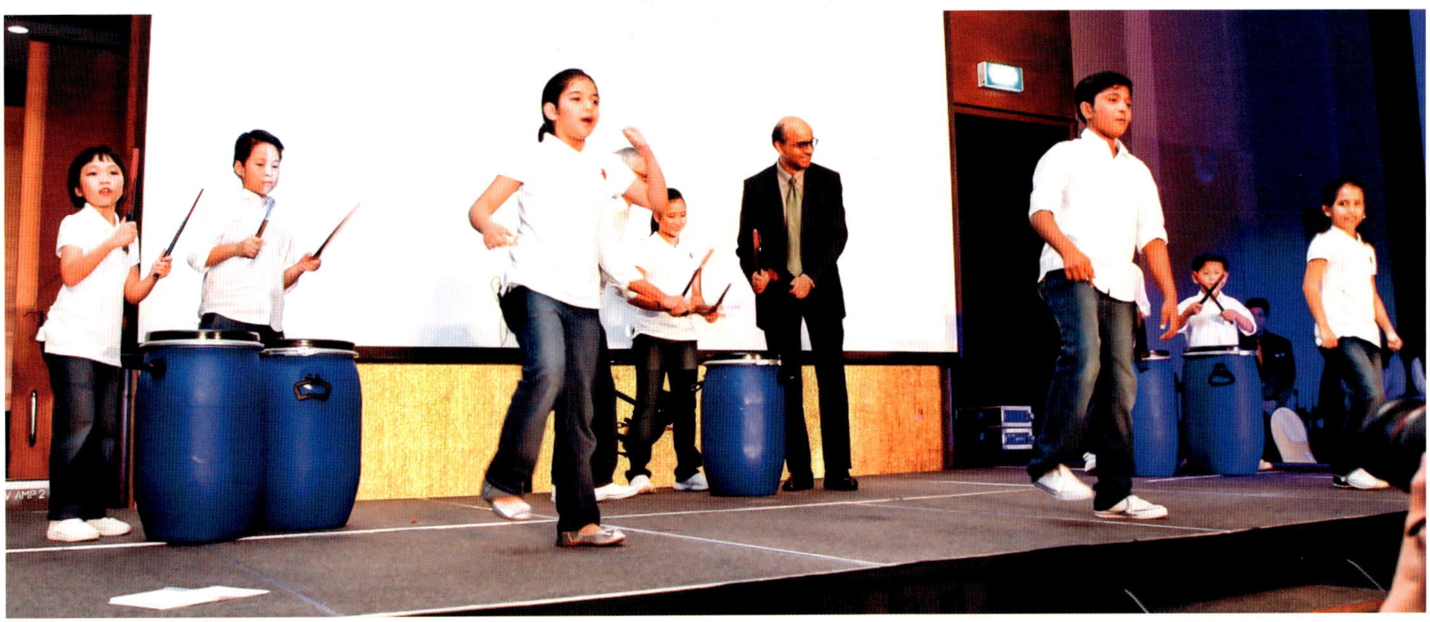

Mr Tharman Shanmugaratnam had a chance to perform with DAS students at the 21st Anniversary Dinner.

2012

SEP Mr Sam Tan, the Mayor of Central Singapore District, declared that he is dyslexic in the Singapore press.

Student enrolment on the main literacy programme stands at 2,300 students.

OCT The Register of Educational Therapists (Asia) or RETA was officially launched at Traders Hotel with guest speaker Dr Kate Saunders, CEO of the British Dyslexia Association. RETA aims to set professional standards amongst practitioners, and members are classified according to their professional experiences and qualifications in the field of educational therapy.

DAS formed the DAS Student Alumni for ex-students to act as mentors to our current students.

NOV DAS held its fourth annual conference themed "Maths Learning Differences and Dyscalculia" and speakers included Professor Angela Fawcett, Mrs Anne Henderson, Professor Brian Butterworth, Professor Steve Chinn and Asst Professor Lee Ngan Hoe.

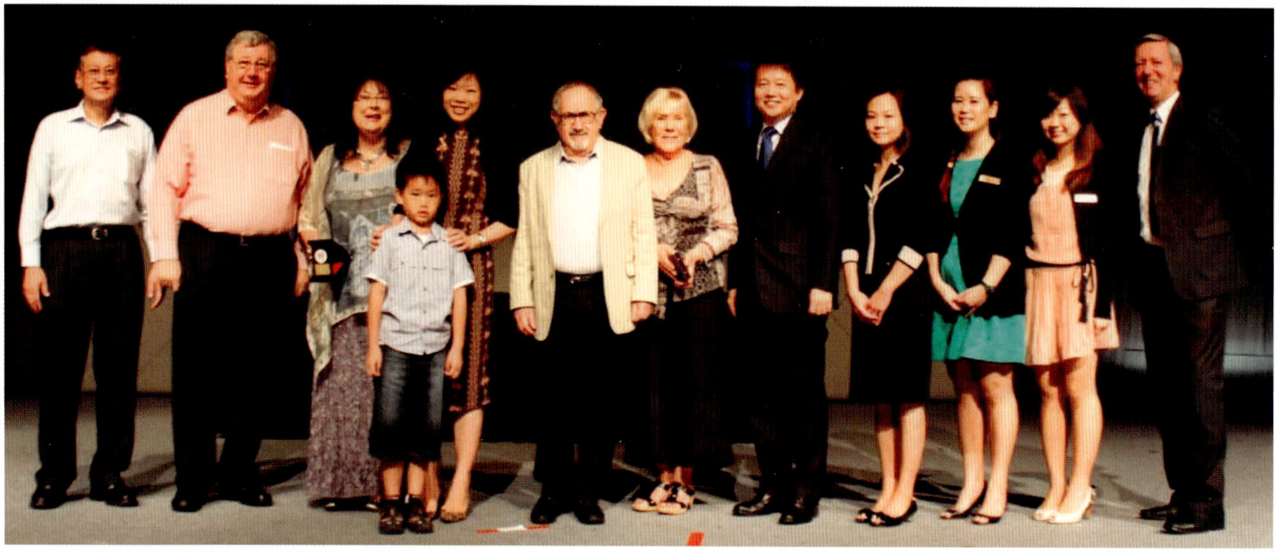

(L to R) Mr Paul Lim, DAS Exco; Mr Robin Moseley, DAS CEO; Professor Angela Fawcett; Benedict Lo, a DAS Student; Ms Sim Ann, Guest of Honour, Senior Parliamentary Secretary, Ministry of Education and Ministry of Communications and Information; Professor Brian Butterworth; Mrs Anne Henderson; Assistant Professor Lee Ngan Hoe; Ms Chang Suo Hui; Ms Claire Yeo, DAS Educational Therapist; Ms Priscillia Shen, Lecturer DAS Academy; and Professor Steve Chinn.

2013

JAN The Chinese Remediation Programme was launched after a pilot study was conducted from 2010 to 2011. The Programme aims to support dyslexic students in their Chinese language studies.

MAR DAS officially opened its 11th centre at Chinatown Point. The centre will serve as a hub for various DAS services to meet the rising demand. The launch event was graced by Mr Sam Tan, Senior Parliamentary Secretary, Ministry of Foreign Affairs and Ministry of Culture, Community and Youth, and Mayor, Central Singapore District.

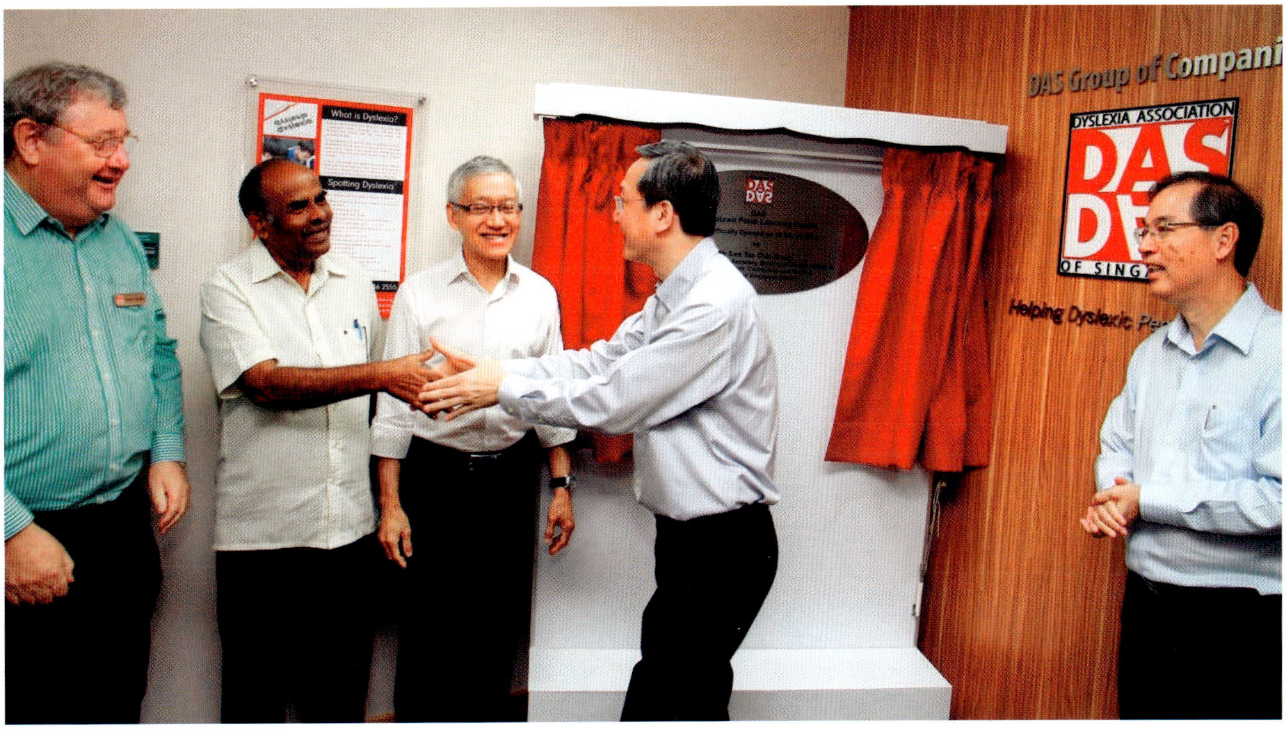

(L to R) Robin Moseley, DAS CEO; Mr Kesavapany, DAS Exco; Mr Eric Lee, DAS Vice President; Mr Sam Tan, Senior Parliamentary Secretary, Ministry of Foreign Affairs and Ministry of Culture, Community and Youth and Mayor, Central Singapore District; and Mr Vincent Chen, DAS Exco.

JUN More than 100 parents and educators attended the first ever DAS Preschool Seminar to learn about specific learning difficulties that preschool children face.

2013

JUN DAS, in collaboration with OCBC's Global Trading & Investment Banking Group (OCBC GTIB), established the DAS-OCBC GTIB Scholarship. The scholarship is awarded to dyslexic students enrolled with the DAS in recognition of their resilient character and outstanding excellence in various areas.

The DAS-OCBC GTIB Scholarship is awarded to DAS students at the Student Graduation Ceremony.

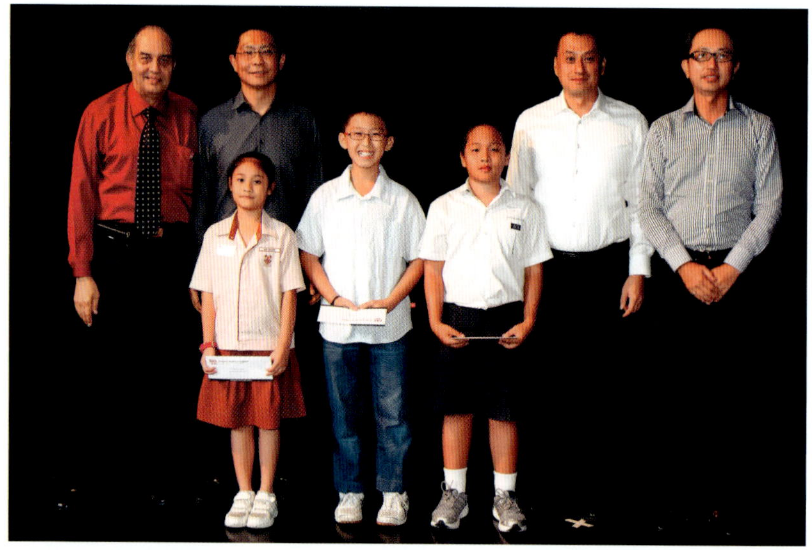

The three $10,000 scholarship awardees Deanna Binte Mohamed Ismail, Law Yong Jun Jabez Mason and Lim You Wei Jonathan are pictured above with (L to R) Dr Jimmy Daruwalla, DAS President; Mr Lam Kun Kin, Senior Executive Vice President, Head Global Treasury & Investment Banking OCBC Bank; Mr Kenneth Mark Lai Chin Kui; and Mr Jason Ho, also from OCBC-GTIB.

JUN The DAC Academy formed a partnership with the University of South Wales, UK to launch the Master of Arts in Special Educational Needs (MA SEN). Accredited by the University of South Wales and jointly delivered by the DAS Academy, this programme has been well received by both educators and caregivers of people with special educational.

JUL The DAS English Exam Skills programme was launched for Primary 5 and 6 students to better prepare them for the PSLE.

AUG A Speech and Drama Arts Programme was launched for primary school students. Besides improving speech and self-confidence of students, this is the only Speech and Drama programme to also focus on literacy.

NOV The fifth DAS conference took the form of a workshop series themed "A Practical Approach to Learning" from 18 to 20 November, for the sharing of the knowledge and expertise of local and international experts such as Ms Susan Lowell and Dr Kate Saunders

2014

JAN DAS published its first research journal, the *Asia Pacific Journal of Developmental Differences*. This was to encourage research into dyslexia and related learning differences. This focus of this journal was to encourage regional research for dyslexia and related learning differences. The journal's editor is Emeritus Professor Angela Fawcett.

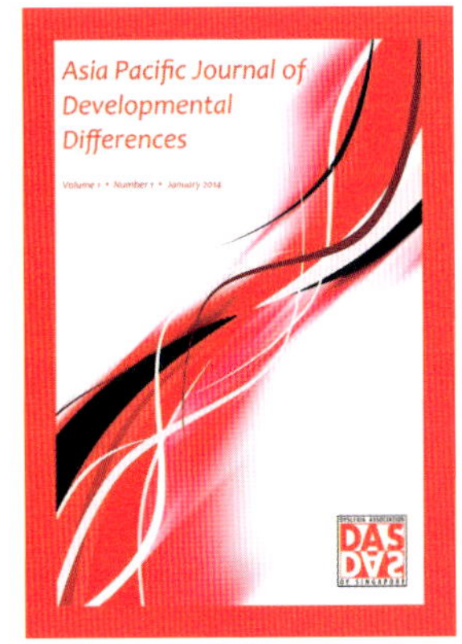

MAR DAS officially opened its 13th centre on 17 March. The Chairman of the Citizen's Consultative Committee, Minister for Health Mr Gan Kim Yong was the Guest of Honour. Mr Rajesh Malkani generously donated $300,000 to the building of the centre in the name of his late mother Mrs Ratna Malkani. Mr Malkani's donation is the largest donation ever from an individual donor.

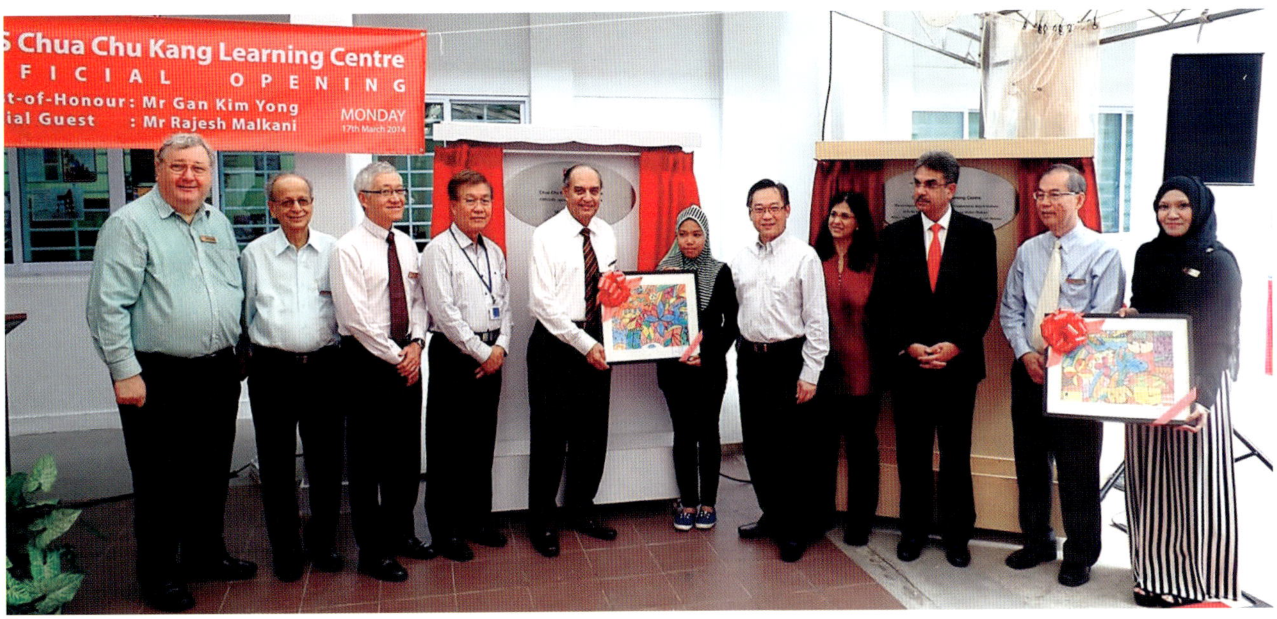

(L to R) Mr Robin Moseley, DAS CEO; Mr Arun Desai, DAS Honorary Asst. Secretary; Mr Eric Lee, DAS Vice President; Mr Ng Hock Lye, Chua Chu Kang CCC Chairman; Dr Jimmy Daruwalla, DAS President; Miss Rosila Rahan, DAS Student; Mr Gan Kim Yong, Minister for Health, and MP for Chua Chu Kang GRC; Special Guests Mrs and Mr Rajesh Malkani; Mr Vincent Chen, DAS Treasurer; and Nur Aisyah Hashim, DAS Educational Therapist.

2014

APR Specialised Educational Services (SES) was launched as a division of the Dyslexia Association of Singapore. SES oversees all programmes not under the main literacy programme and aims to uncover the true strengths of individuals with learning differences and empower them with the necessary skills and strategies to succeed.

Specialised Educational Services
UNLOCKING POTENTIAL

JUN Starhub donates $160,500 for children from lower-income families to attend the DAS SES Essential Maths Programme.

The largest student graduation ceremony to date was organised with 165 students graduating from the main literacy programme. Ten students received the DAS-OCBC GTIB Scholarship of $5000 each, to be used to further their education.

SEP CEO Succession.
After 12 years of sterling service at DAS, Mr Robin Moseley retired from the post of Chief Executive Officer and the baton was handed over to Mr Lee Siang, who is also a long-serving staff member. Mr Lee Siang joined DAS in 2001 and has played a key role in the rapid growth of DAS.

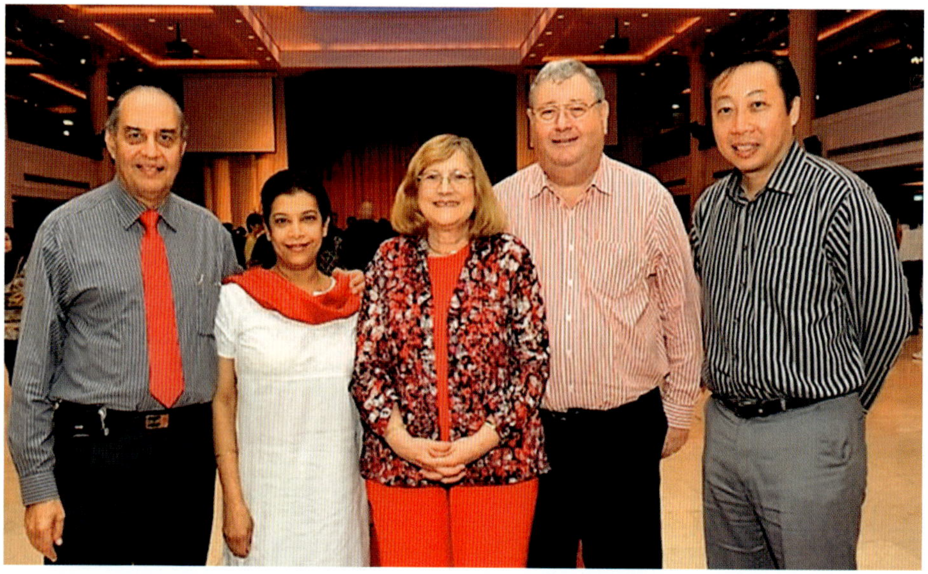

(L to R) Dr Jimmy Daruwalla, DAS President; Mrs Jothy Daruwalla; Mrs Glynis Moseley; Mr Robin Moseley, Retiring DAS CEO; and Mr Lee Siang, DAS COO.

2014

NOV DAS launched EMBRACE DYSLEXIA, a campaign that seeks to bring greater awareness of dyslexia to Singapore and garner greater support for students and families. The campaign consisted of events such as the Embrace Dyslexia Dinner and Seminar in November with famous guest speakers such as Thomas G. West, who is dyslexic himself. The campaign also included a call for adults who are dyslexic and willing to share their personal stories as a form of encouragement and inspiration to people with learning differences.

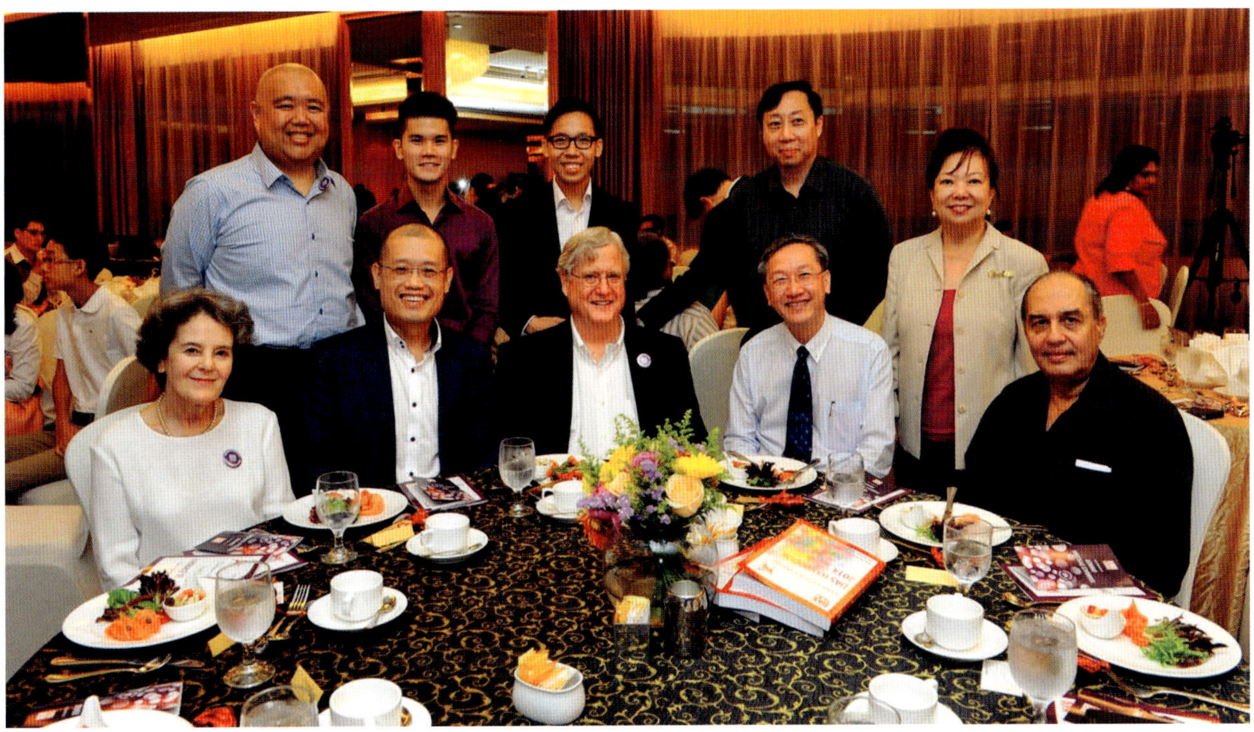

At the Embrace Dyslexia Dinner the VIP guests with our special guest speaker Mr Thomas G. West and Guest of Honour Mr Sam Tan, Minister of State, Prime Minister's Office, Ministry of Culture, Community and Youth. (L to R) Seated Mrs Margaret West; Mr Chua Weng Foo; Mr Thomas G. West; Mr Sam Tan; Dr Jimmy Daruwalla, DAS President. Standing (L to R), Dr Thomas Sim, Executive Director of DAS Academy; Mr Louis Liow, DAS Student Alumni; Mr Edward Yee, DAS Student Alumni; Mr Lee Siang, DAS CEO; and Mrs Corina Lai, DAS CFO.

2015

JAN Our former CEO, Mr Robin Moseley, was awarded an OBE in the 2015 New Years Honours List for his services to children with dyslexia and to education in Singapore. Robin worked for the Dyslexia Association of Singapore for 12 years, rapidly expanding the reach and services of this social enterprise for people in Singapore, and even launching projects in other parts of Asia. Robin is pictured here holding his award with his wife Glynis and his son Matthew.

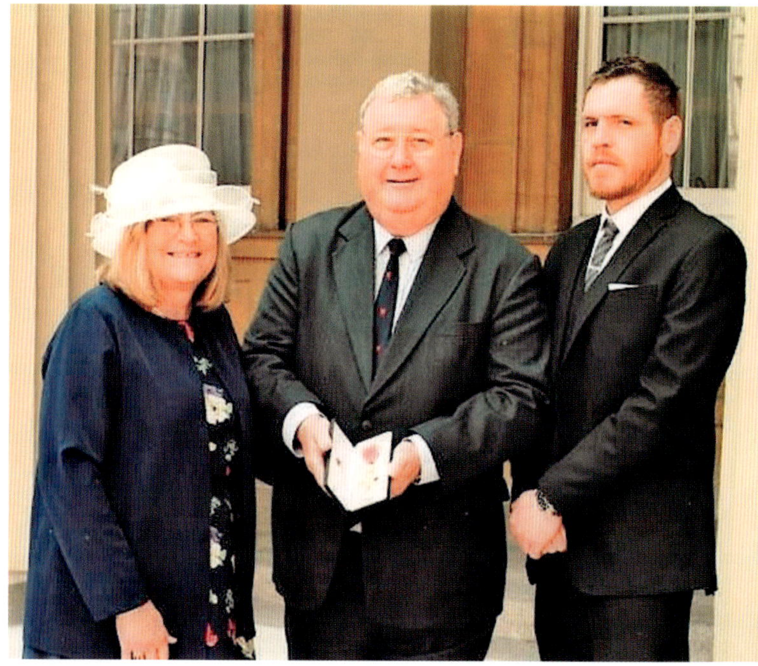

FEB DAS saluted the Rotary Club of Raffles City (RCRC) by unveiling a plaque to commemorate their setting up of DAS 25 years ago and their continuing support to help students with dyslexia. At the event, RCRC also announced their donation of $34,000 to DAS.

Ms Sim Ann, Minister of State, Ministry of Education and Ministry of Communications and Information, and Ms Denise Phua, MP for Moulmein-Kallang GRC, Mayor Central Singapore District, and President of the Autism Resource Centre visited DAS's Rex House Learning Centre on 26 February. A wide range of topics regarding developments for the support of children with dyslexia was discussed.

APR For the second year running, DAS organised the Preschool Seminar to a sold-out crowd of preschool educators and parents. The seminar was extremely well-received, garnering praise from participants, and for the first time featured an overseas guest speaker, Dr Hugh Catts, from the USA.

2015

JUN

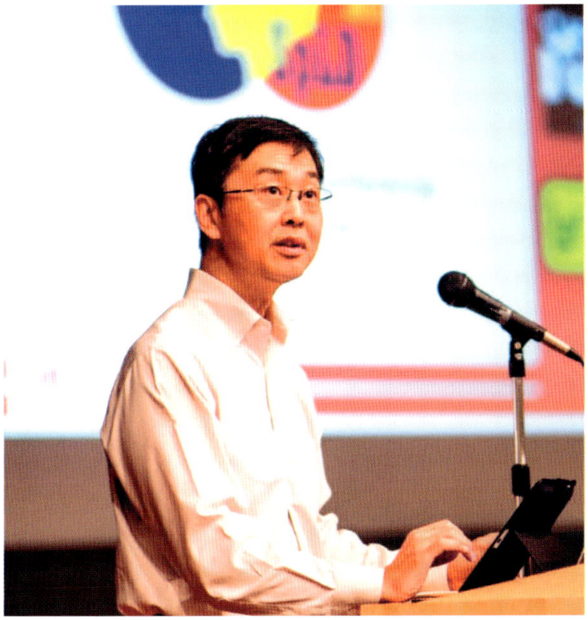

Uniting Ideas in Teaching Excellence: Specific Learning Differences (UnITE SpLD) 2015 was the first ever conference organised by DAS Academy.

Attendees came together to share and discuss ideas in supporting children with learning needs and encourage a community of practice in this area.

The Guest of Honour was NCSS CEO Mr Sim Gim Guan.

JUL

Singapore Cruise Centre (SCC) commenced a 3-month fundraising campaign for DAS. At the official opening of the campaign the Guest of Honour was Mr Lee Yi Shyan, Senior Minister of State, Ministry of Trade and Industry and Ministry of National Development. Singapore Cruise Centre raised $50,000 for DAS.

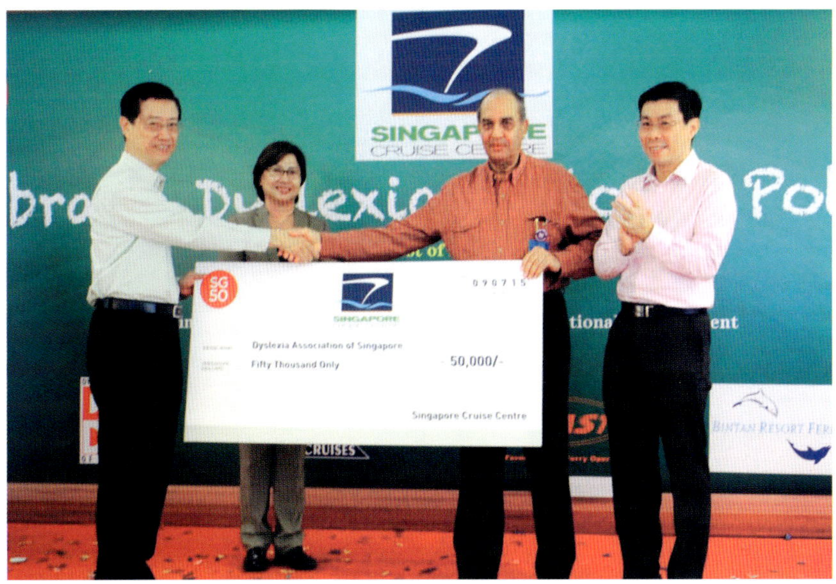

SCC Chairman Mr Soo Lok Len shaking hands with DAS President Dr Jimmy Daruwalla, looking on are Mr Lee Yi Shyan, Senior Minister of State Ministry of Trade and Industry and Ministry of National Development, and Ms Christina Siaw, SCC CEO.

2015

AUG In conjunction with EZ-Link, DAS organised an art competition for its students where the winning designs would be printed on EZ-Link cards to be sold islandwide. A portion of the proceeds amounting to $50,000 was donated to DAS.

The Guest of Honour was Mr Sam Tan, Minister of State, Prime Minister's Office, and Ministry of Culture, Community and Youth.

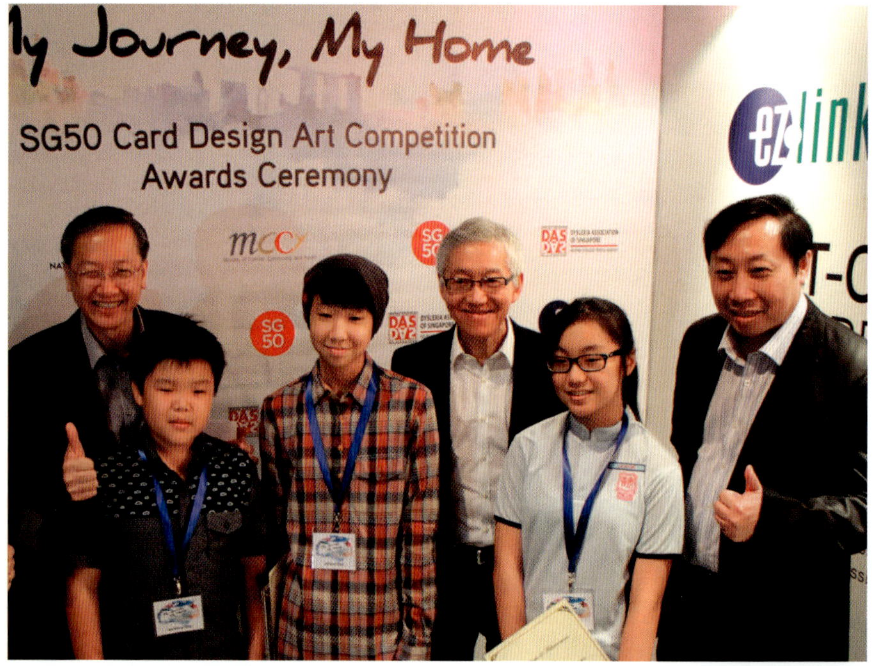

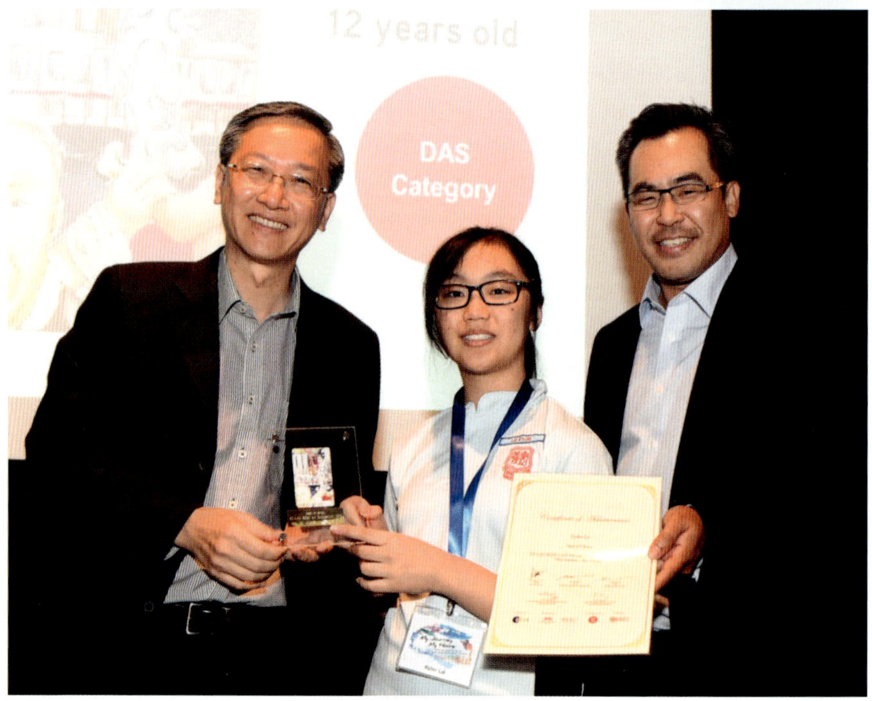

Pictured above right (L to R) Mr Sam Tan, DAS Winners Matthew Tang and William Choo; Mr Eric Lee, DAS Vice President; Kyler Lai, who was one of the 20 Best-of-Show winners, and Mr Lee Siang, DAS CEO.

Pictured right is Kyler Lai with her Best-of-Show entry. Mr Sam Tan (L) and Mr Nicholas Lee, EZ-Link CEO. (R)

2015

AUG Specialised Educational Services (SES) crossed the milestone of 1,000 students enrolled as of 22 August. The SES Maths Programme led the way with 269 students while the SES Preschool Programme had 266 students. Other SES programmes include Chinese, Exam Skills, Speech and Language, Specialist Tutoring, and Speech and Drama.

SEP DAS Academy celebrated its largest graduating cohort yet with their 2015 Graduation Ceremony. Held at the Lifelong Learning Institute, more than 80 students graduated from DAS Academy's higher-education courses such as Specialist Diplomas and Master of Arts programmes. The Guest of Honour was Mr Hawazi Daipi, Senior Parliamentary Secretary for Education and Manpower.

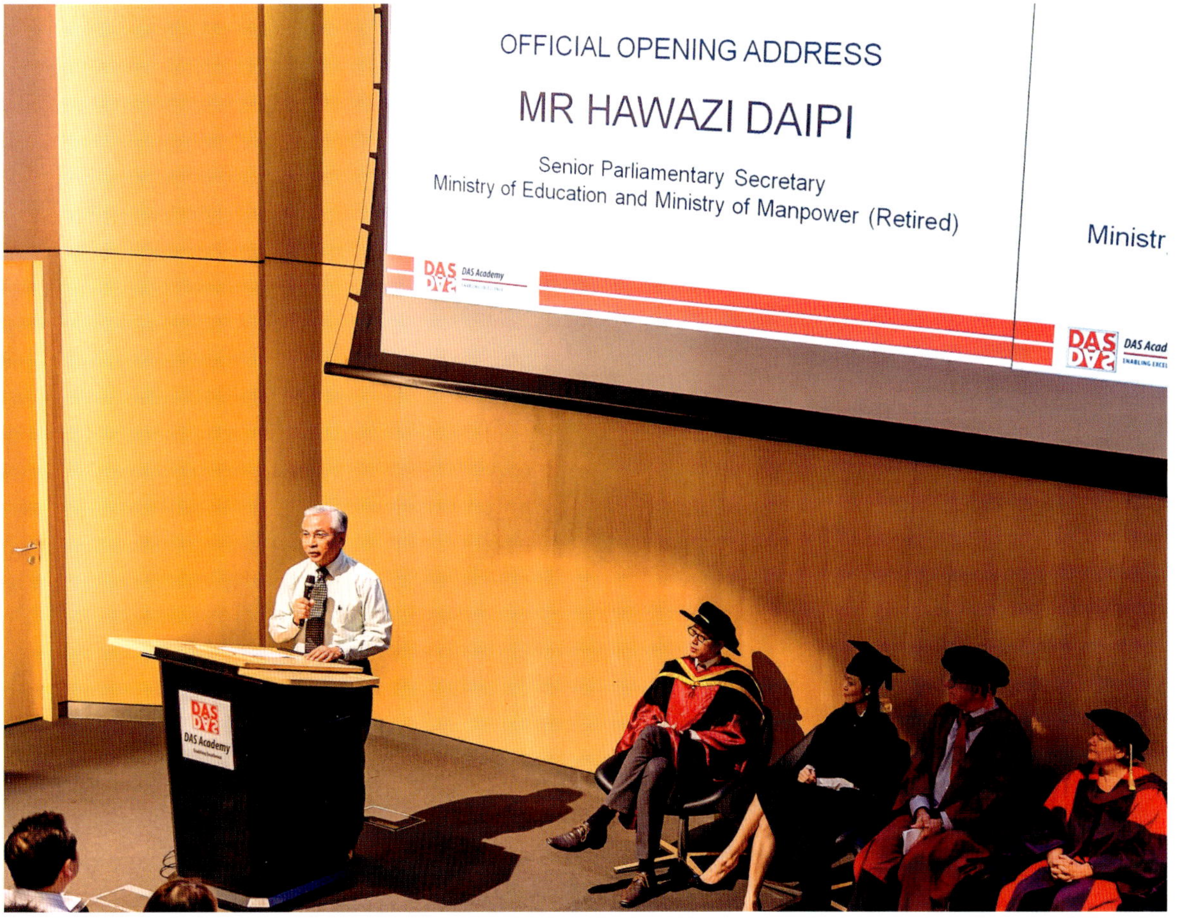
OFFICIAL OPENING ADDRESS
MR HAWAZI DAIPI
Senior Parliamentary Secretary
Ministry of Education and Ministry of Manpower (Retired)
DAS Academy

2015

OCT MOE-aided DAS Literacy Programme (MAP) achieved a significant milestone by crossing the 3,000 student enrolment mark as of 17 October (3,007 to be exact).

NOV *"Embrace A Different Kind of Mind: Personal Stories of Dyslexia"* is published containing more than 50 stories of local heroes who have risen above their learning differences to make their mark in Singapore and beyond.

At the official launch individuals who had their story featured in the book came together to celebrate.

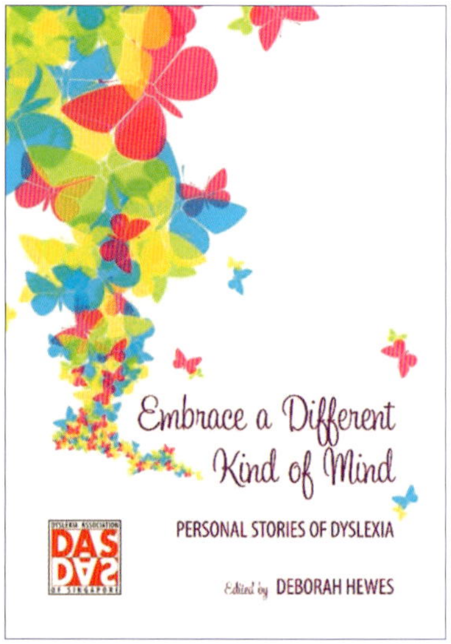

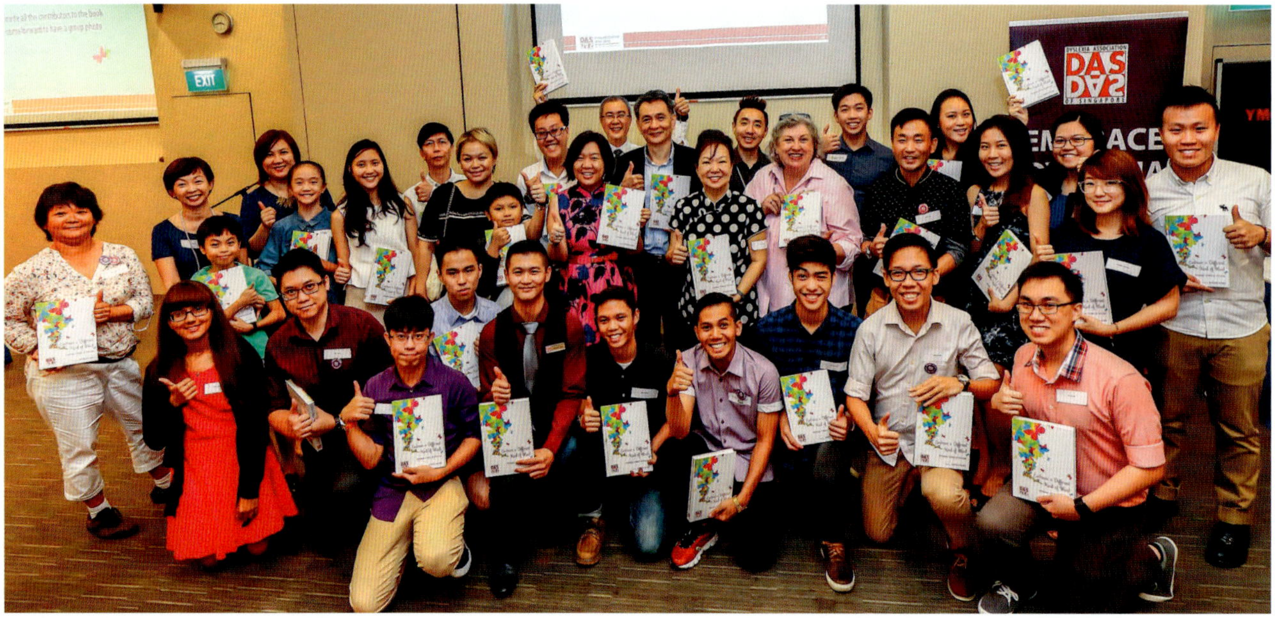

2015

NOV The DAS Student Graduation and Awards Ceremony was graced this year by our patron, Mrs Goh Chok Tong, as well as Guests of Honour Ms Sim Ann, Senior Minister of State, Ministry of Finance & Ministry of Culture, Community and Youth, and Associate Professor Muhammad Faishal Ibrahim, Parliamentary Secretary, Ministry of Social and Family Development, and Ministry of Education. This was the largest graduation ceremony yet with a total of 238 graduates from our MOE-aided DAS Literacy Programme (MAP). There were also Special Awards for excellence. For the first time, DAS recognised the role of our Educational Therapists by introducing the MAP Educational Therapist of the Year award.

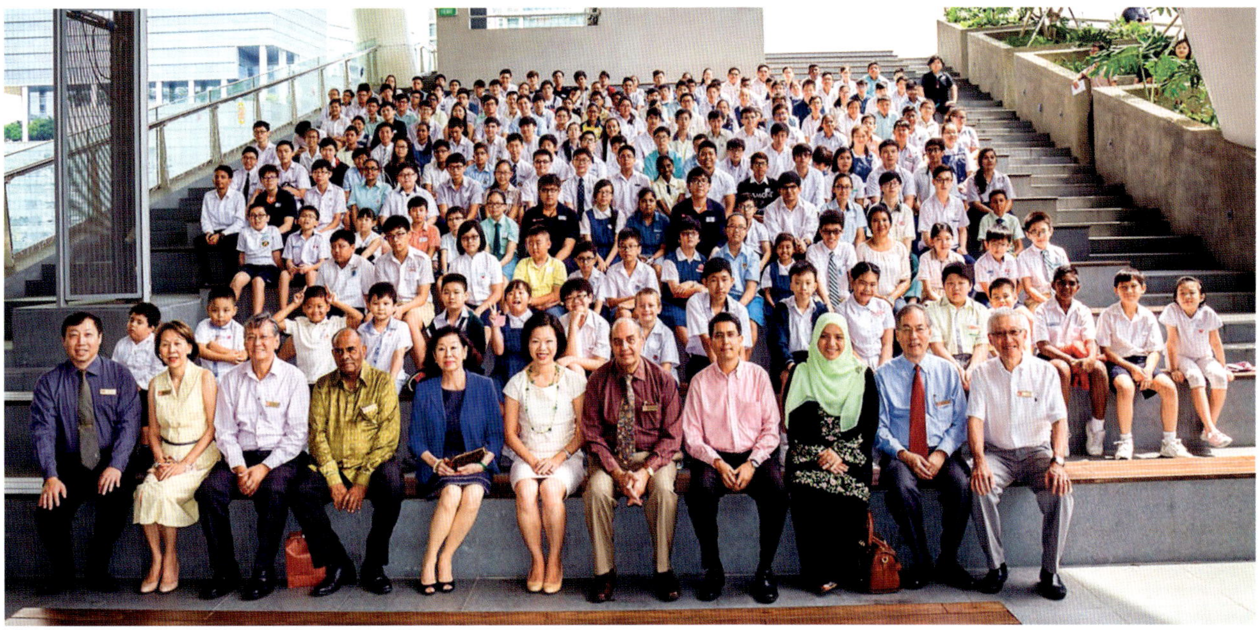

Seated in front of the DAS graduating students, (L to R) Mr Lee Siang, DAS CEO; Ms Cynthia Tan, DAS Exco; Mr Paul Lim Boon Tong, DAS Exco; Mr K Kevasapany, DAS Exco; Mrs Goh Chok Tong, DAS Patron; Ms Sim Ann, Senior Minister of State, Ministry of Culture, Community and Youth and Ministry of Finance, Deputy Government Whip; Dr Jimmy Daruwalla, DAS President; Associate Professor Faishal Ibrahim, Parliamentary Secretary, Ministry of Social and Family Development and Ministry of Education; Dr Sharifah Mariam Aljunied, Ministry of Education; Mr Vincent Chen, DAS Exco; and Mr Eric Lee, DAS Vice President.

2015

NOV Speech and Drama Arts Production 2015 – The Singapore Story, SG50. Thirty-five children, aged between 7 and 13, from across three DAS Learning Centres performed in a 45-minute staged play at the MDIS Auditorium. Paying attention to the many intricate details and character traits of our forefathers, the Speech and Drama Arts students gave their all in portraying the various roles given to them. It definitely no simple task to portray the heroes of this era.

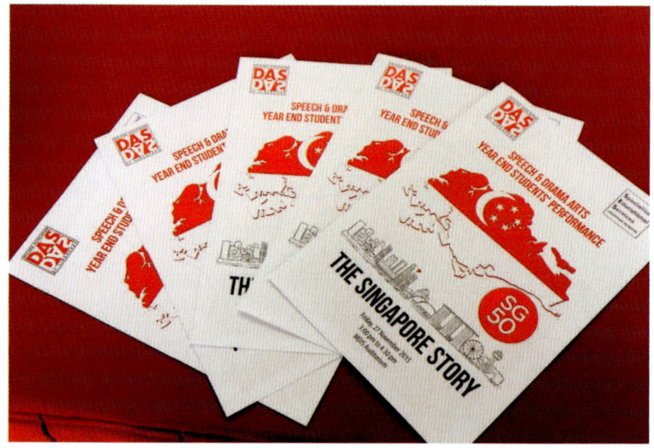

The performance consisted of 24 scenes depicting Singapore's story from how Singapore got its name and Sir Stamford Raffles establishing Singapore as a trading post, to the struggles and challenges Singapore faced after independence in 1965. The play ended with a display of our national identity reflecting 50 years of independence.

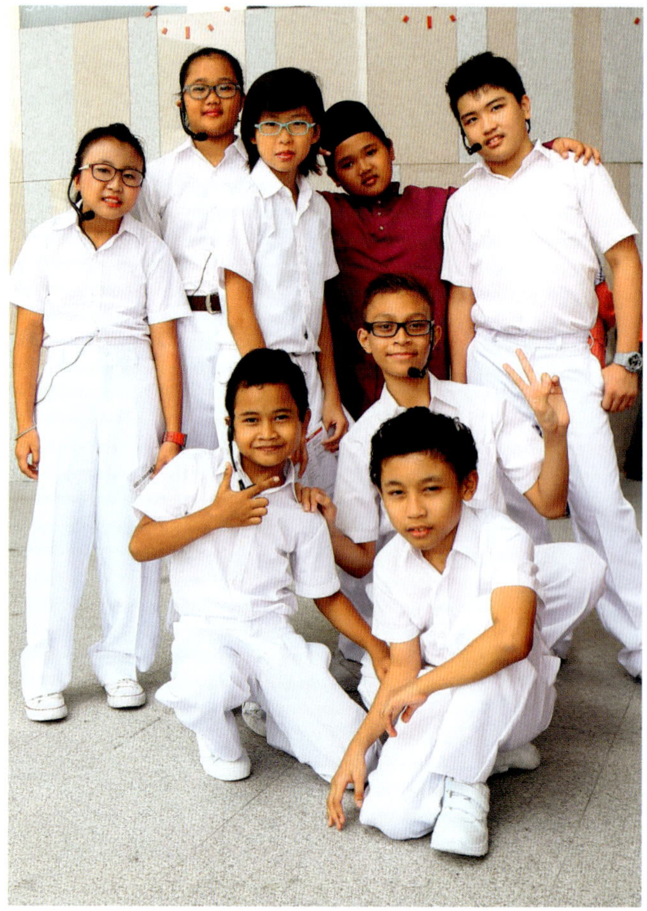

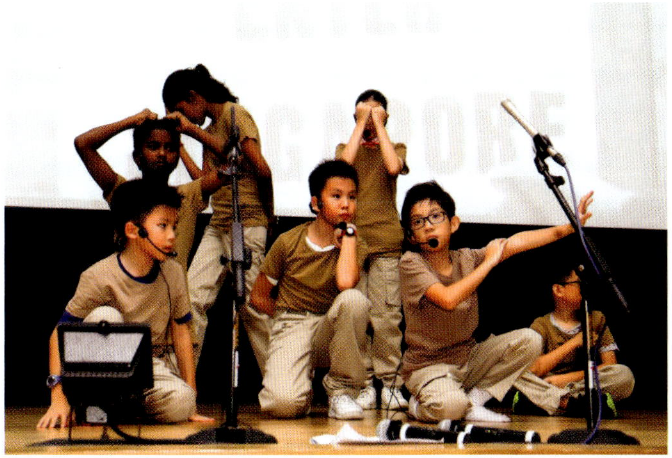

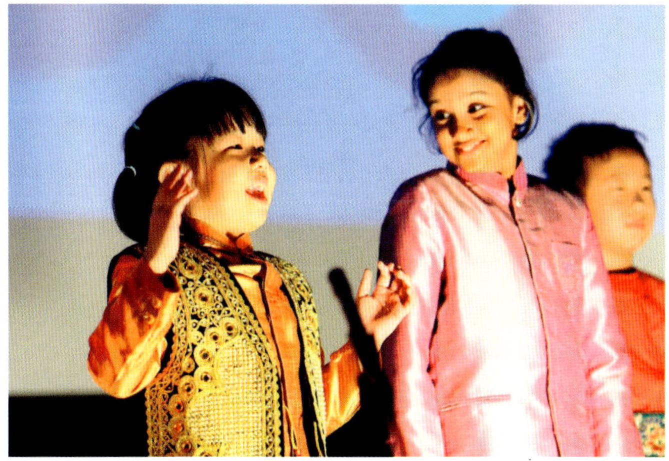

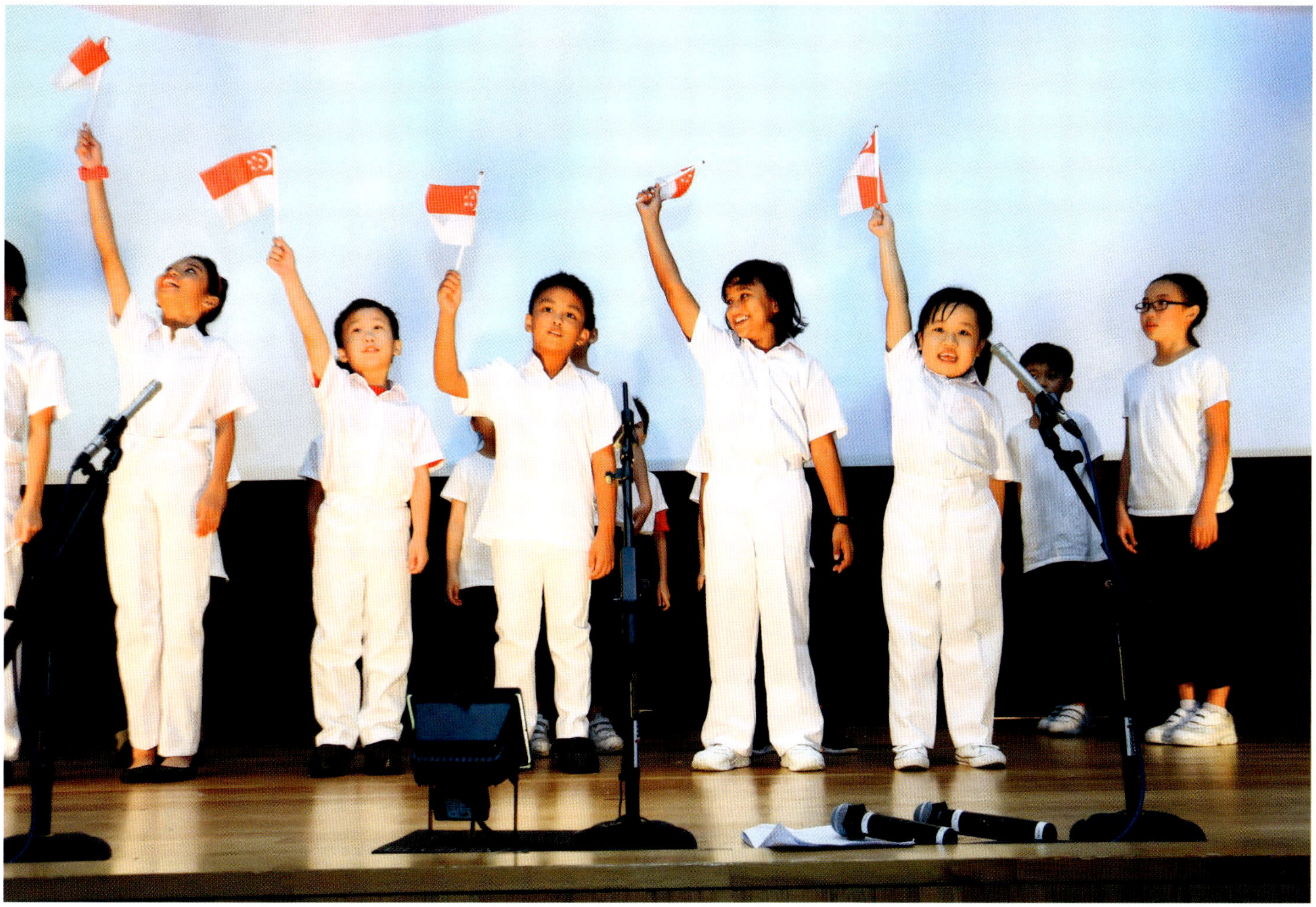

2015

NOV DAS CEO Mr Lee Siang was appointed to the Board of the International Dyslexia Association (IDA), which reflected the increasing international reputation of the DAS. Mr Lee Siang is also chair of the IDA's Global Partners Committee. The Global Partners consist of 27 dyslexia organisations from all around the world and the committee seeks to highlight and share the efforts and challenges of these organisations.

2016

MAR The annual Preschool Seminar held concurrent workshops filled with practical tips and strategies for educators and parents. The Guest Speaker was Dr Charles Haynes (USA). The seminar was sponsored by NTUC Income OrangeAid who expressed admiration for DAS's continuing efforts to support preschool children with literacy difficulties.

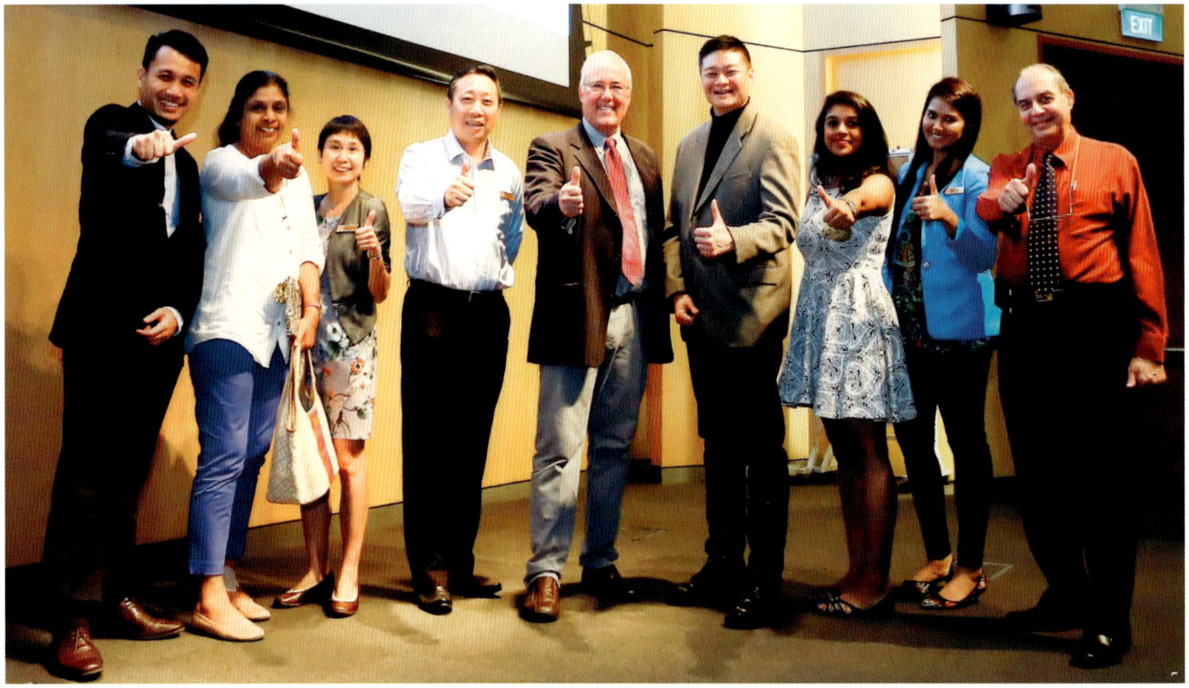

(L to R) Mr Nor Ashraf Bin Samsudin, Director of DAS Specialised Educational Services; Ms Nirmala Vijayarengan, Principal of PCF Ulu Pandan @ Ghim Moh Link; Ms Wong Kah Lai, DAS Preschool Programme Manager; Mr Lee Siang, DAS CEO; Dr Charles Haynes, Special Guest Speaker; Mr Theodore Teo, Senior Manager & Head of Corporate Social Responsibility, NTUC Income; Ms Rathika Shanugham, NTUC Income; Ms Hema Krishnan, DAS Fundraising Officer; and Dr Jimmy Daruwalla, DAS President.

2016

MAY Computerised Curriculum Based Assessments (CBA). MAP fully launched their one-of-its-kind computerised CBAs to monitor the progress of their 3,000 students.

JUN The second Unite SpLD Conference and the first International Symposium was unique in that it was the first research-focused conference organised by DAS. With over 33 presentations delivered in three concurrent sessions in short 20-minute presentations, the conference provided a rich learning environment to inspire educators to continue to work with students with leaning differences.

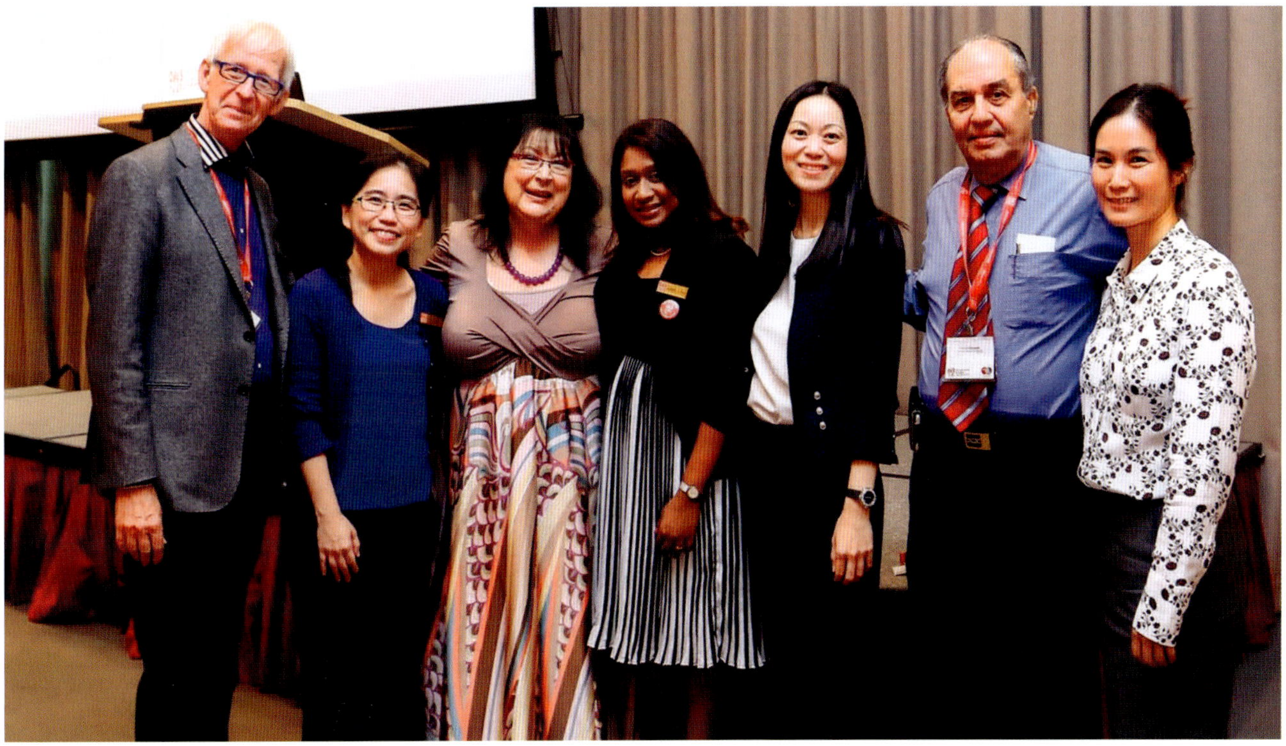

(L to R) Mr David Fawcett; Ms Lois Lim, DAS Lead Psychologist; Emeritus Professor Angela Fawcett, DAS Research Consultant; Ms Geetha Shantha Ram, Director of MOE-aided DAS Literacy Programme and Staff Professional Development; Ms June Siew, Head of DAS Academy; Dr Jimmy Daruwalla, DAS President; Mrs Connie Beng, DAS Exco. This was the last DAS event that Dr Jimmy Daruwalla attended before his untimely death two weeks later.

2016

JUL It was a sad period for DAS when founding President Dr Jimmy Daruwalla passed away. Dr Daruwalla was part of the team who founded the association and had always taken a close interest in DAS events and happenings. He was well respected by all staff and will be fondly remembered as his legacy continues to guide the work at DAS. A Memorial Service was held in memory of Dr Daruwalla. Mr Eric Lee, Mr Rajaram, Mr Lee Siang, Ms Janitha Panicker and Dr Zubin Daruwalla gave moving tributes to their friend, colleague and father.

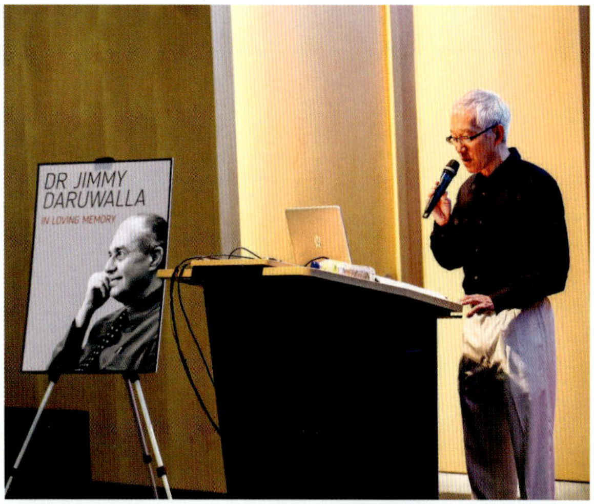

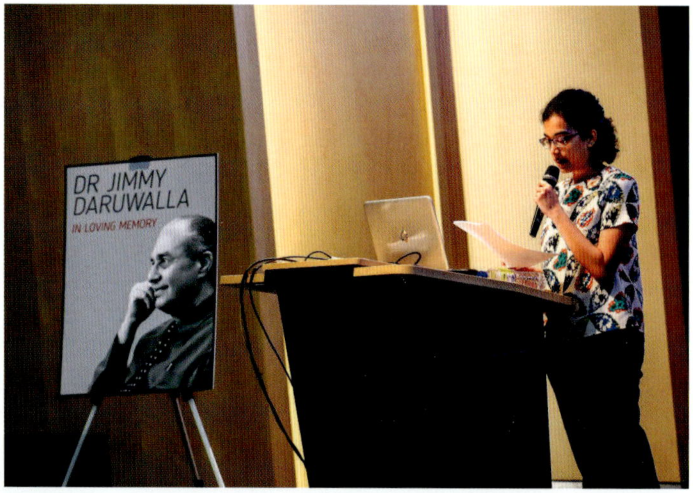

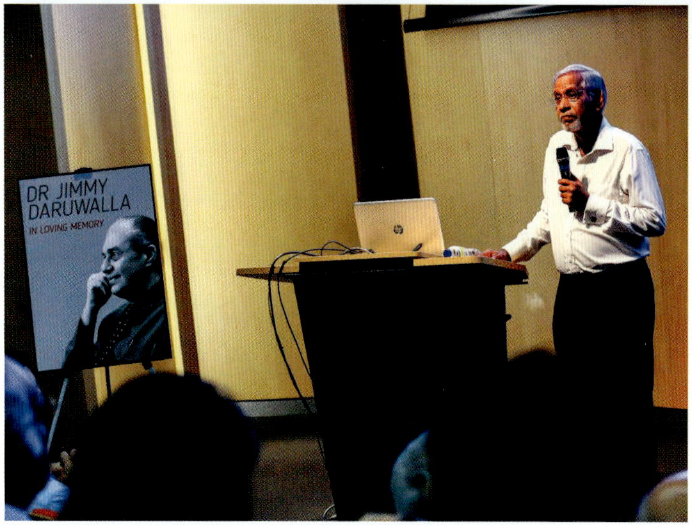

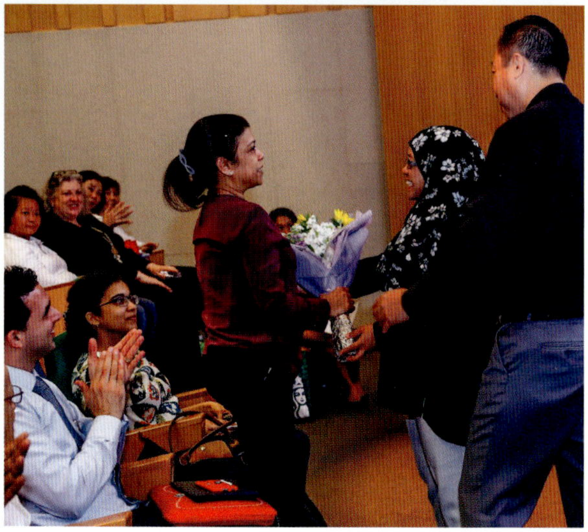

2016

JUL Dr Daruwalla was the driving force behind DAS and his commitment to helping our dyslexics achieve didn't just enable us—it propelled us to greater heights. Since 1991, when DAS was first registered, until his passing, Dr Daruwalla was never deterred from his goal of making learners with dyslexia equal and important members of our society.

We owe him our thanks.

As of 2016 and under his leadership, more than 9,500 children have been identified as dyslexic, around 6,500 received intervention, at least 30,000 people were reached through awareness talks and upwards of ten programmes are now available to support the varying needs of our students with dyslexia.

He wholly embraced dyslexia and marched its acceptance into thousands of households and improved the lives of countless children. And with that he marched straight into our hearts.

Nothing stopped him.

If anything, the challenges we faced only spurred him onward with renewed spirit. We have been inspired by how much commitment he brought to DAS and we could see the fire in his eyes whenever he spoke about the importance of support for our children with dyslexia.

He was their strongest advocate.

He honoured us with his passion and we will miss him greatly.

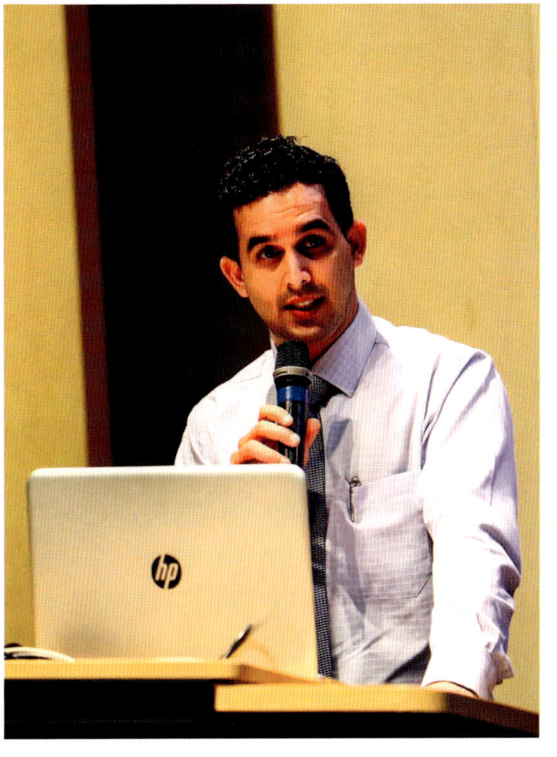

2016

OCT DAS's 25th Anniversary Carnival was held at the Toa Payoh HDB Hub and saw over 1,000 members of the public participating and celebrating DAS's 25th birthday. Live performances, stage games, exhibitions and booths allowed the public to engage with our staff to learn more about dyslexia and the range of services that DAS offers. The carnival was opened by Mr Eric Lee, DAS President.

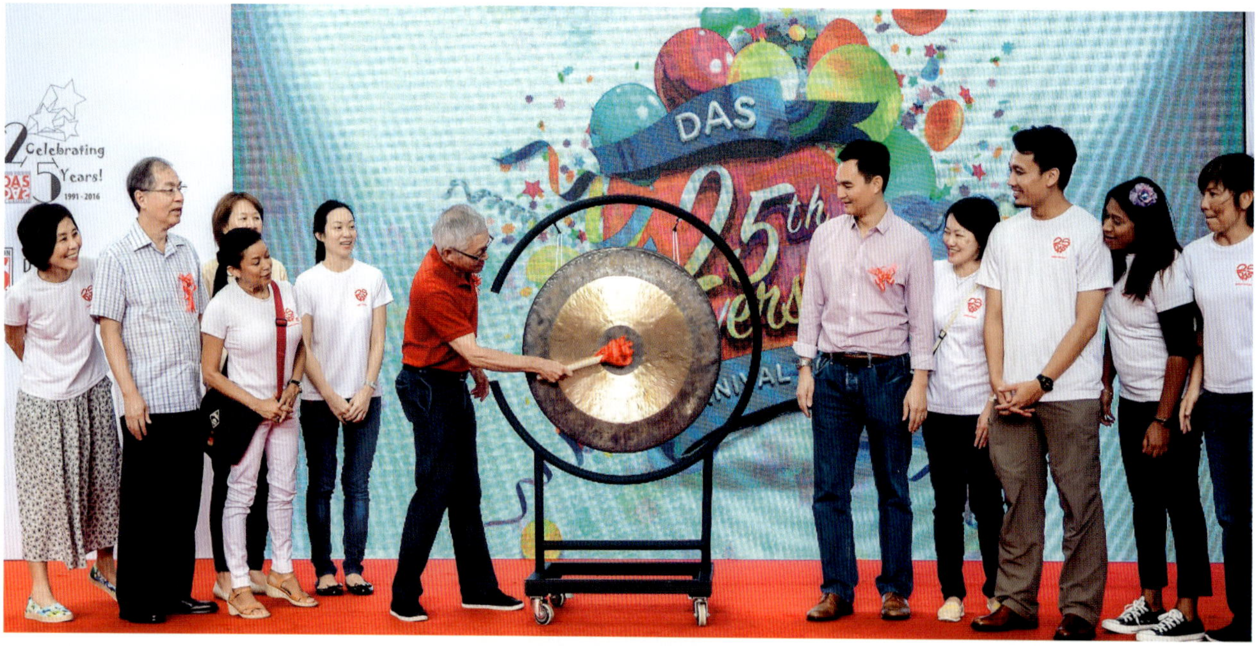

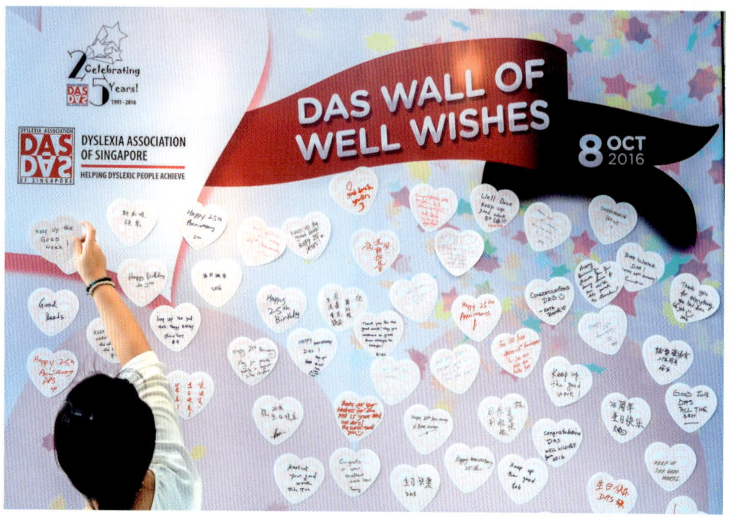

(L to R) Ms Quek Gek San, DAS Director of Corporate Services and HR; Mr Vincent Chen, DAS Exco Asst. Honorary Treasurer; Ms Anaberta Oehlers-Jaen, Head of DAS International and Programme Director of SES Maths, Specialist Tutoring and Assessments; Ms Cynthia Tan, DAS Exco; Ms June Siew, Head of DAS Academy; Mr Eric Lee, DAS President; Mr Kevin Kwee, DAS Exco Honorary Secretary; Ms Chai Soo Chiao, DAS CFO; Mr Nor Ashraf Bin Samsudin, Director of Specialised Educational Services; Ms Geetha Shantha Ram, Director of MOE-aided DAS Literacy Programme and Staff Professional Development; Ms Fanny Foo, Director of Learning Centres and Outreach.

2016

OCT On a high from a successful carnival in the heartlands, DAS again celebrated its 25th Anniversary with a charity dinner. Funds raised from the dinner were added to the "Jimmy Daruwalla Fund". The charity dinner raised $500,000 for the fund.

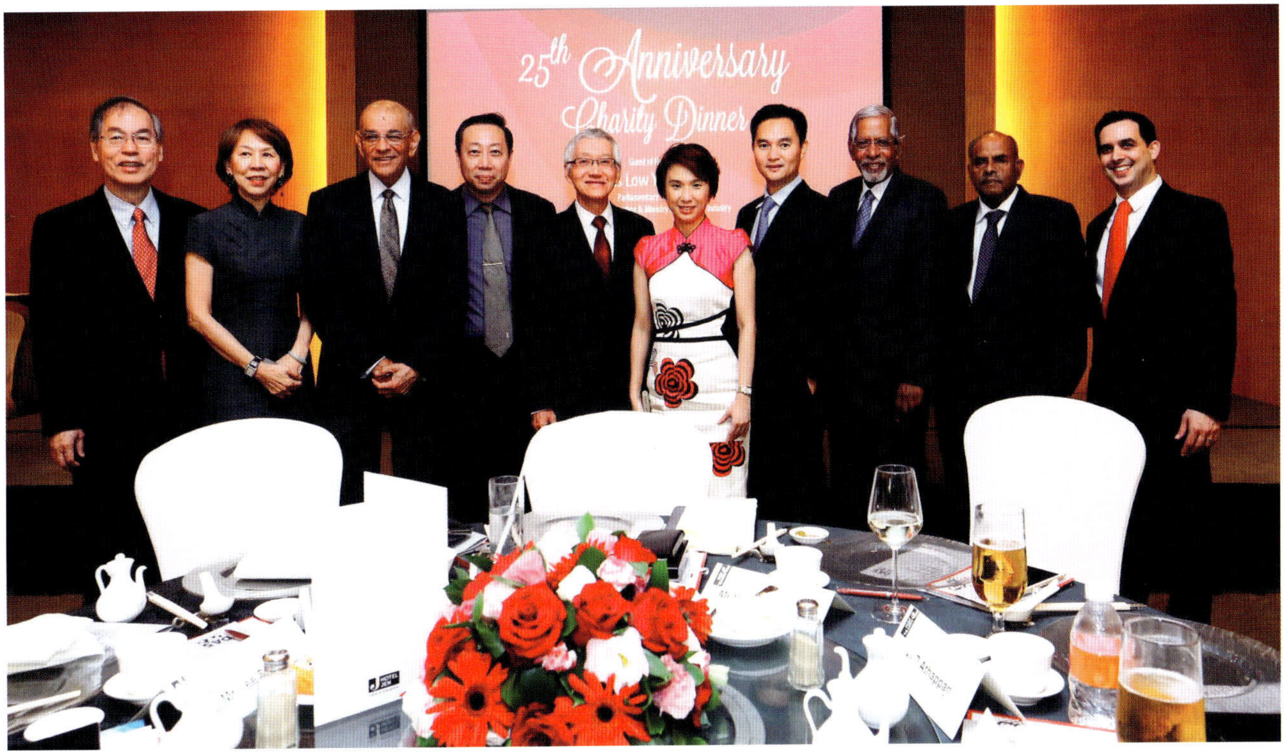

Above: DAS Executive Committee (L to R) Mr Vincent Chen, Exco Asst. Honorary Treasurer; Ms Cynthia Tan, Exco Member; Mr Kaka Singh, Exco Honorary Treasurer; Mr Lee Siang, DAS CEO; Mr Eric Lee, DAS President; Ms Low Yen Ling, Parliamentary Secretary, Ministry of Education, and Ministry of Trade and Industry, Mayor, South West CDC; Mr Kevin Kwek, Exco Honorary Secretary; Mr Rajaram, Vice President; Mr Kesavapany, Exco Member; and Dr Zubin J Daruwalla, Exco Member.

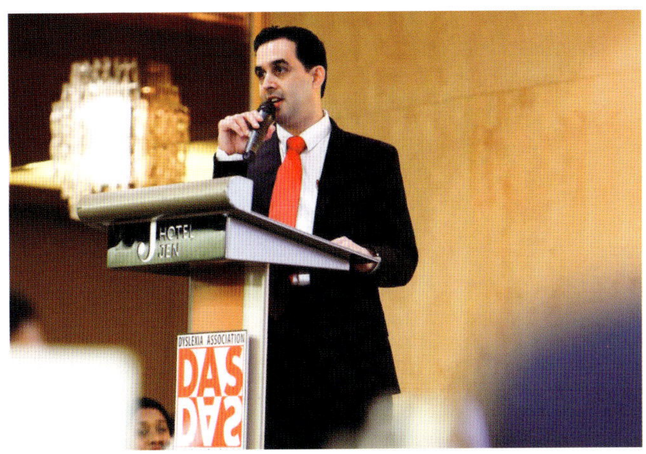

Right: Dr Zubin J Daruwalla gave a tribute to his father, Dr Jimmy Daruwalla, at the 25th Anniversary Dinner.

2016

OCT At the 25th Anniversary Dinner a loving tribute was made in memory of Dr Jimmy Daruwalla and his work at the DAS was celebrated. A condolence book of messages was also presented to Mrs Jothy Daruwalla on the night.

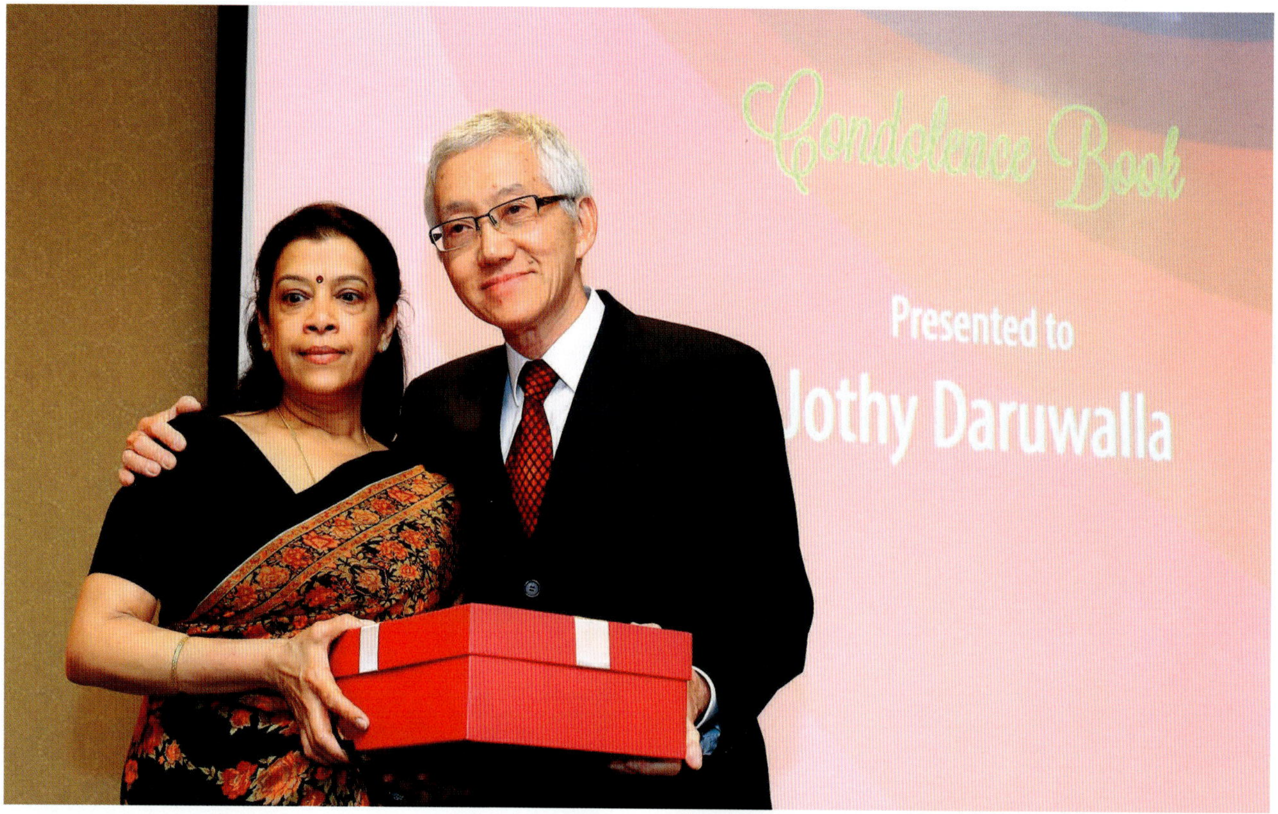

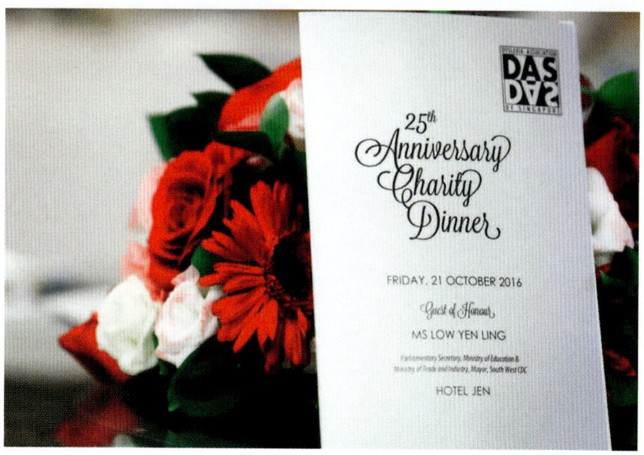

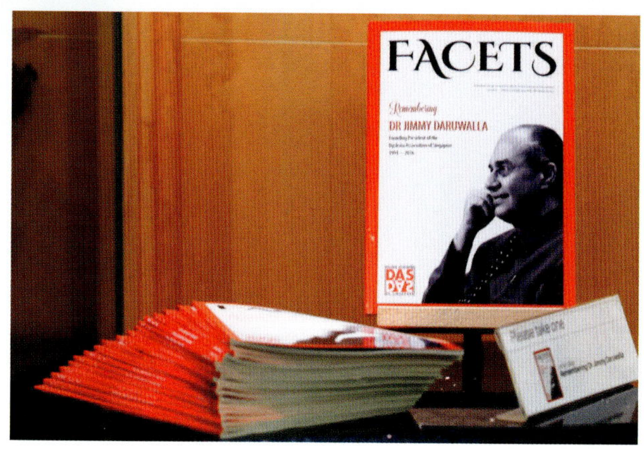

2016

Mr Kevin Kwee (right), successfully bid for the autographed Lee Kuan Yew Book—*My Lifelong Challenge,* auctioned on the night and his donation took the total raised for the Jimmy Daruwalla Fund to over $500,000.

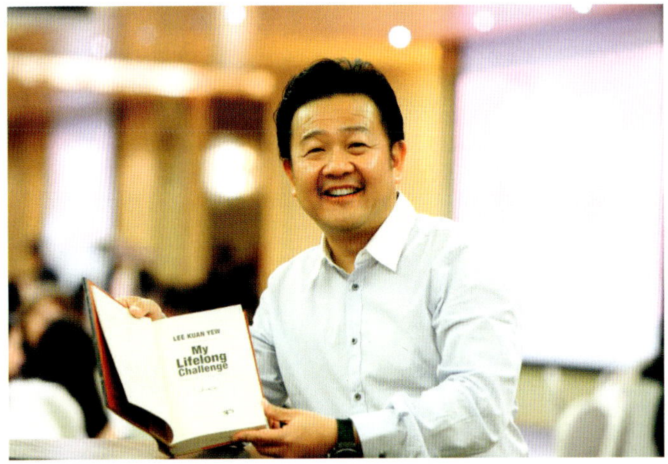

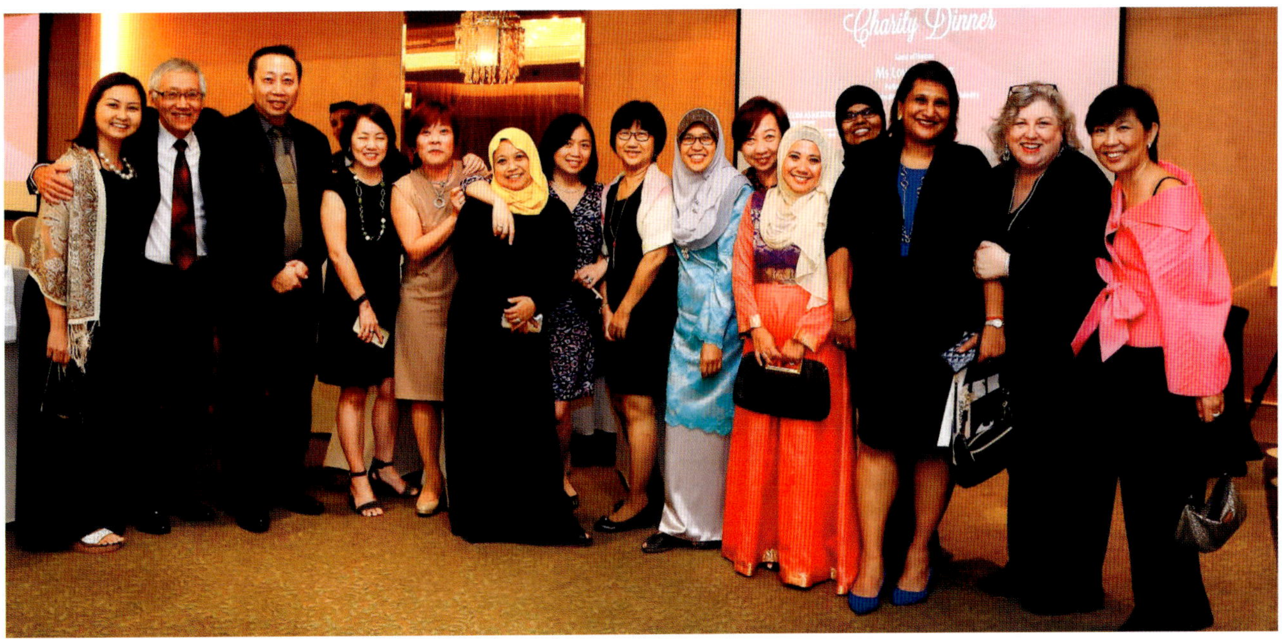

Above: DAS Staff at the 25th Anniversary Dinner, (L to R) Ms Chris Chia, Assistant Director DAS Learning Centres; Mr Eric Lee, DAS President; Mr Lee Siang, DAS CEO; Ms Chia Soo Chiao, DAS CFO; Ms Tey Ching Ching, DAS Head of Logistics; Ms Kharyati Kamsani, Office Manager and PA to DAS General Management; Mrs Marcel Ortiguerra, Assistant Director, Finance; Ms Betty Lee, Senior Bursary Officer; Ms Suzana Bte Fizal, Senior Academic Services Officer; Ms Jacqueline Song, Head of Fundraising; Ms Surjati Soekraman, Assistant Director of Outreach; Ms Bowshiya Begum, DAS Learning Centre Manager for Ang Mo Kio and Yishun; Ms Deepam Gnaneswaran, DAS Learning Centre Manager for Bishan; Mrs Deborah Hewes, Head of Publicity and Publications; and Ms Fanny Foo, Director of Learning Centres and Outreach

2016

OCT The DAS Academy Graduation saw 88 graduates receive their qualifications. The first Master of Arts in Special Needs degrees were awarded at this ceremony.

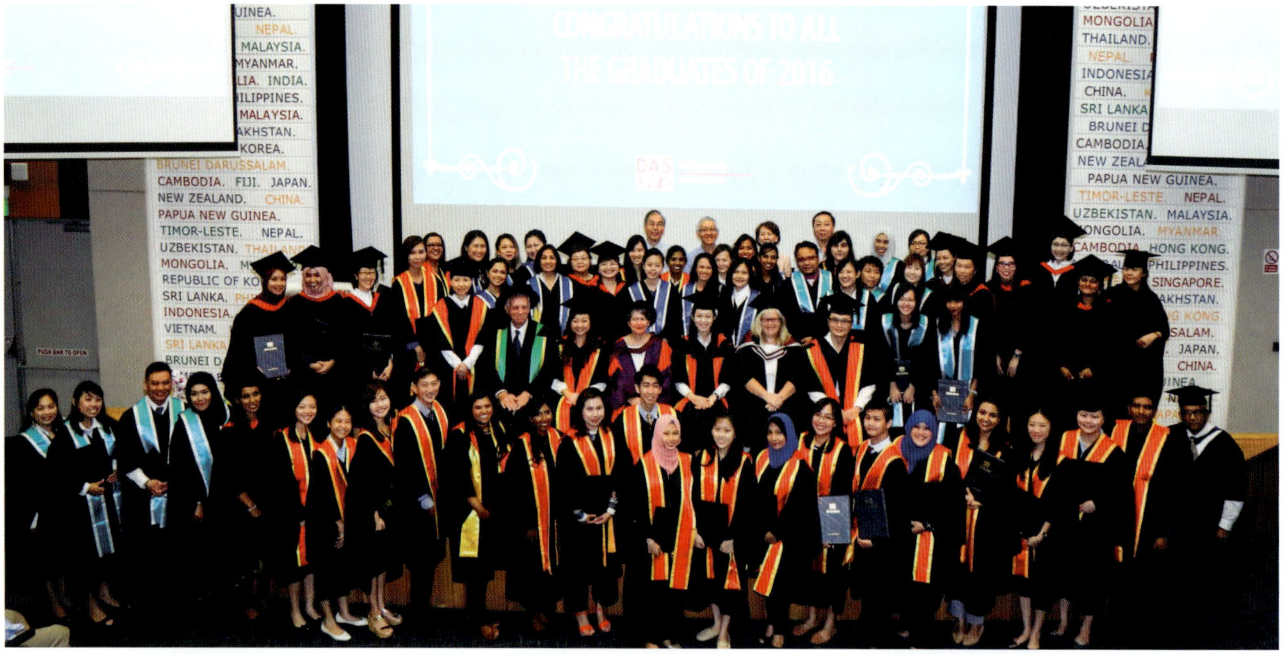

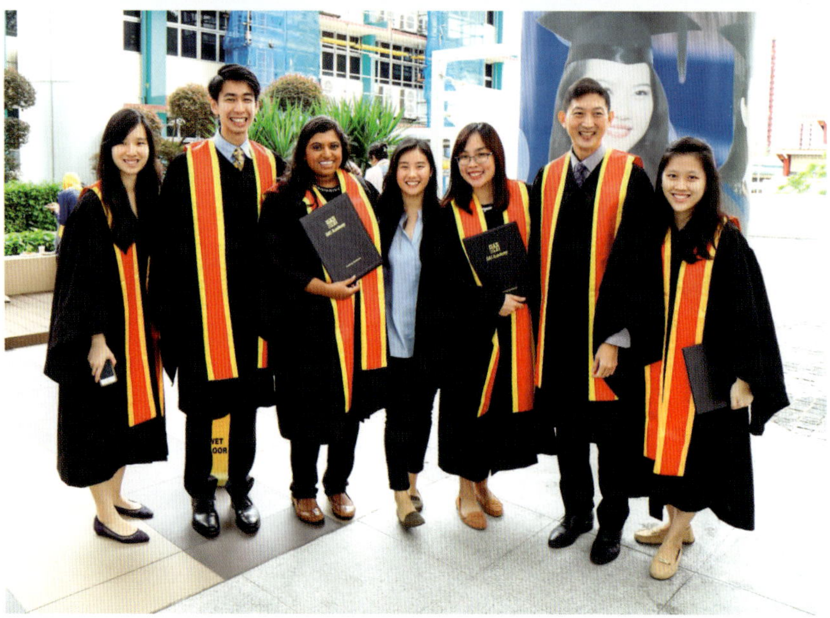

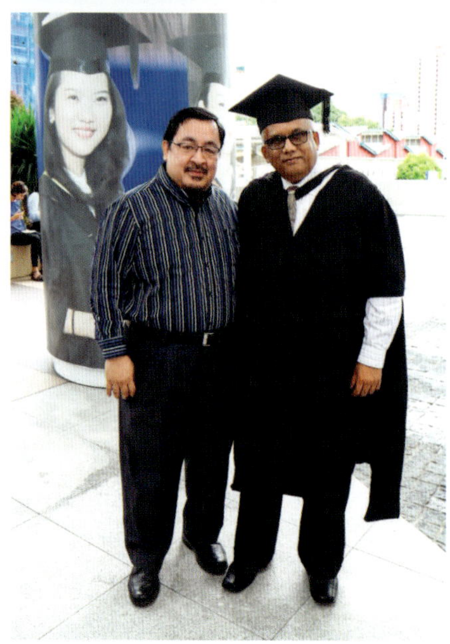

2016

NOV Speech and Drama Arts Production 2016 – Shakespeare 400. The SES Speech and Drama Arts Programme performed their second end-of-year production at Genexis Theatre to a crowd of 200. Forty-six students of the SDA programme from three learning centres presented adaptations of the playwright William Shakespeare's works, and were featured in the local news for their efforts.

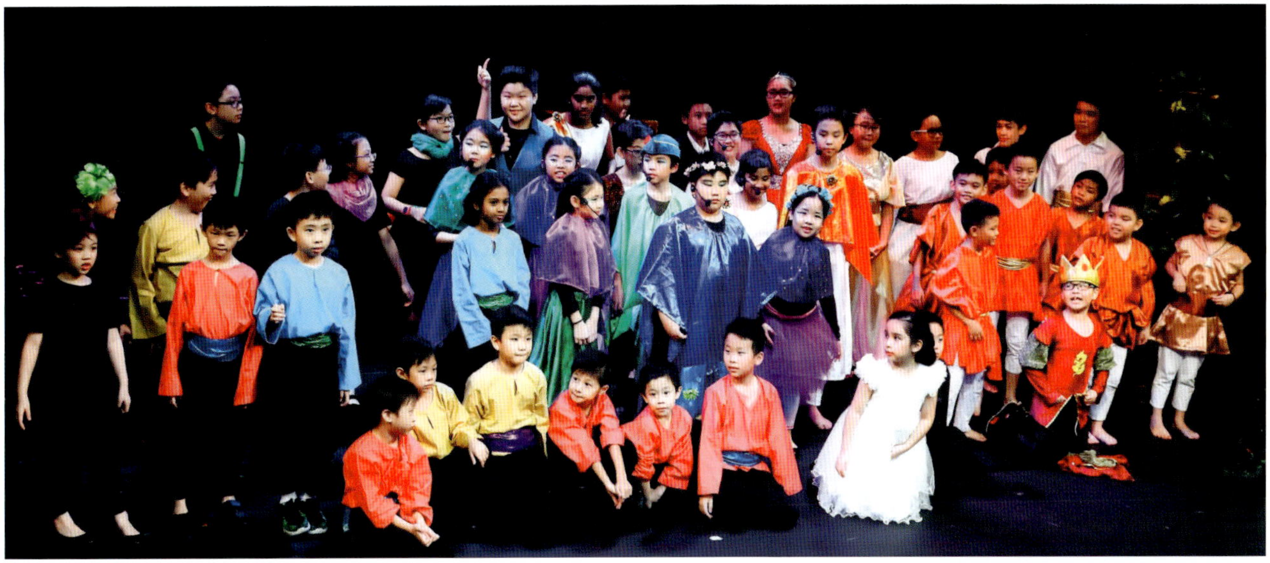

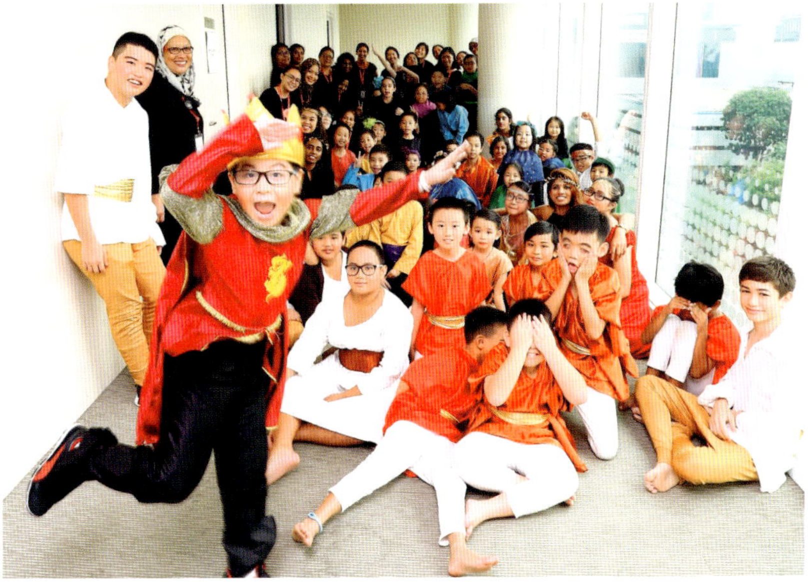

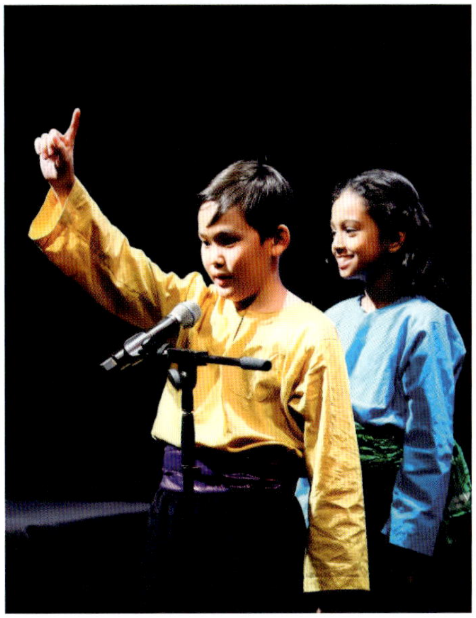

2016

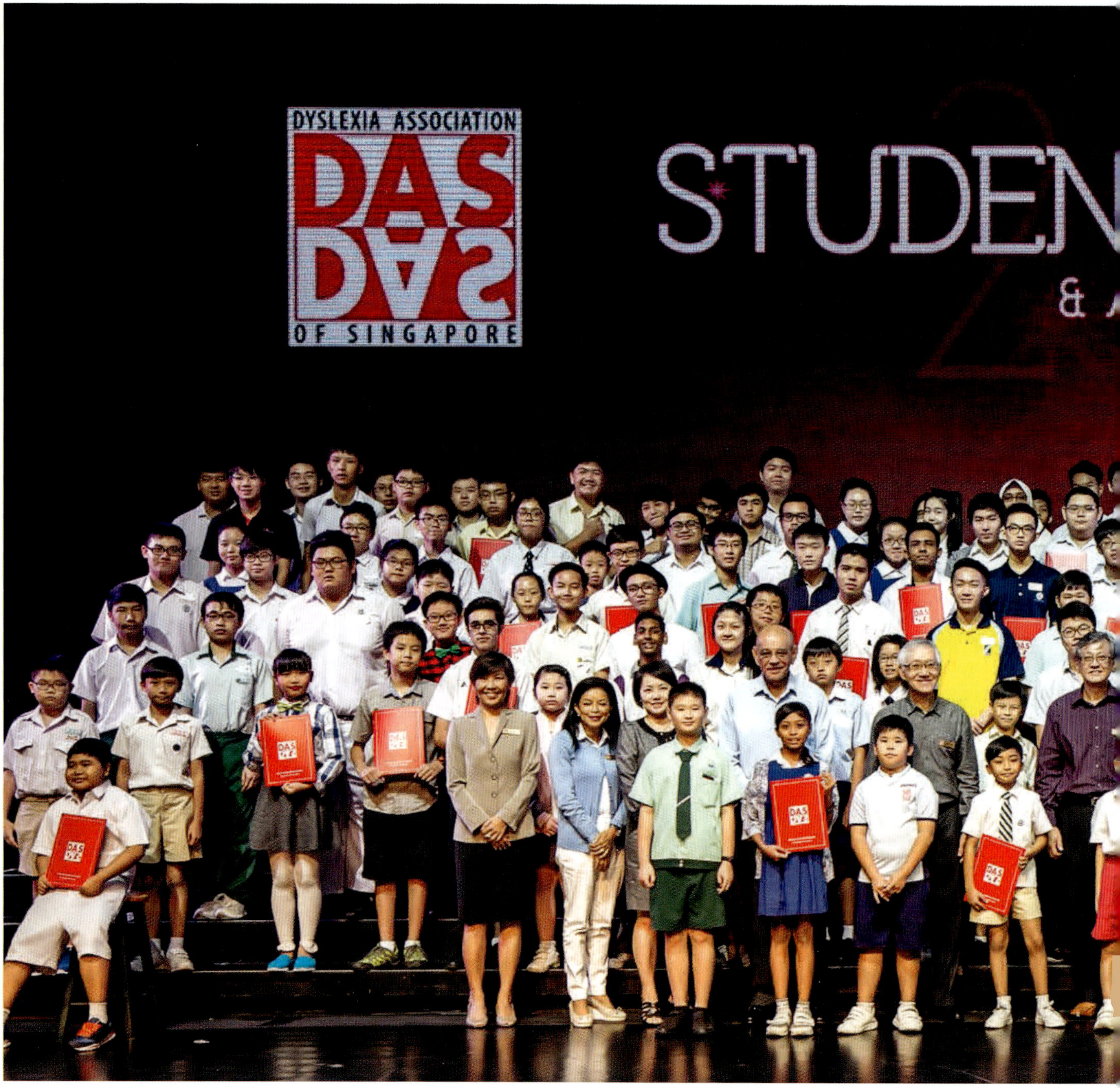

NOV The DAS Student Graduation and Awards Ceremony 2016 was held at Kallang Theatre with 219 graduating students and more than 50 award winners who were celebrated for their achievements.

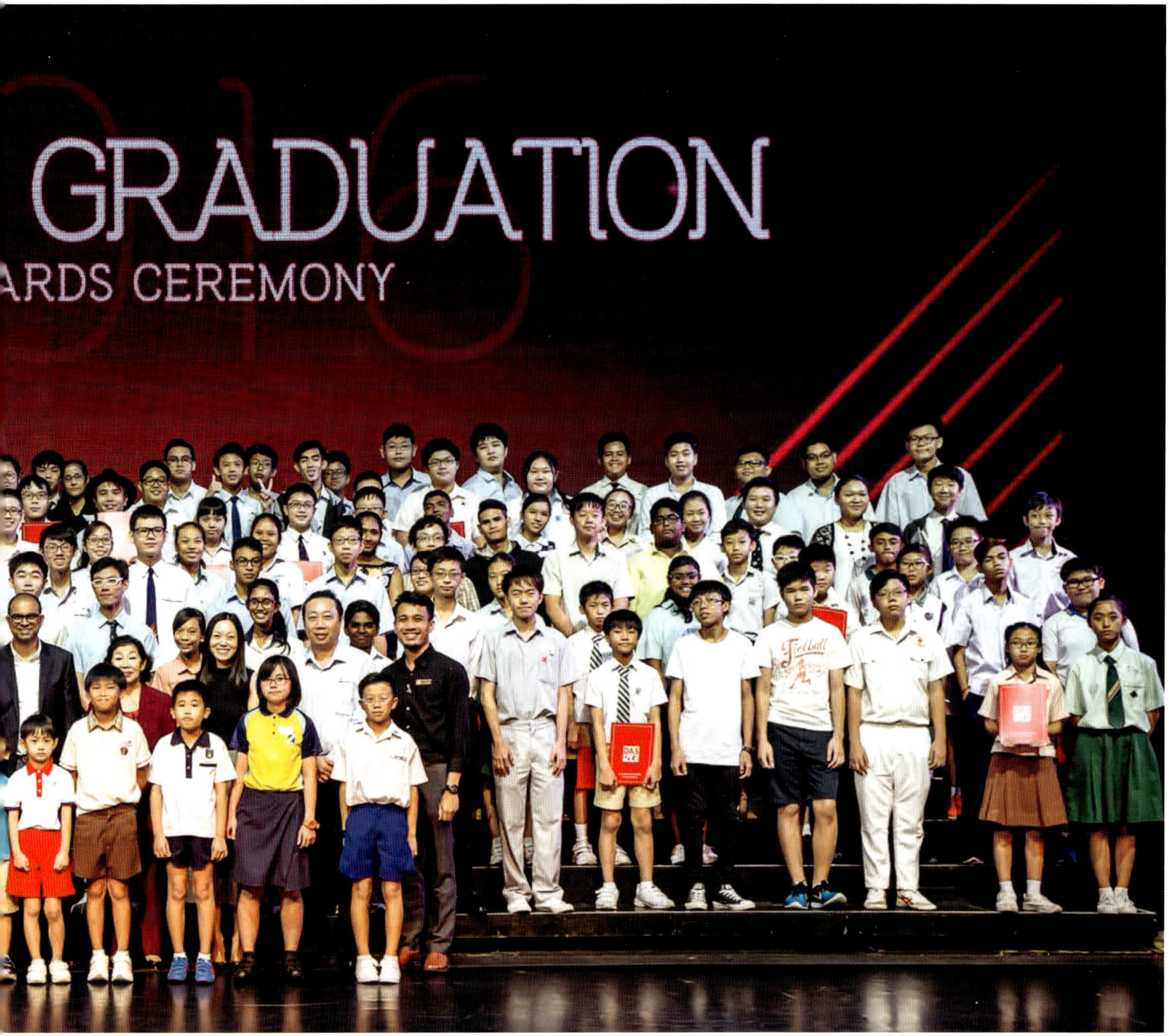

The event was graced by DAS Patron, Mrs Goh Chok Tong and Guest of Honour Mr Janil Puthucheary.

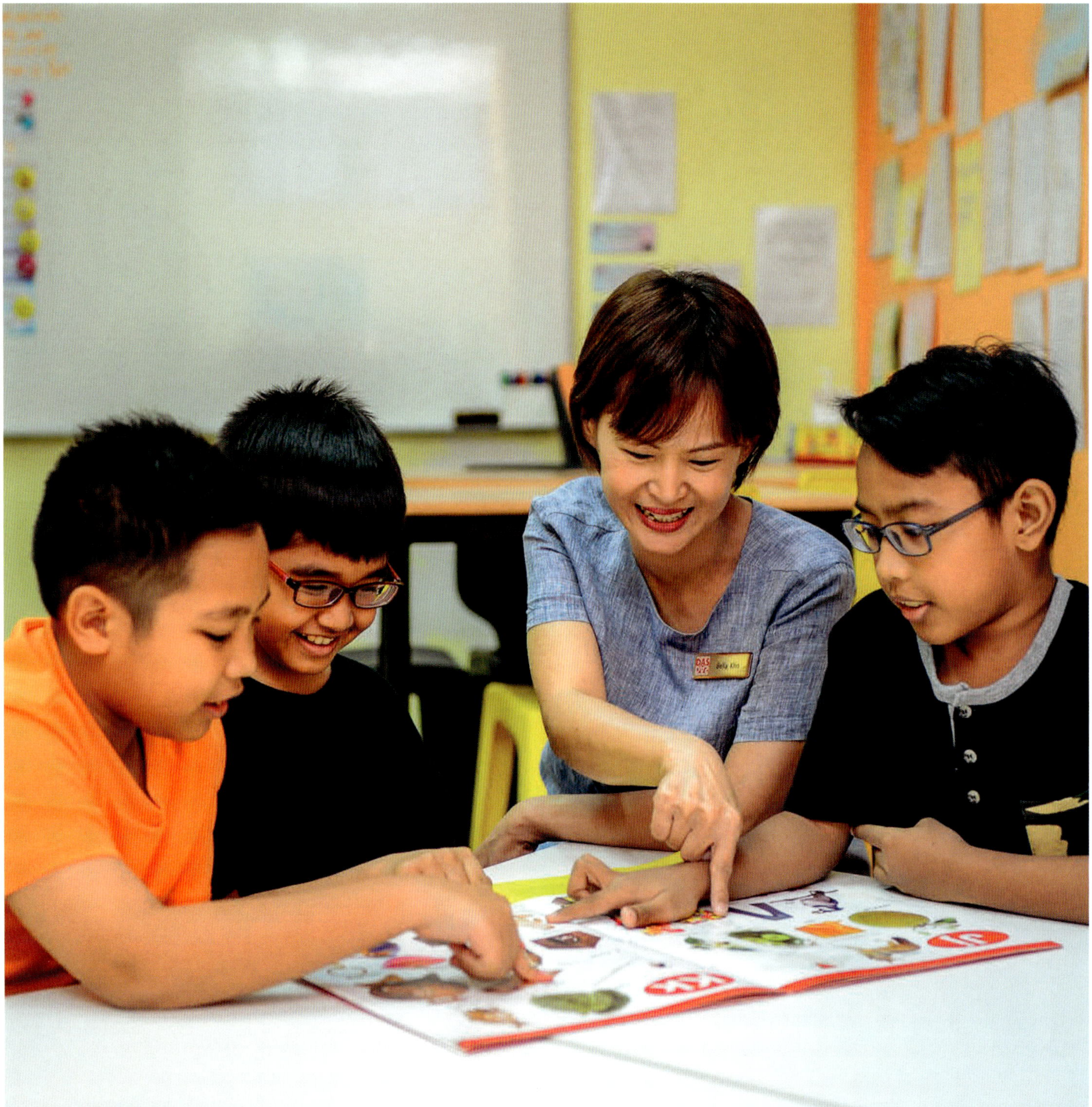

3

SPECIAL PEOPLE, SPECIAL STORIES

When a child knows that he or she is dyslexic, that it's the way their brain is programmed, and it's not their fault, that makes all the difference in the world.

Philip Schultz
Author of My Dyslexia

OUTSIDE THE BOX

When talking to dyslexics, several common threads stand out. Most go through a bewildering period in their childhood when they grapple with acquiring various skills that seem to just elude them. For some, their dyslexia remains undiagnosed and they struggle on through delinquency and petty crime until the law catches up with them. For others, though, there is a moment of epiphany when their parents / teachers / guardians realise that they are not lazy / stupid / naughty / unmotivated. They are simply dyslexic.

That is when the light at the end of the tunnel begins to glow brighter. With a pedagogy that accommodates their learning challenges, most dyslexics can be helped to fulfil their potential and go on to excel in areas such as entrepreneurship, science, design, writing, music, arts, sports and a host of other professions.

They are better able to think out of the box precisely because their minds function outside the box already.

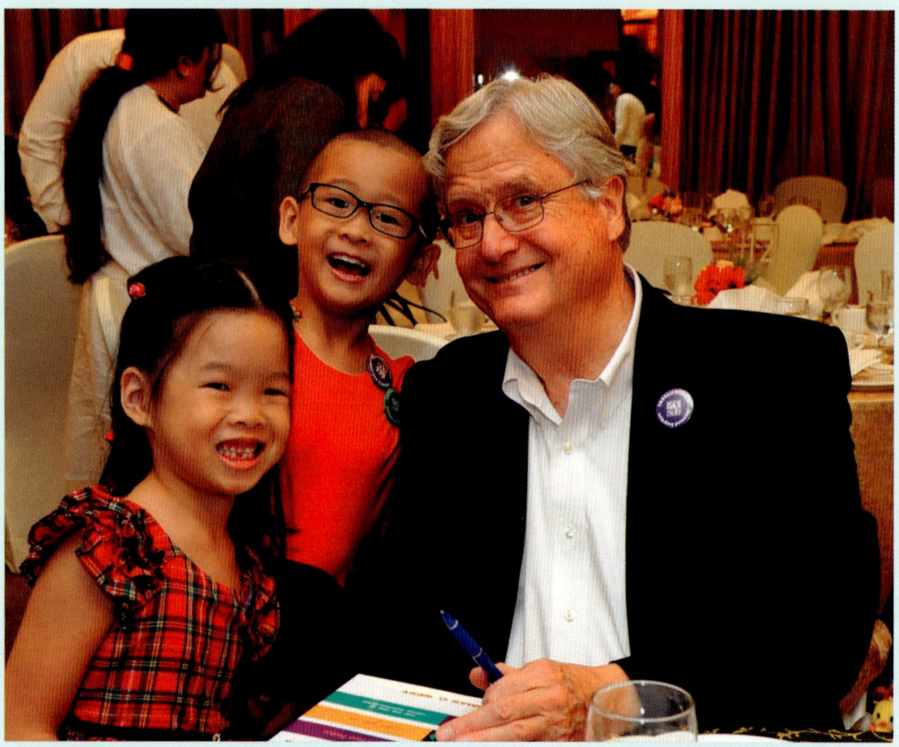

As one highly successful dyslexic pointed out, it is not hard for a dyslexic to think "out of the box" because, as he says, "they have never been in the box."

Mr Thomas G. West
Author of *Thinking like Einstein*, *In the Mind's Eye* and *Seeing What Others Cannot See*

Mr Thomas West autographing his book, In the Mind's Eye, *for two fans, "Dr JiaJia" (aka Chua Jin Sen) and his little sister Chua Jin Zhu.*

"IT IS A GREAT TIME TO BE DYSLEXIC"

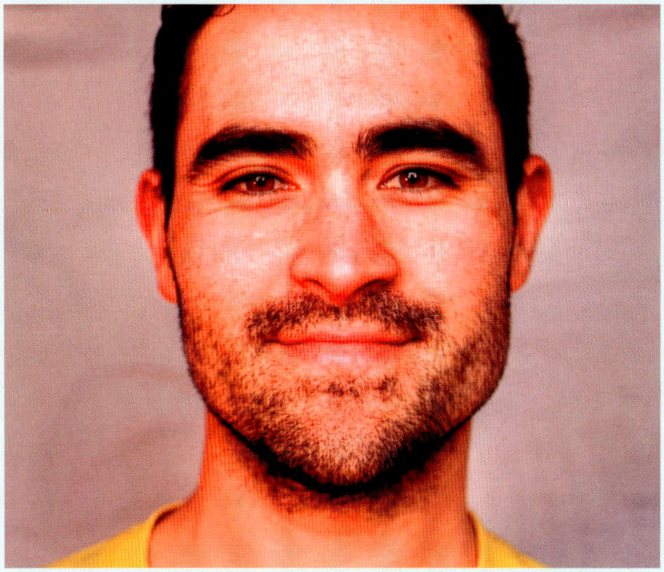

"I have always stood out, even before attending kindergarten and frustrating my teachers by not understanding numbers and how certain letters were meant to face. I remember being held behind in kindergarten because I didn't know how to fill out an addition table. I recognised a pattern and worked from there: 10, 20, 30, 40, 50, 60, then 11, 22, 33, 44, 55, 66, etc., but this was not how my teachers wanted me to complete the task. They were trying to make me understand after 10, it was 11, then 12, etc. All the teachers gathered around, one by one trying to explain how addition worked. And I, sitting in silence, alone, with adults on the verge of shouting at me, upset.

I always found my past poor ability to read, write and comprehend a minor detail; what was the big deal with a few incorrect letters? The meaning is still present. Now, thanks to technology, the minor details can be taken care of: auto-correct, voice recognition, typing and artificial intelligence have solved or will solve all these pattern recognition problems. It is a great time to be dyslexic. Having said that, this doesn't give anyone the licence to be lazy. I used that card many times and it doesn't help you.

Thank you, Uncle George, the father of my best friend, Ajit Abraham, who lived next door to me at Jalan Kasau. Thank you for reaching out to experts around the world and speaking your mind about finding a better way to help.

You planted the seed which has become the Dyslexia Association of Singapore, an organisation that has touched the lives of thousands of kids who might have otherwise pretended to finish reading just so they wouldn't be last again."

Mr Erin Khoo
Project Manager, Mobile Implementation @Indeed.com

"DYSLEXIA IS NOT A DISABILITY"

"Before I learned about my condition and mastered the techniques, I did not do well in English throughout my early years of schooling. I could achieve over 80-90 marks for Chinese and other subjects. But no matter how hard I tried, my English grades were still poor. I even failed my GCE 'O' level and 'A' level English oral examinations. Back then, nobody in my family had a clue about dyslexia. As a result, I always received red marks in English and I suffered many canings from my mother who was a strict disciplinarian.

Recently, a parent wrote an email to me saying that his son has just been assessed to be possibly dyslexic. He was concerned and worried like any other parent would be about his son's future.

I told this father that we must adopt the right mind-set when dealing with dyslexia. Firstly, dyslexia is not a disability. It's just that a person with this condition needs to find a different method of learning and reading. I also suggested that the parent approach DAS for assistance as DAS offers many programmes and has the professionals who can provide useful advice and suggestions. Finally, I shared with this parent that the journey of overcoming dyslexia can be long and winding.

I ended my email with this sentence — someone once said this: 'He who does not hope to win has already lost.' So it's crucial that you and your wife must always have the hope that your son will overcome the condition and do just as well as any other person in life. If both of you hold up this hope, your son will succeed one day."

Mr Sam Tan

Minister of State, Prime Minister's Office, Ministry of Manpower & Ministry of Foreign Affairs, Deputy Government Whip

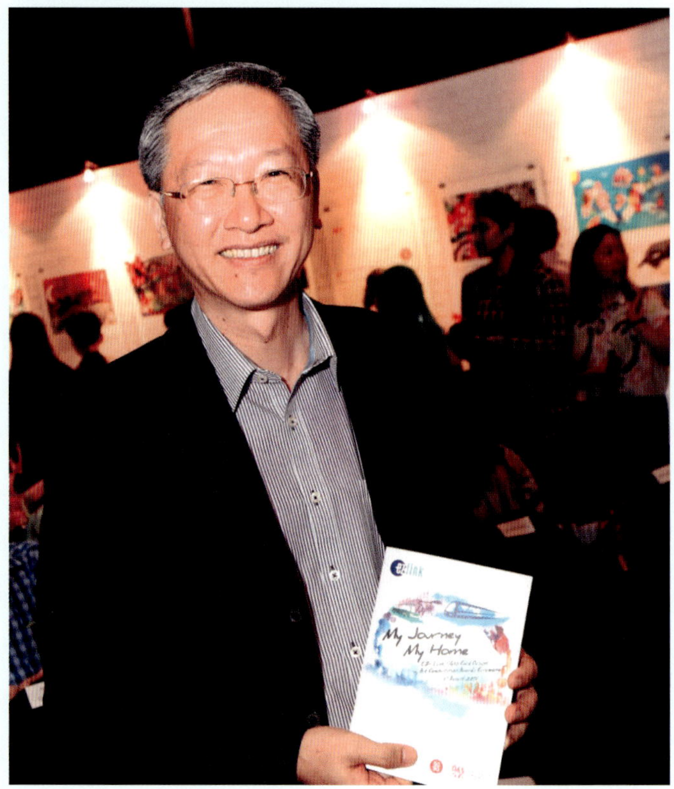

"I FELT LIKE THE TORTOISE IN 'THE TORTOISE AND THE HARE'"

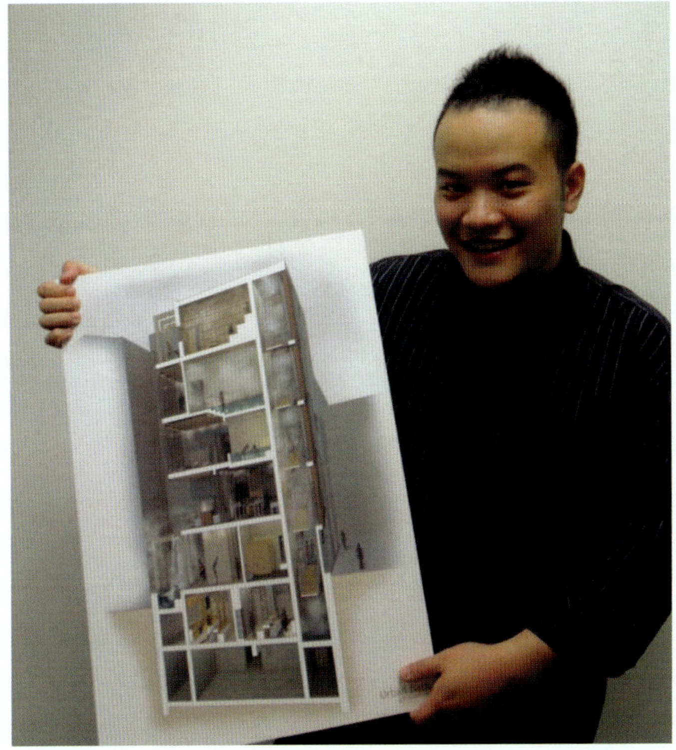

"When people look at me, they see a fairly successful young person. At 26, I've attained my Masters in Architecture with a High Distinction (University of Melbourne), worked at a firm, set up my own interior design business, W5A, and have more plans in the pipeline. Seventeen years ago, nobody would have thought this possible.

Like most Singaporean families, my parents and my three older brothers placed a high value on education. Nagging, scolding, tuition, homework, and occasionally, the cane with the neon-coloured tip would make its appearance. Everyone around me was trying his or her best to help me, and I was trying hard, really hard. No results. I felt like the tortoise in 'The Tortoise and the Hare', except this tortoise could never win the race. After confiding in my mother, my brother's close friend, a teacher, advised my parents to get me tested for any form of learning disabilities that were hindering my progress in school. Tested, I found that I am, indeed, dyslexic.

Initially, at DAS, I was a little apprehensive. If all other help had failed, what made these people so sure they could help me? It wasn't as if life after the discovery was a breeze. I struggled with the same things and pressures in school. Perhaps, what made the difference were the skills I had acquired through the sessions at DAS. I didn't feel so helpless anymore. I was able to bask in the joy of my little successes, despite not doing exceedingly well.

I had always known that I was different from my peers. Dyslexics are known to be more able to visualise concepts in 3D, and I capitalised on my strengths in this area. In Secondary 4, I worked hard on my Design and Technology to achieve the 'Tan Kah Kee Young Inventors Award'. It was one of those life-changing moments that added to my dream of being an architect."

Mr Patrick Siah
Interior Designer and Entrepreneur

"WE'RE JUST DIFFERENT"

"Diagnosed with dyslexia at the age of 7, Shun did not understand what the word meant until much later. 'I thought I was stupid,' he said, recalling his primary school days when reading was an uphill task and his classmates could read much faster than he could.

From the relentless negativity around him, he soon lost confidence in himself and started to believe that he was indeed stupid. He went through a period when he was a youth delinquent as he felt that nobody understood what he was going through and nobody could support him. He smoked and played truant. In a world governed by words, it seemed as though he was the only one who did not speak that language.

Coming from a non-musical family, Shun had always seen music creation as a special talent. 'Music to me was this divine thing that only divine people created, it was very abstract to me.' His parents noticed his interest and bought him a guitar for Christmas. He started to learn music and his passion grew. Although he continued to struggle in school, Shun started to look forward to going home to his guitar every day.

At the age of 16, he decided to drop out of the traditional Singaporean academic route to pursue music. Shun experimented with different music genres during his time in the Singapore Polytechnic and explored them with the acoustic guitar. He went on to serve his National Service with the SAF Band, doing band arrangements and performing as its guitarist.
Shun was subsequently accepted into the prestigious Berklee College of Music with a scholarship. In his second year, his talent and passion were acknowledged and he was selected for the highly coveted Berklee Artist Diploma, a two -year individualised programme for further specialised training. Although studying at Berklee was highly enjoyable, Shun left the college after two semesters to pursue a full-time career in music as he was already making a name for himself. He was signed on by a management company and booking agent and was performing far and wide, including Japan and Singapore.

To young dyslexics, Shun has a message: 'We are all different. Dyslexia is seen as a disability, but it isn't, we are just different. We think differently, work differently, and we learn differently. Everyone has a talent and a passion for something; the trick is searching for it and, more importantly, knowing that it's okay to chase your dream and no one can tell you that you are not good enough. Embrace your dyslexia, it's because you are dyslexic that you have your talent.'"

Mr Shun Ng

Fingerstyle Guitarist, Vocalist and International Performer

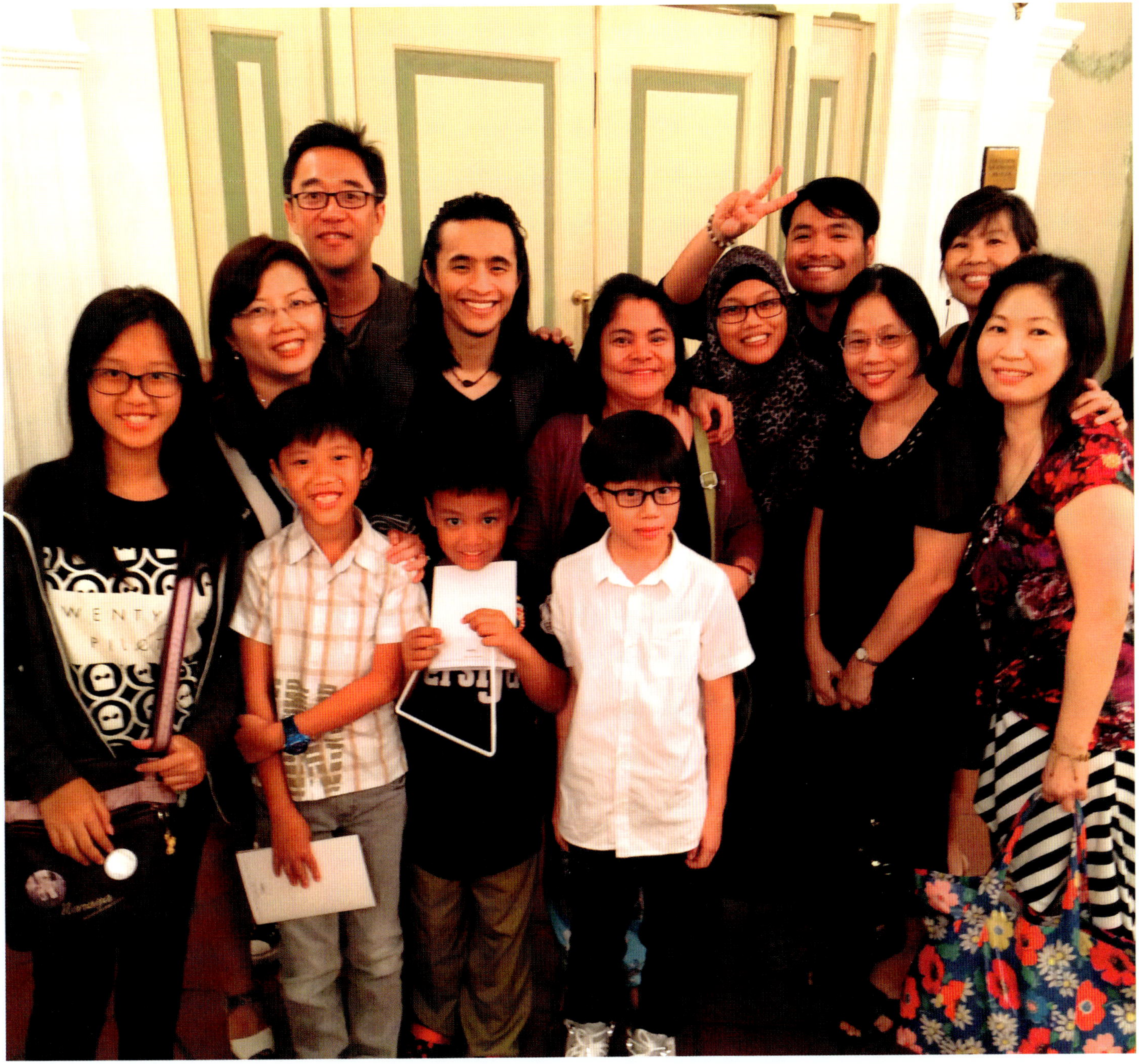

Guitarist Mr Shun Ng pictured with DAS students and staff who were treated to complimentary tickets to the "Rhythm of Christmas" Concert, held at Jubilee Hall in December in 2015. Shun is standing fourth from the left wearing a grey jacket and black t-shirt.

"MORE CREATIVE IDEAS AND SOLUTIONS"

"I could never quite tell my left from my right, or my M's from my W's. You will never hear these sounds from me: p, t, n, k. 'Huh?' is probably the most common reaction I get from anyone, because I mumble and my thoughts are never ordered in the way that you would be familiar with.

Being dyslexic might explain why I am visually attracted to shapes a lot more than others people. Think about it — b, p, q, and d are all the same shape rotated and flipped. To us, they're one and the same…so can everyone calm down please?

I wear my dyslexic badge with honour. I saw it as a brilliant reason for getting to take my time in exams, and for not having to take Chinese. I also used my dyslexic badge as an excuse not to focus and work hard. Sure, concepts were hard to follow and grasp, but that wasn't a reason not to work at it.

It's not going to be easy. It still isn't. You might have to take a couple of extra years…but look at the world that you're in! Thank God for the world today and the technology — little red zigzag lines will point out when the word is spelt wrong, and searching for a word or definition is as easy as looking for it in Google. YouTube holds a wealth of education so that you can find out what the teacher is talking about in a more visual manner. (Crash Course is a brilliant place to start.)

Will it ever leave you…? Probably not. I still get distracted very easily — but this also means that I'm exposed to a lot more ideas than others normally would. I take hours crafting coherent emails, and a couple of hours more ordering my thoughts for meetings. I never can quite remember how some words are spelt, which means that I'm constantly trying out new ways of solving things. And because I see things differently, this might have resulted in a lot more creative ideas and solutions.

Lastly, there will be plenty of people out there like you, and there are plenty of people who will be willing to help. They might not understand what being a dyslexic is, so explain very nicely, and ask for help. Find something you love to do, and you will find the focus that you never thought you had. Till then, don't worry, work hard, and have fun."

Ms Grace Au Yong
Social Media and Content Specialist

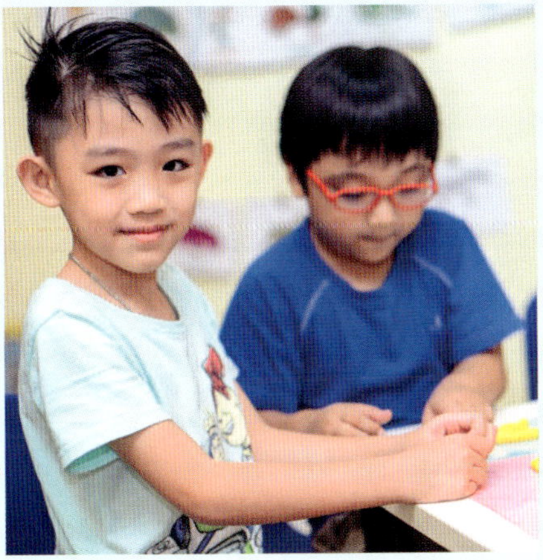

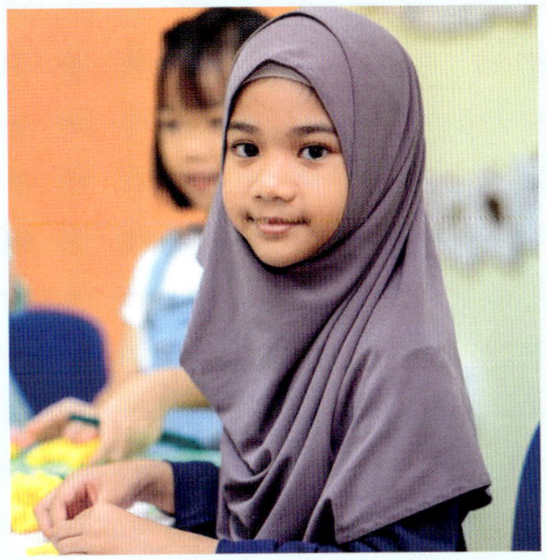

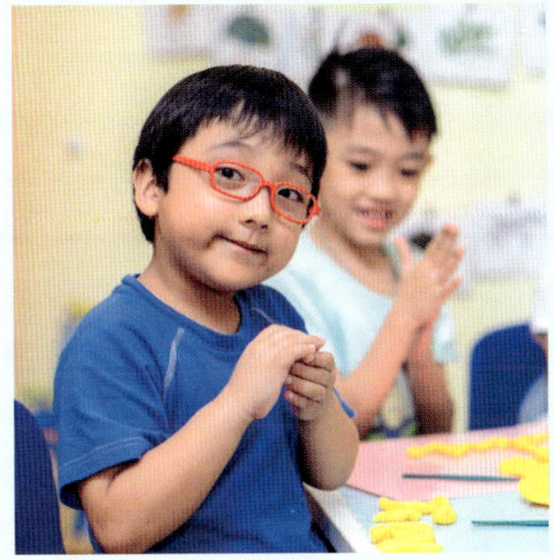

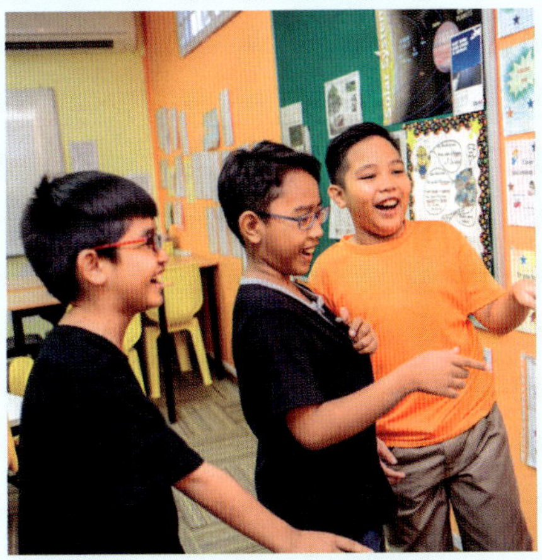

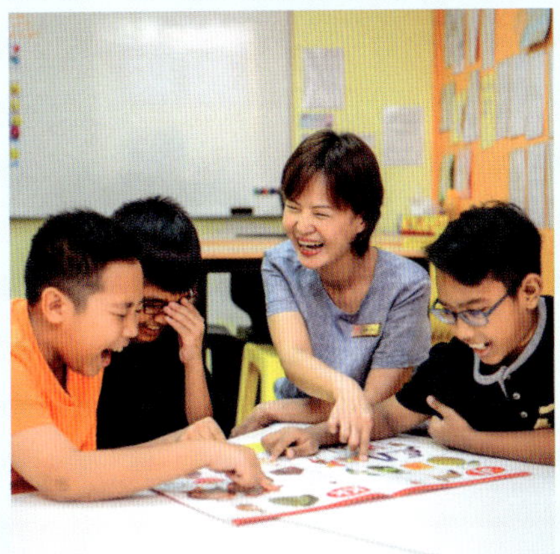

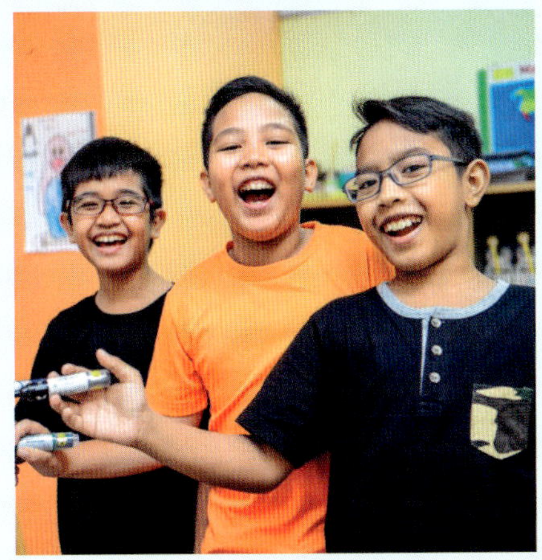

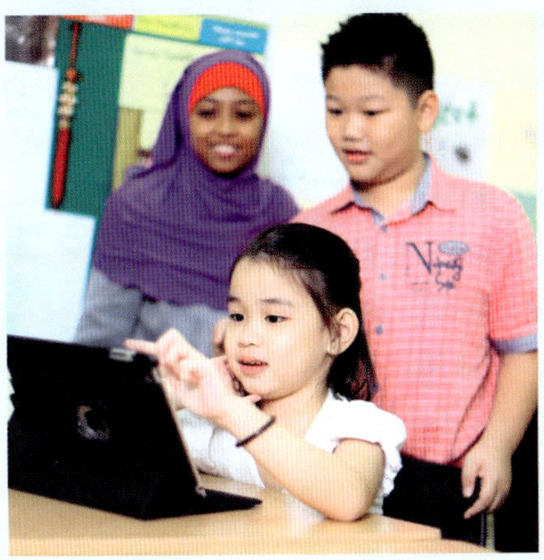

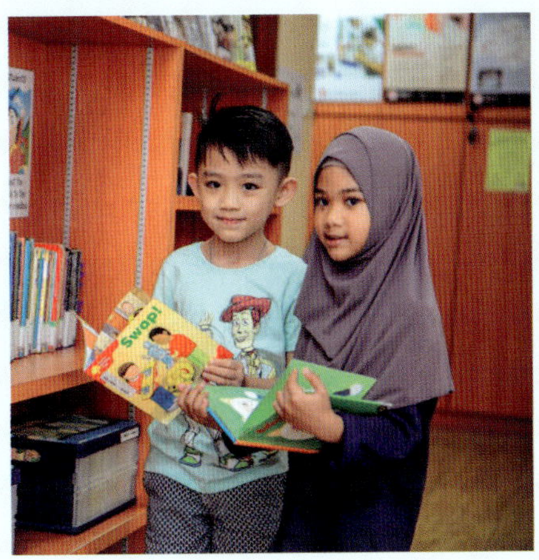
Swap!

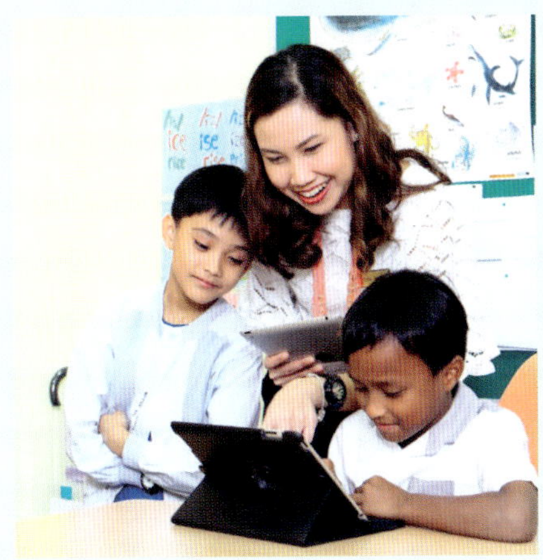

PSYCHOLOGICAL-EDUCATIONAL ASSESSMENTS

Specific learning difficulties such as dyslexia are normally diagnosed through an assessment by an educational or specialist psychologist. A psychological educational assessment provides an objective measurement of your child's abilities in a variety of areas.

An assessment is vital to identify individual strengths and weaknesses, and provide recommendations for intervention and support. Comprehensive assessment reports will contain detailed practical recommendations for parents and educators involved in supporting the child's education.

During an assessment, the child is tested for intelligence, literacy abilities and ability to use psychological processes of imagination, creativity, and reasoning with language. As no two children with specific learning difficulties are the same or have the same type/severity of difficulties, an assessment is vital.

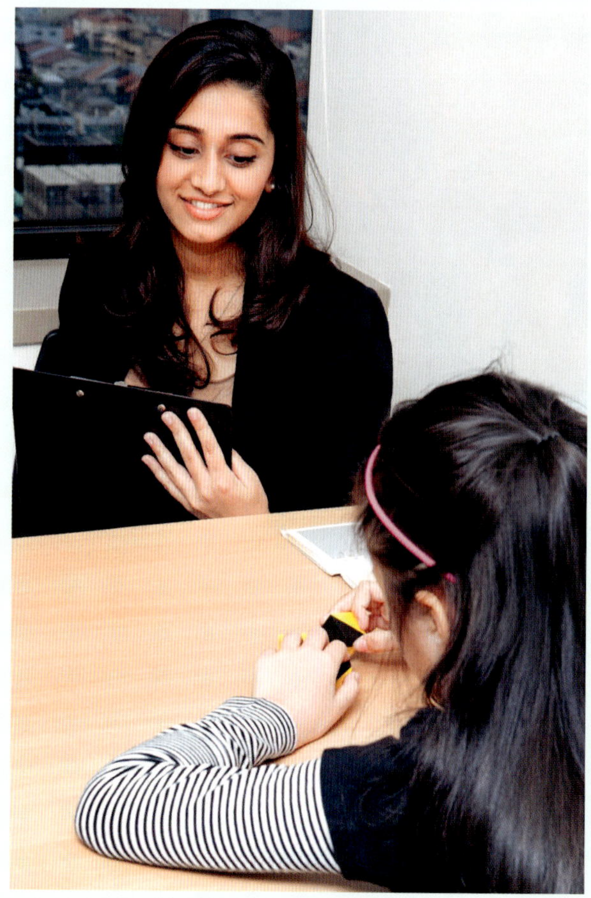

BENEFITS OF AN ASSESSMENT

The main aim of the assessment is to find the best way of helping your child. It provides recommendations on how to support your child. An assessment:

1. Provides useful information about your child's cognitive abilities, memory and literacy skills which you can share with your child's teacher and others that work with your child.

2. Gives greater insight into the nature and extent of the difficulties that your child may have or if other forms of therapy may be of benefit.

3. Helps you identify the appropriate learning programme based on your child's learning needs.

4. Helps you identify your child's profile of strengths which he/she can make use of in learning as well as give an indication of pathways to success in education and in future careers.

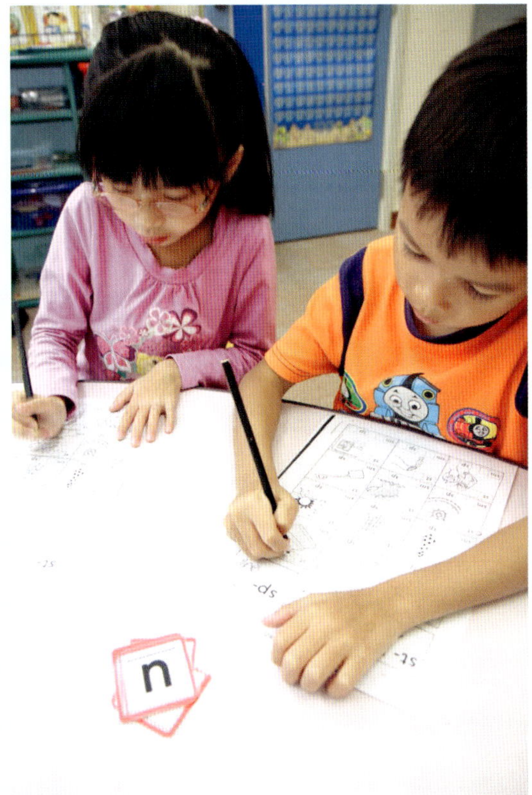

If we find that your child would benefit from our learning programme, then the assessment will help guide the ways in which we teach your child. In the case of review assessments, the information can also be useful in determining how much your child has progressed following intervention. Furthermore, the assessment results will help us recommend how you could support your child at home.

ASSESSMENT REPORTS

DAS psychologists will give you a personal explanation on the results of the assessment together with a written report. The DAS assessment report is recognised by most Singaporean organisations and government bodies such as the Ministry of Education.

An assessment report is required when requesting for access arrangements for your child in school or during national examinations. The written report can be given to those who care for or teach your child so that they are aware of your child's needs. Access arrangements are recommended based on evidence of needs and your child would typically need to receive a diagnosis of dyslexia before they are granted them.

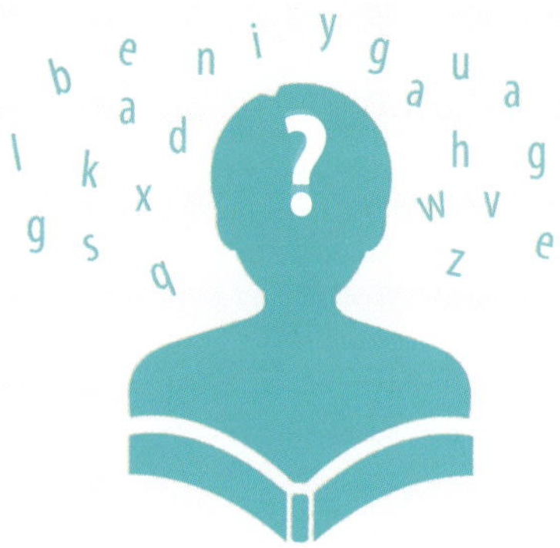

10 MYTHS OF DYSLEXIA

You are unable to determine if a child has dyslexia just by looking at them. Children with dyslexia might start out fine in school, but gradually, schoolwork can become a struggle for them. If left unsupported, dyslexia may lead to low self-esteem, behavioural problems, delinquency and withdrawal from friends, family and school. Here we explore some myths and the facts about dyslexia.

Myth 1: Dyslexia is a sort of mental retardation.

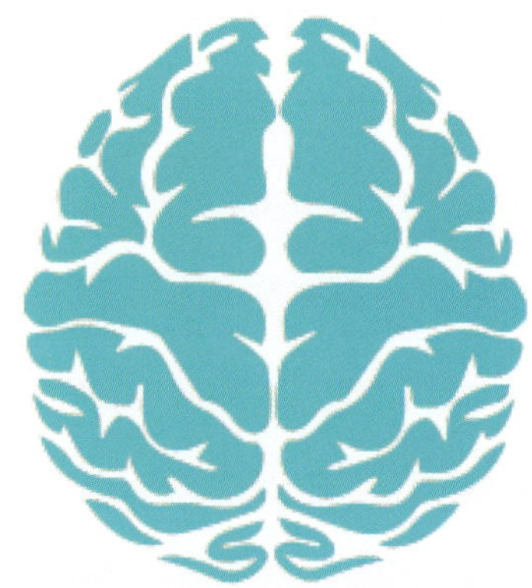

THE FACTS: Dyslexia is a difficulty in learning to read, write and spell, despite traditional teaching, average intelligence, and an adequate opportunity to learn. It affects the brain's ability to translate information received from the eyes or ears into understandable language. It does not result from vision or hearing problems. It is not due to mental retardation, brain damage, or a lack of intelligence.

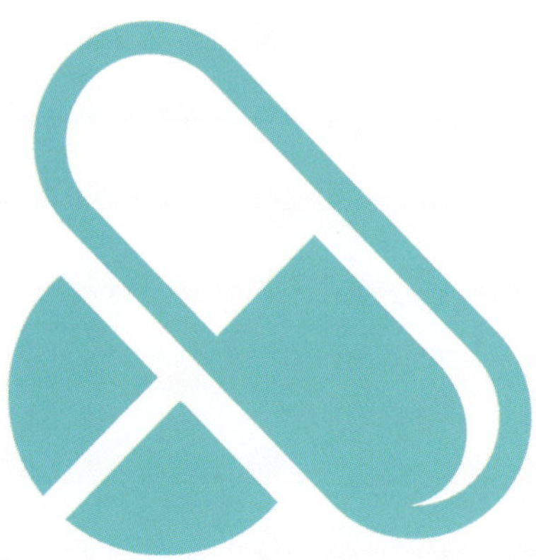

Myth 2: Dyslexia is a disease.

THE FACTS: Dyslexia is NOT a disease. It is a learning difference that is lifelong. Children with dyslexia become adults with dyslexia. If they are identified and given the right kind of help early, individuals with dyslexia can learn to compensate for their learning difference and read accurately. Given the appropriate specialist teaching, children with dyslexia can successfully learn to read and spell. Even so, they may continue to read slowly and not automatically.

Myth 3: Everyone with dyslexia has letter reversals.

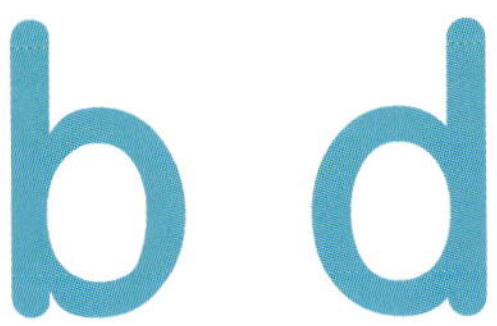

THE FACTS: Backwards writing and reversals of letters and words are common among young children learning to write whether or not they have dyslexia. Only about 10 percent of people with dyslexia reverse letters. In general, letter reversals become an area of concern if it persists beyond eight years of age.

Myth 4: Dyslexia only affects the use of the English language.

THE FACTS: Dyslexia has been shown to affect native Dutch, Israeli and Portuguese speakers as well as speakers of other languages. Dyslexia primarily affects the processing of speech sounds, otherwise known as phonological awareness. Dyslexia is also known to affect languages that are orthographically based like Chinese.

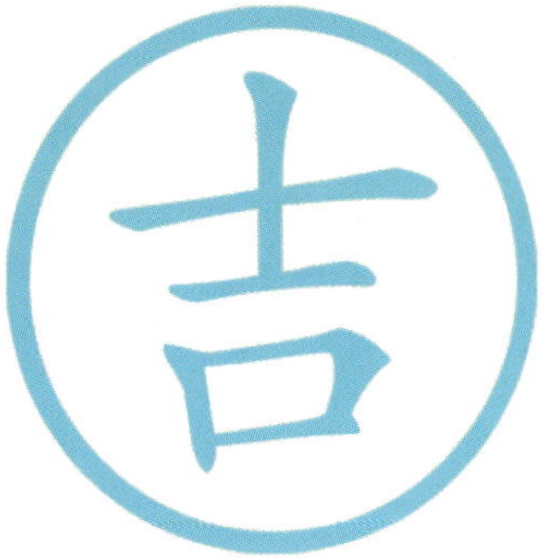

Myth 5: Smart people cannot have dyslexia.

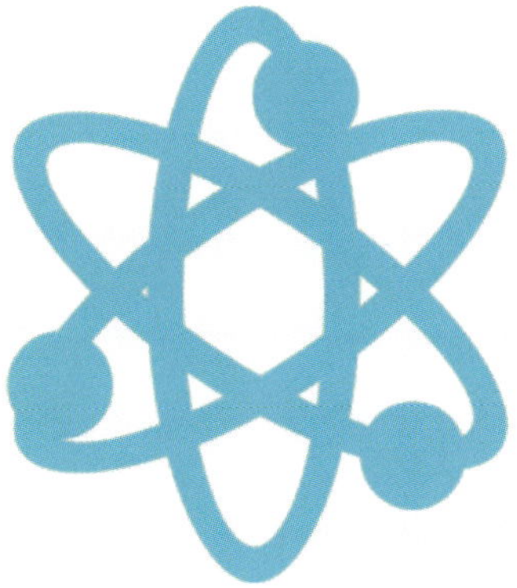

THE FACTS: Repeated studies have shown that there is very little relationship between dyslexia and intelligence in young children. Dyslexia occurs across a whole spectrum of intelligence and is as likely to be found in the gifted and talented population as it is to be present in those with low ability. Most people with dyslexia fall in the middle. However, if people with dyslexia do not learn to read, their IQs tend to fall behind as they get older.

Myth 6: My child can't have dyslexia. No one else in the family has it.

THE FACTS: Beware. In some families, one or both parents are obviously dyslexic and all, or most, of their children have learning differences. In other families, dyslexia is not apparent in either parent and the other children are unaffected.

Myth 7: He can't have dyslexia because he can read.

THE FACTS: All children with dyslexia can read — up to a point. But the problem they have with processing speech sounds prevents them from hearing all the individual sounds in a word. So they generally do not read by sounding out. With poor ability to detect and manipulate speech sounds, people with dyslexia tend to have inadequate knowledge and application of how sounds are linked with their written form.

This weak letter-sounds link affects their ability to read and spell. They often use alternative strategies such as memorising familiar stories, recognising words by their shapes or guessing based on the first letter or two. But their memories can hold only a limited number of words. It may take until Primary 3 or 4 for the reading struggles to become obvious. Without the right type of help, they cannot progress any further — no matter how smart they are and how hard they try. Their difficulties with spelling, however, are obvious very early. Poor spelling is highly related to poor reading.

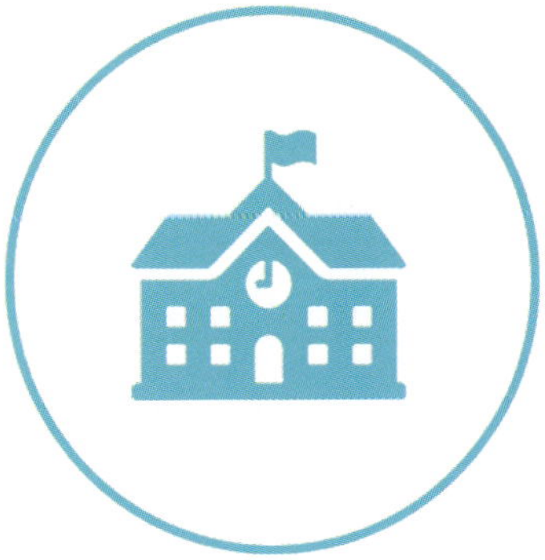

Myth 8: All children with dyslexia must go to a special school.

THE FACTS: Children with mild to moderate dyslexia are able to do well in mainstream classes as long as they are taught the appropriate coping techniques and are diligent in their work. Children with severe dyslexia can also study in mainstream classes with added support from professionals who can aid in their learning.

Myth 9: Individuals with dyslexia are just plain lazy.

THE FACTS: Research has shown, through brain mapping, that those with dyslexia use a different part of their brains when reading and working. The process is not as efficient, with much more effort and time required than is typically used. This extra time needed for processing does not mean they are slow or lazy. The learning process for them is exhausting, and until they are taught the way their brains need to learn to make these connections to the automatic language centre, it will always be a laborious process for them.

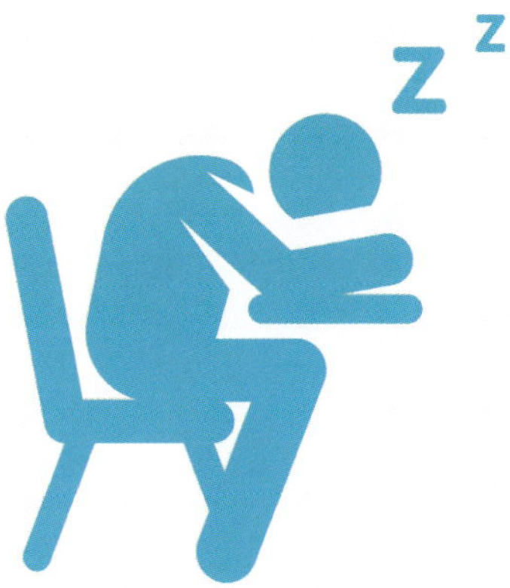

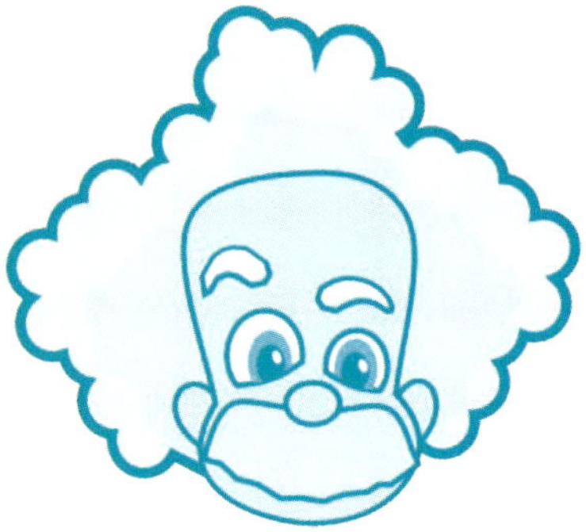

Myth 10: People with dyslexia will not succeed in life.

THE FACTS: A great majority of people with dyslexia are successful in their life endeavours. Some famous and accomplished people with dyslexia include Albert Einstein, the late Minister Mentor Lee Kuan Yew, Steven Spielberg, Richard Branson, Agatha Christie and Tom Cruise, to name a few.

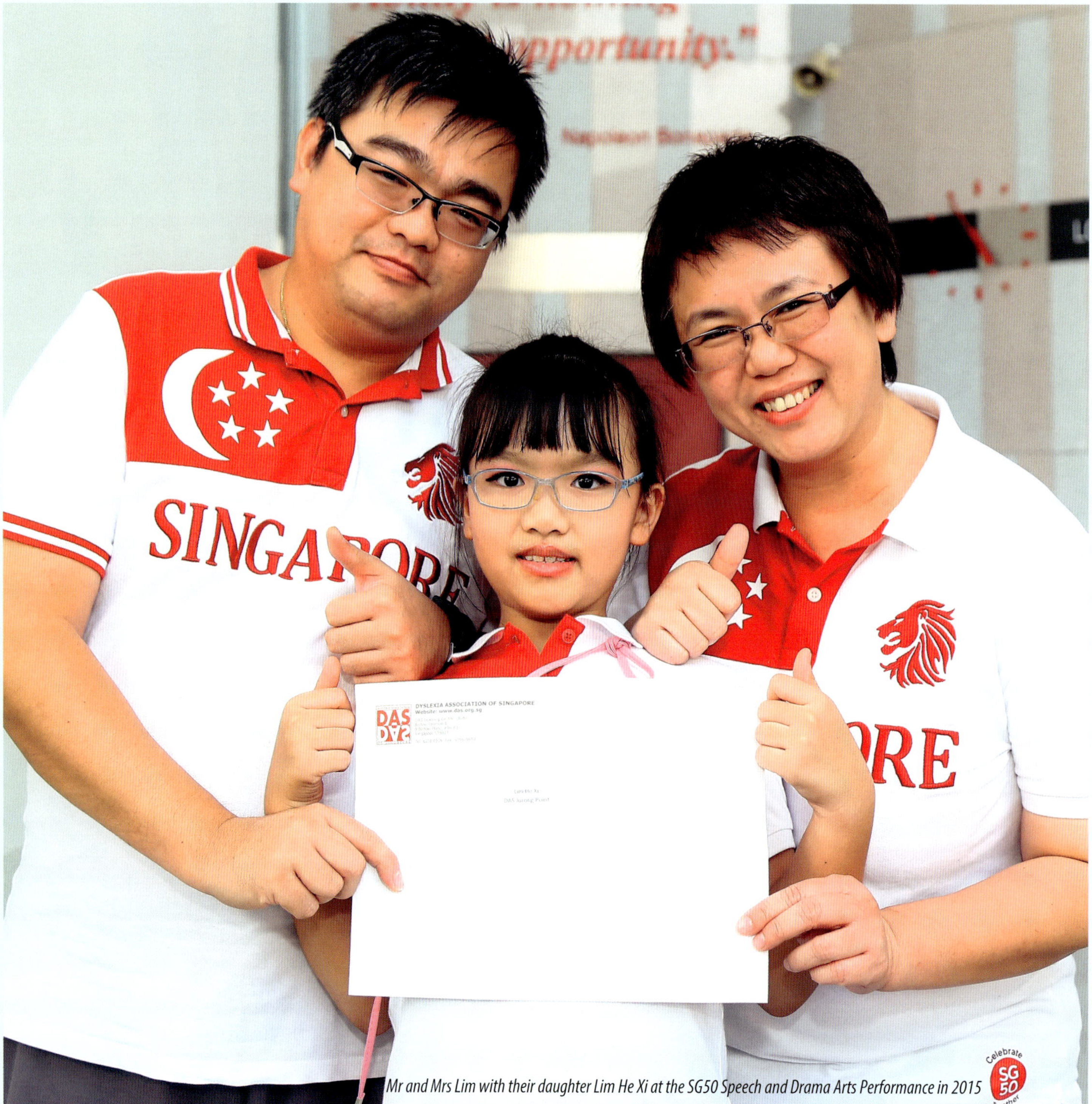

Mr and Mrs Lim with their daughter Lim He Xi at the SG50 Speech and Drama Arts Performance in 2015

4

FAMILIES OF SIGNIFICANCE

My mother rephrased dyslexia as a gift in my mind early on. She constantly told me when I didn't do well in school not to worry about it. Her attitude was, 'You have a wonderful imagination and you'll fill in the blanks.

Barbara Corcoran
Real Estate Mogul

SIGNIFICANT OTHERS

Parents and siblings of dyslexics are often the first to notice their learning differences. Some parents are more sensitised because they themselves are dyslexic. In many cases, however, the parents discover that they are dyslexic only after their children have been diagnosed. Dyslexia is a hereditary condition and although, rarely, it does skip a generation, it is normative that one parent or both are dyslexic. DAS's former CEO, Robin Moseley, had a dyslexic father, was himself dyslexic, and has a dyslexic son. That probably contributed in large measure to how sensitive he was to learning differences and how passionately he went about championing the cause of dyslexics.

While more and more educators from mainstream schools have received training to spot the signs of learning differences, not all are equipped to do so. And whether they are sensitised to learning challenges or not, not all have the time to provide individualised attention. So, parents remain a key resource in our efforts to identify those who need help.

Early identification and intervention are vital. Children with dyslexia are often unable to reach their full potential due to their learning differences and may be frustrated with learning. Early identification and intervention can enhance their learning experiences. For parents, nothing can be more satisfying than seeing their children beam with confidence because they have experienced a more positive learning experience and had their self-esteem boosted.

GIVING PARENTS A VOICE

Knowing how isolated and bewildered parents can feel when their children are diagnosed with dyslexia, DAS formed a Parent Support Group (PSG). Inspirational sharing sessions by successful dyslexics, and fun-filled activities for DAS students, their parents and even the whole family are organised to help parents to be better informed and involved in their child's learning journey. They also have more opportunities to build rapport with the DAS educators who are helping their children.

Being part of a network makes parenting a child with learning differences less challenging. The PSG therefore provides a platform for sharing ideas, concerns and experiences with other parents. Parents also gain valuable experience in how to support their children more effectively.

PSG meetings are held regularly and parents are kept informed through the monthly Parents' Newsletter. There is also a private PSG Facebook group that allows for more timely interaction among the parents who are members. The privacy of this group, together with the smaller number of members, allows for a deeper level of sharing and connection among the parents.

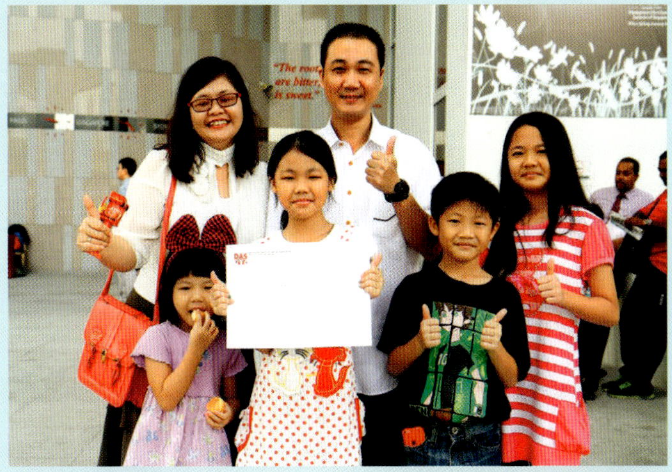

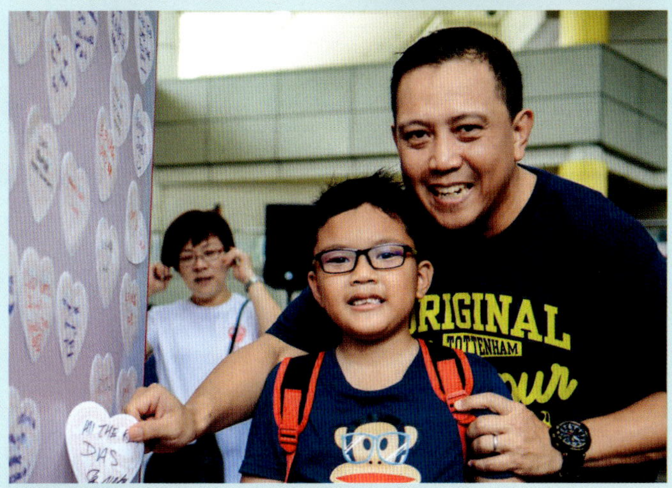

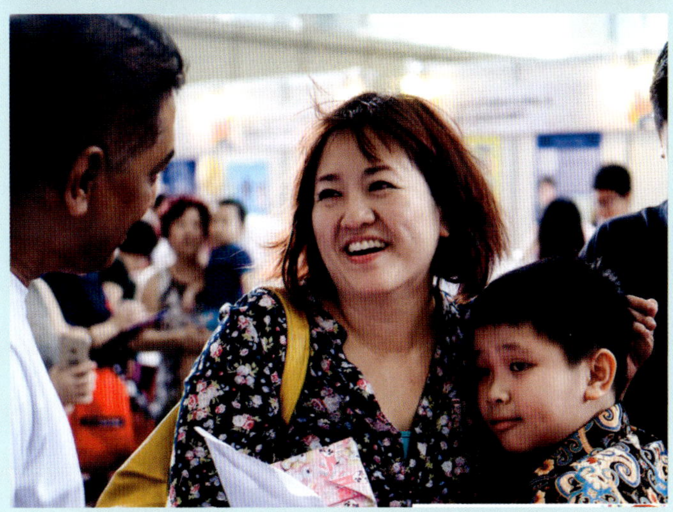

WHAT SOME PARENTS AND SPOUSES HAVE TO SAY

"DON'T TRY TO DRIVE A ONE-LITRE CAR LIKE A TWO-LITRE CAR"

"My Kenrick never failed in his school exams, but he barely scraped through. He used to say, 'I passed, mum. Why are you scolding me?' But I knew he was capable of doing better. He was an intelligent, bright boy, yet when it came to his results, they were never as good as we would have expected. Like so many others in similar situations, he had a hidden handicap. He enjoyed reading, so he was still able to understand enough of his schoolwork to get by. But he couldn't spell. So when he had to write sentences or essays, he would choose the simplest words that he could remember. This explains why his grades were below par.

I often tell my friends that Kenrick talks a lot. If you interview dyslexics, more often than not you will find that they are very verbal. When he was three years old, he would talk and talk. Even in his sleep, he would talk. So I asked him one day, 'Son, why do you talk so much in your dreams?' He said, 'In the day, my brain talks to me. At night, I talk to my brain!' The typical response from my friends when I relate this to them is, 'He's so bright.'

Unfortunately, the schools are not always very supportive. For the first two years in primary school, I would let the Form Teacher know that Kenrick is dyslexic. The response I received was, 'I'm not taught to handle dyslexic children'. Fortunately his Primary 3 teacher was very interested in special education. He said, 'I've not taught dyslexics, but let me see what I can do'. I'm convinced that was when my son began to be interested in reading.

But as parents, we also need to know our limits when it comes to helping our children. I remember how Kenrick and I used to drive each other mad! All because I was trying to help him do better. So, it is very good advice when DAS tells parents, 'Try not to tutor your son unless you are a teacher or are trained'. You can't help it, you have your mother's hat on and you tend to say things that turn out all wrong. That leads to resentment. My wake-up call came when a close friend said to me, 'Corina, don't try to drive a one-litre car like a two-litre car'. It finally sank in and I changed the way I interacted with Kenrick. That was an important turning point in our relationship and I'm so glad that things are now much better."

Mrs Corina Lai
DAS Chief Financial Officer (2001–2014),
Mother of Kenrick Lai

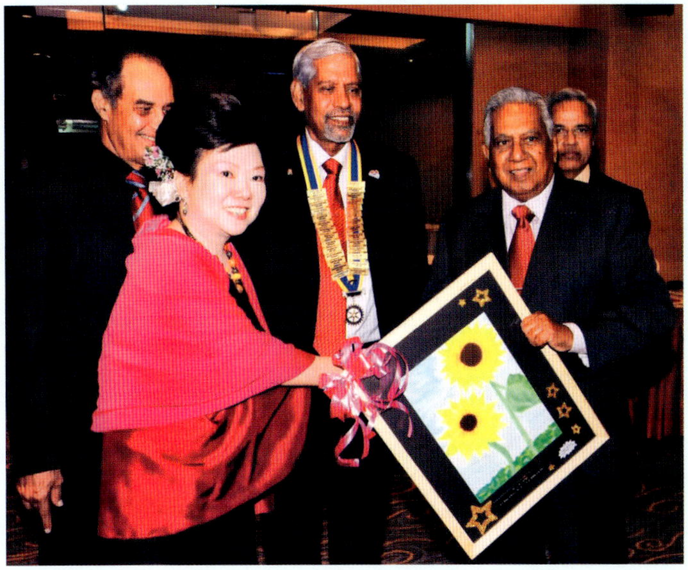

Rotary Club of Raffles City installation and charity dinner. The former President of Singapore, Mr S. R. Nathan, was the Guest of Honour. (L to R) Dr Jimmy Daruwalla; Mrs Corina Lai; newly installed RCRC President Mr Rajaram; President S R Nathan; and Rotarian Hanif from Rotary Club of Kuala Lumpur Di-Raja.

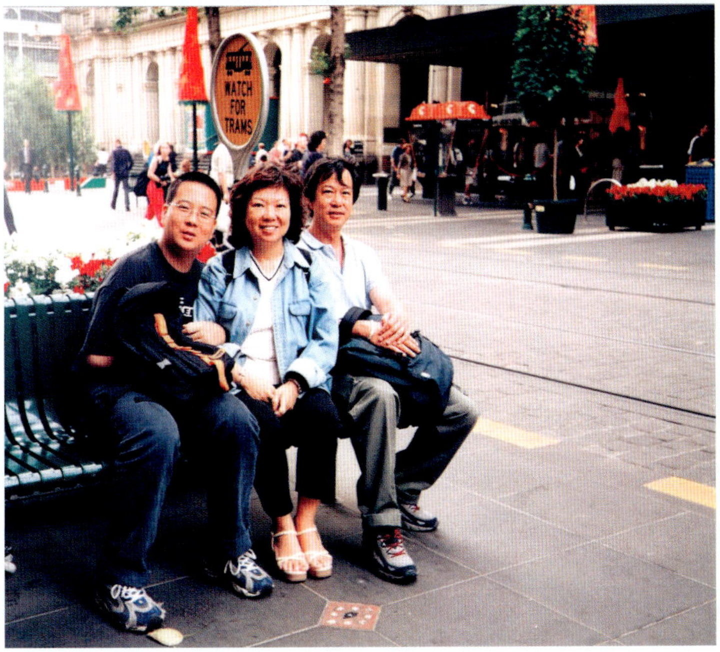

Corina and her husband Richard, together with Kenrick in Hobart, Australia.

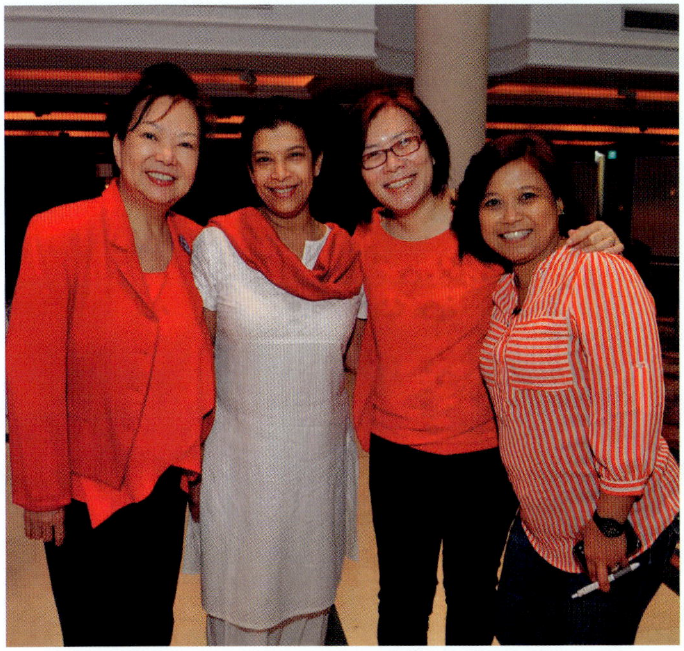

Mrs Corina Lai with Mrs Jothy Daruwalla, and two long-term employees of DAS, Ms Tey Ching Ching and Ms Kharyati Kamsani.

"SOMETHING WAS PREVENTING HER FROM REACHING HER FULL POTENTIAL."

"Deanna is the middle child between two brothers. Being the only girl, she always found it difficult to get her brothers to join her in the games that she would prefer to play. She was therefore elated when she started attending school, just before she turned five. Deanna was confident and chatty and very happy in school until her late nursery years. She grew less chatty and was not as eager to go to school. I did not worry too much about it then, as I assumed that the rigour of a Montessori syllabus was taking its toll on her, especially since she was also trying to cope with Mandarin as a second language.

On days when I came home late from work, I would find Deanna fast asleep with her spelling list as her constant companion. No matter how hard she tried, she could not retain the words for longer than an hour, resulting in her usually failing her weekly spelling exercises. This greatly discouraged her and she became more reserved and hesitant as the days went by. I highlighted these changes in Deanna to her teachers but was informed that there was nothing amiss. They commended her for her conscientious attitude towards her school work and advised me not to worry unnecessarily and to let things be.

As the days passed, Deanna became less confident and would usually keep to herself. The last straw was when Deanna came up to me one day in kindergarten and asked me why she was so stupid. I fought hard to hold back my tears and valiantly extolled her merits and intelligence, but to no avail. I could see in her eyes that she did not believe me. She commented on how all her classmates had moved on to the higher colour scheme in reading while she was the only one still stuck in the lower level. She said she couldn't understand why no matter how hard she tried, things just would not fit together.

I decided to take things into my own hands and got her an appointment at the Specialist Clinic at Kandang Kerbau Women's and Children's Hospital. Every step forward brought us two steps back. After assessing Deanna, the consultant told me that she could be a 'late bloomer' and that I should just let her be so that she could develop at her own pace. But I knew my daughter better. I could sense her frustration. It felt like she had so much inside that was just dying to be set free. Something was preventing her from reaching her full potential.

After further consultation, it was suggested that we go for an assessment at DAS. At our wits' end, we decided to give it a try. That decision changed Deanna's life forever. Reading the psychological report after Deanna's assessment made me cry. Although she was functioning at a high intellectual level, her reading and spelling did not match up. Her inability to clearly express all that was going on in

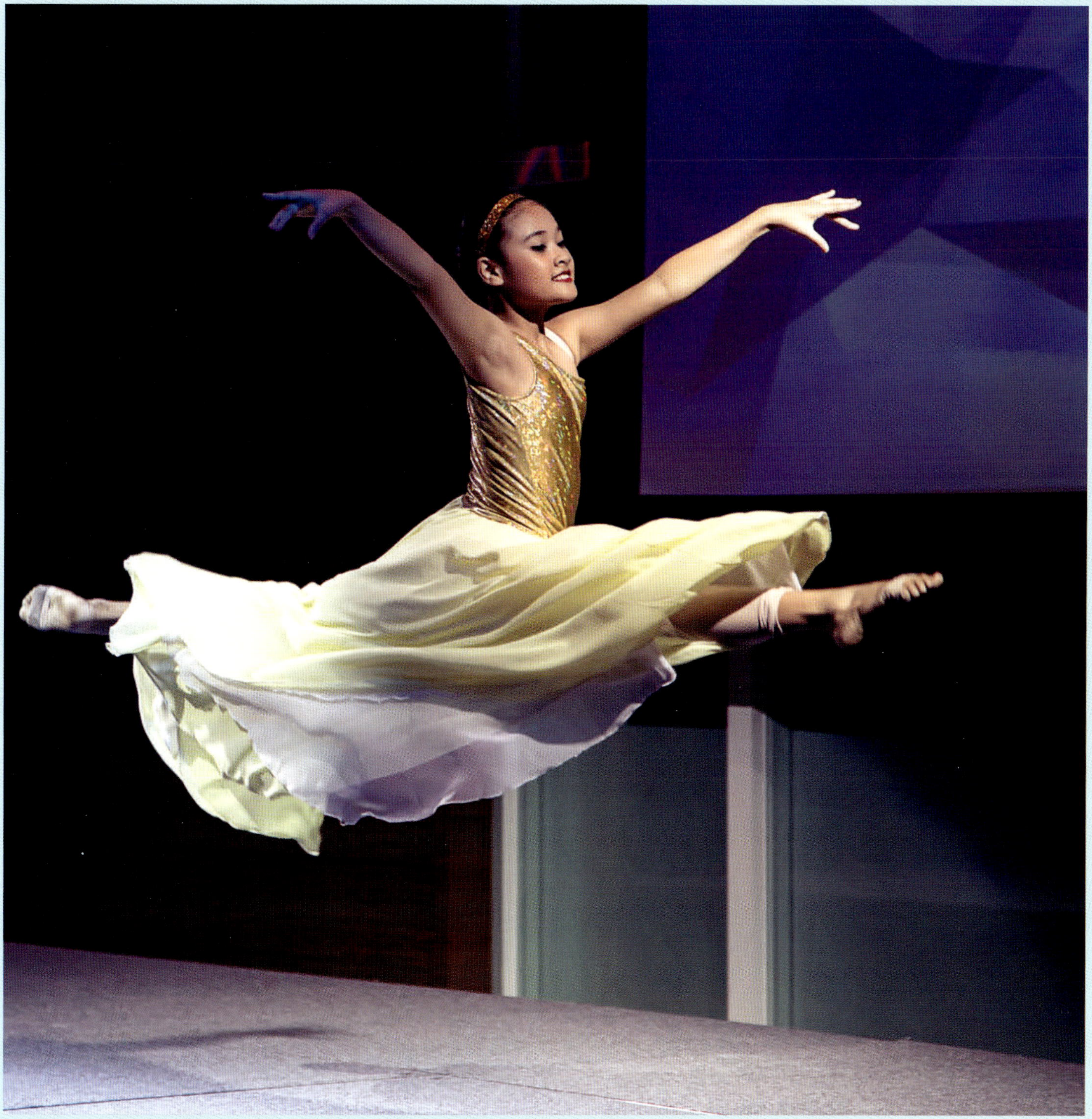

her mind left her frustrated and feeling incompetent, ravaging her self-esteem and confidence along the way.

After learning about her dyslexia, my husband and I vowed to do all we could to pick up the pieces and slowly but surely build up her esteem again. Her love of dance was clear, so we allowed her to develop her talent in that area. By God's grace, and with a lot of hard work and sacrifice, Deanna has won a number of local and international dance awards, the most recent being the inaugural Asia's Got Talent competition in 2015 where her group, Dance Thrilogy, was the only grand finalist from Singapore.

Every parent wants the best for her child. To me, the development of character takes precedence over academic excellence. Deanna has a passion for dance and is amazingly blessed with the talent for it. Nevertheless, the choice of allowing her to participate in Asia's Got Talent and missing a month of school in the PSLE year was not an easy one. However, she has gained so much from the experience and has developed into a more disciplined and determined individual."

Ms Zalina Zakariah-Ismael
Mother of Nur Deanna bte Mohd Ismael
(member of Dance Thrilogy, grand finalist of the inaugural Asia's Got Talent)

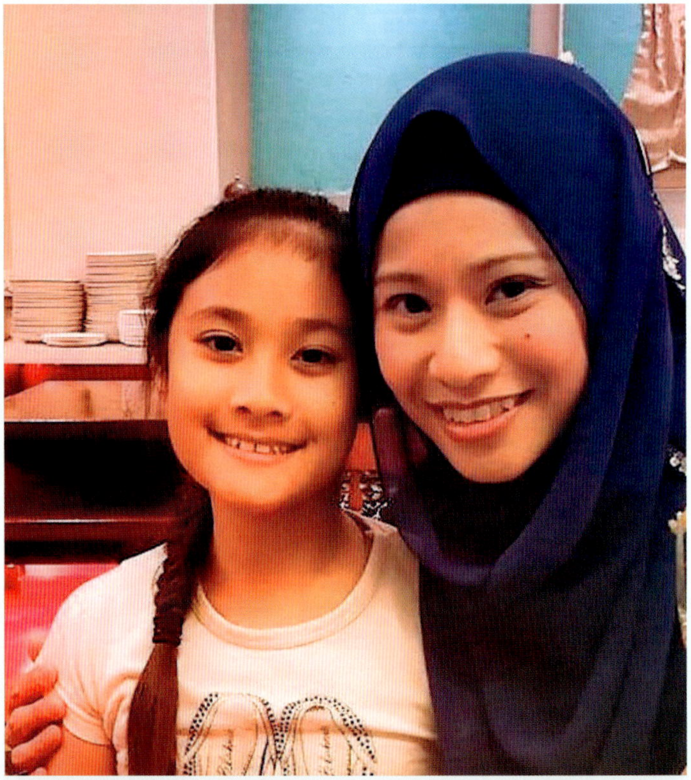

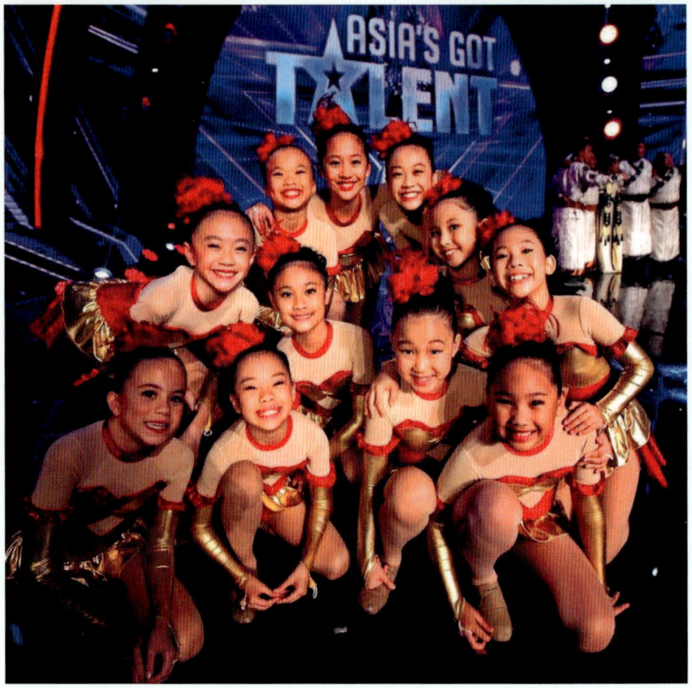

"WE FOUND A SIGNIFICANT MISMATCH BETWEEN MY SON'S INTELLIGENCE AND HIS ABILITY TO READ AND WRITE."

"Many may see dyslexia as a stumbling block, but it only causes difficulties when we try to see things the way everyone else sees them. When given free rein, dyslexics shine because we see and think differently, and that creativity is a huge asset in a profession like engineering.

When my son was young, he told us that the words moved about when he tried to read them. We found a significant mismatch between my son's intelligence and his ability to read and write. Our suspicion that he might have Attention Deficit Hyperactivity Disorder was ruled out after a test proved that he was, instead, dyslexic. After my son's diagnosis at DAS, I realised that I face similar problems and found out that I am dyslexic too.

As a child, I was very curious and had a vivid imagination. To satisfy my curiosity about how things worked, I would dismantle appliances and toys, even though I would be punished for spoiling them. At school I had problems memorising words, texts, the multiplication tables and names. Even when I was studying in the polytechnic, copying information from the board, which was a breeze for my peers, was an extremely tedious exercise for me, as I was copying letter by letter instead of phrases. I remember overhearing a neighbour commenting that my future was bleak and that spurred me to work even harder.

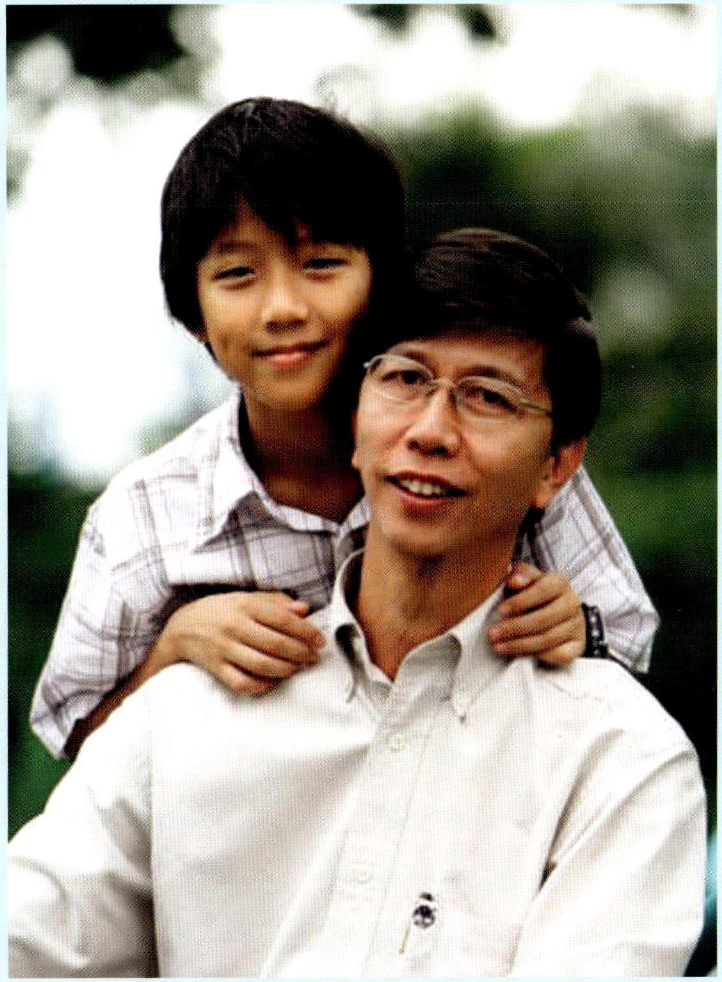

Richard Kwok with his son Kwok Ting Yu in 2006. Ting Yu is now studying in Melbourne at Monash University, and is pursing an Actuarial Science & Econometrics degree.

Fuelled by passion and with a keen understanding of my strengths, I decided to pursue a career in engineering, where my creativity would be valued and where I could contribute to Singapore's development and improve the lives of others. It was tough at the start because I had to attend night classes after working all day. But it was worth it.

Ultimately, I chose to be a defence engineer, as I am always excited by new technologies and feel immense satisfaction when I see my work helping to make a difference.

Back in the 80s, not many of my colleagues believed that we could develop an indigenous armoured vehicle. However, I was very determined. My team and I developed the first ever made-in-Singapore armoured fighting vehicle, now known as BIONIX. From this success, our team used this prototype to develop more armoured platforms.

I often share the mantra 'IDENTIFY-ACT-BECOME' with young people such as my son to encourage them to identify or envision what they want, to act on their passion, and to persevere until they become who they want to be to achieve their goal.

The diagnosis of my son's learning differences was important as it helped my wife and me, as his parents, to know how to help him deal with it, to provide him with relevant support, and to help him improve. It was also good for his self-confidence and enabled him to obtain extra time and be excused for poor spelling during high-stake examinations.

Parents who see their child struggling academically should get them diagnosed as early as possible. Unlike certain physical challenges that can be seen, learning differences can be frustrating as you don't know what you're dealing with. I hope that as a society, we will support, help recognise, and foster the natural gifts and abilities of children with dyslexia, as their potential can be limitless. Just look at Sir Isaac Newton, Albert Einstein, and Thomas Edison, three dyslexic heroes who are celebrated around the world for their ingenuity in science and engineering."

Mr Richard Kwok
Father of Kwok Ting Yu
(Actuarial Science & Econometrics undergraduate, Monash University)

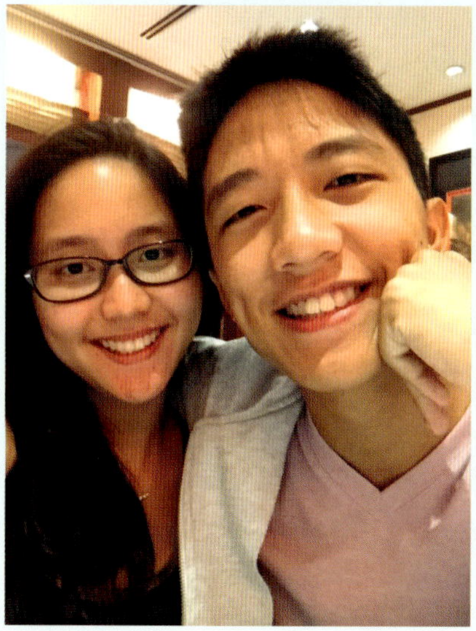

Siblings Kwok Fuyu (L) and Kwok Ting Yu (R). Fuyu is a PhD candidate in the department of Psychology at the Nanyang Technological University. Her interest in dyslexia was sparked by her brother, who is dyslexic and was an ex-student of DAS.

"IN MY EYES, HE'S JUST A NON-SPELLER."

"When Gary was approached to share his journey with dyslexia, he was eager to accede, but only on one condition — that I help him write it. I instantly agreed, thinking that it would be just another piece of writing. Little did I envisage that penning his story would be an emotional roller coaster of ups and downs for me.

In the '80s, ours was a long-distance relationship — he was working in China and I, in Singapore. We would communicate via snail mail. I often noticed the spelling and grammatical errors in his letters, but love was blind. I had assumed it was due to him coming from a predominantly Chinese-educated environment. But it all makes sense now.

I grew up a classic bookworm. A perfect Sunday was one spent reading a thick book at Starbucks. Gary would bring along his book to join me. But shortly after his fourth page, I would often find him doodling on the napkins.

Gary has a very detailed eye for design and beauty. He designed my wedding dress. At my first fitting, he flew into a huge rage. He was shooting off a string of instructions to the designer — 'The neckline should be 5mm lower; the flower applique should tilt a few degrees to

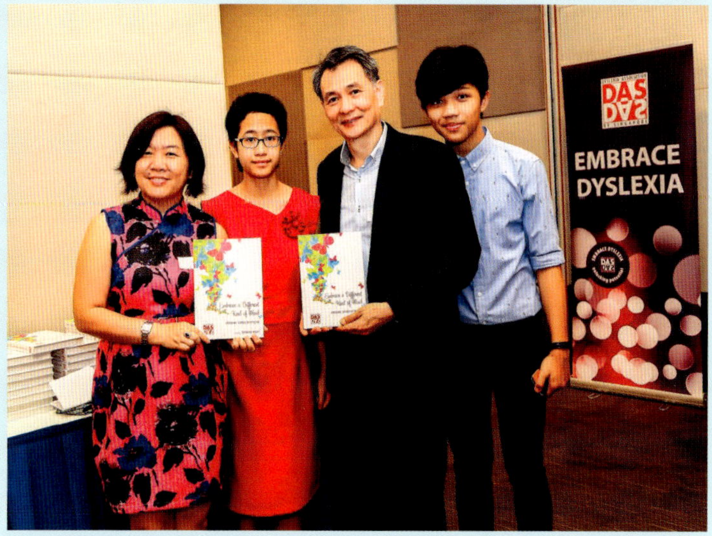

Carrie Chan with daughter Tyshae, husband Gary Seow, and son Skylar at the launch of Embrace a Different Kind of Mind.

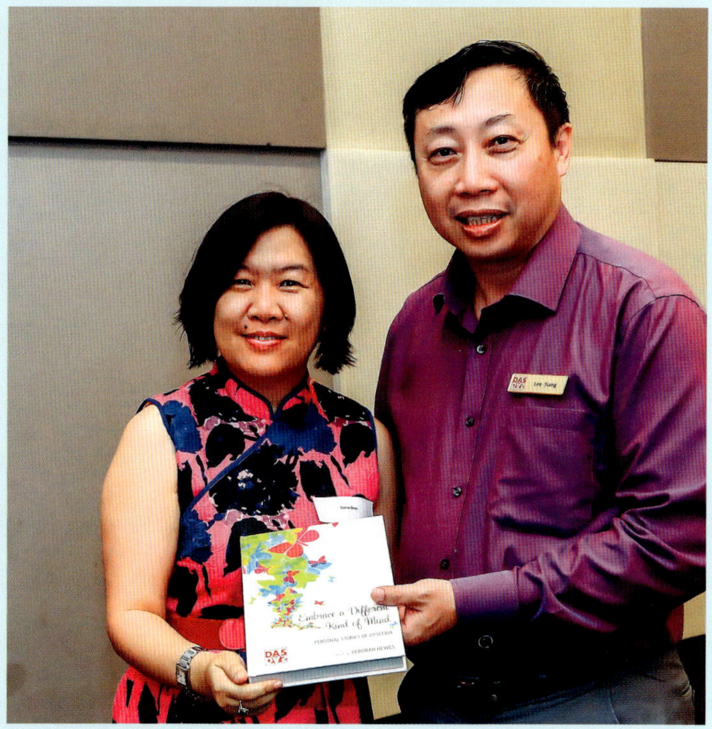

Carrie receiving her copy of the book from DAS CEO Mr Lee Siang.

the left; the pearls on the sleeves are hanging too low.' Neither the designer nor I noticed any of these 'flaws'. In the end, the studio agreed to tailor a new dress according to Gary's exact specifications. The final product was so gorgeous that it was featured in a magazine.

When Gary was diagnosed with dyslexia in his early 40s, my two children and I did not make a big deal of it. Instead, the diagnosis came as a great relief to me. There was now an explanation for all his 'idiosyncrasies'. We could talk openly about it. The diagnosis allowed us to bond more tightly as a family unit.

Until this day, he will misspell even the simplest of words: big duel (deal), paintful (painful), stri (straight). He also has difficulty with long words. I eventually became his personal spell-checker, vetting every important email and document that he drafts. He still shouts for help across the room if he needs me to spell a word for him.

Through the years, dyslexia has shaped the way we communicate. I do not receive long love letters or poems from him. Instead, Gary designs novel toys and dedicates them to me. At times, when I asked for clarification of the descriptions and specifications of his inventions, Gary would get frustrated because he felt that he was not being understood.

In recent years, however, Gary has become an expert in providing descriptions with minimal words.

I now see that I have been selfish and intolerant. I can't draw. I can't visualise in 3D. I can't sing. I can't play any musical instruments. I don't excel in sports. But it didn't matter to him. He didn't think of me as being any less intelligent. There was never a time when he would say to me, 'You have to be able to draw' or 'By now you should have perfected at least one instrument if you had practised every day'. Not once did he criticise me for my lack of creativity.

In my eyes, he's just a non-speller. To me, more importantly, Gary is an extremely creative person, a driven entrepreneur, and a man with amazing tenacity. I am proud of him because I know many of his accomplishments have been hard won. These are his gifts that have richly blessed my kids and me."

Ms Carrie Chan

Wife of Gary Seow (Founder of KYDZ International)

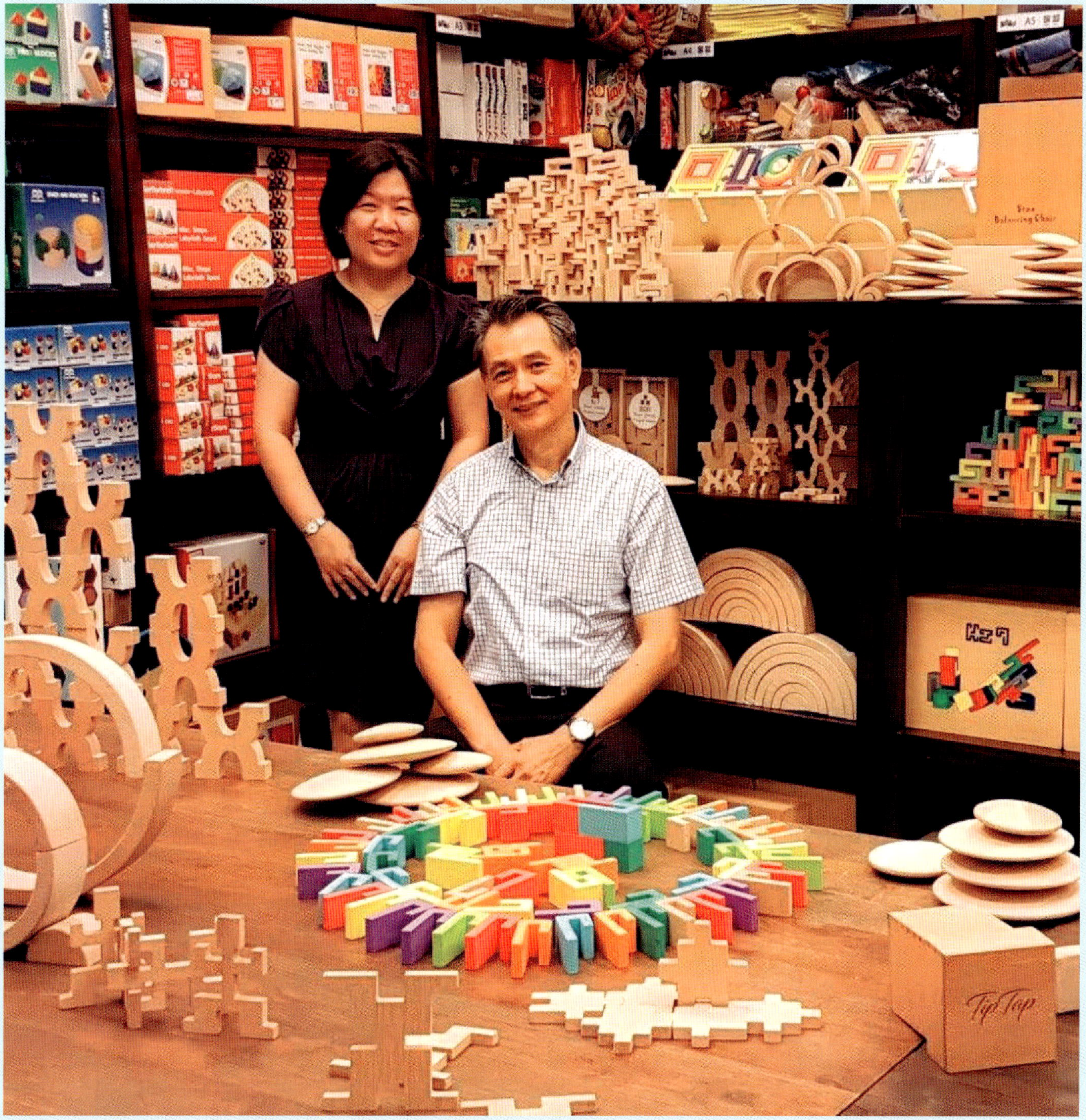

"A SILVER LINING TO EVERY CLOUD"

"My daughter, Kayla, who is 11 years old, was only diagnosed with dyslexia last year. In July 2016, she started at DAS, so she's completed four terms already.

Her spelling had always been good. And even though her grades were not so great, she managed to get by. Last year, when I was going through one of her CLOZE passages, I discovered that for one of the answers which should have been "DEPOSIT", all the letters were there, but they were mixed up. So I asked her what she was trying to write. She said DEPOSIT. I asked her to spell it and I broke down the syllables DE-POS-IT. She could spell it.

Also, because the usual concept of dyslexia is bad handwriting, I never connected it to Kayla. She has very neat handwriting. So I used to put it down to not paying attention, perhaps. And she reads a lot. In fact she's a reading ambassador in school. So then I began to think, 'What are you reading?'

I knew that her vocabulary is not that great either. So it all began to add up. I also realised that her spelling was done from memory. When you study science, it also involves spelling, so she was always getting low scores for poor spelling.

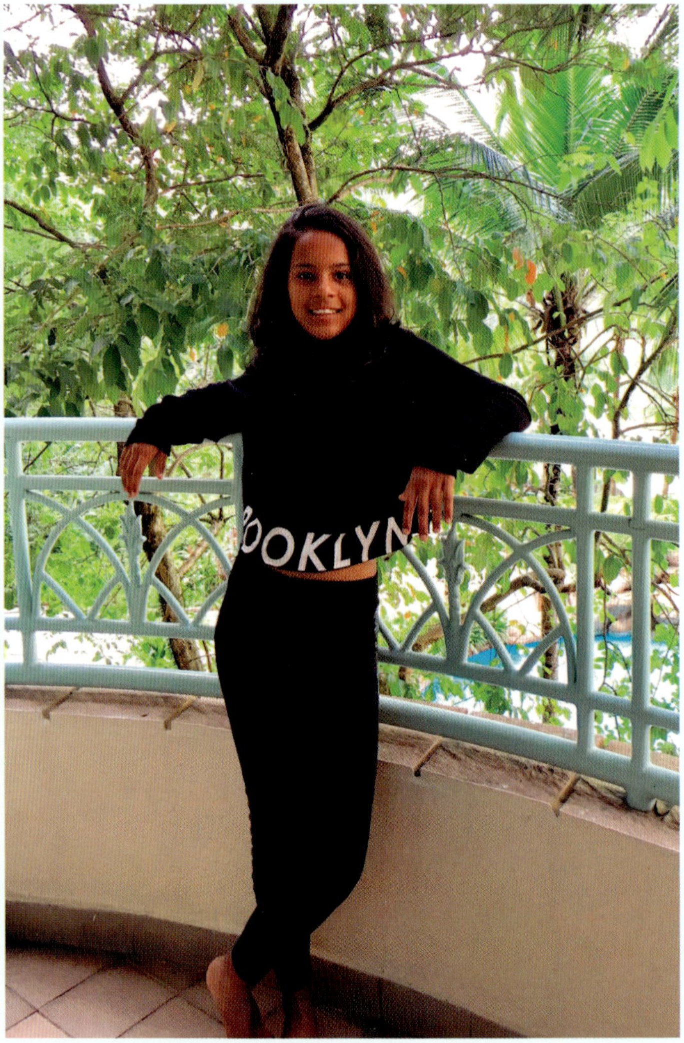

Kayla Morton

I decided I wanted to get her tested. Also, she had to take mother tongue and her mother tongue was pretty bad. She takes Chinese. I felt that it really wasn't fair if she has dyslexia and I'm forcing her to take Chinese. So I googled to see where I could get her tested and I found DAS.

I mentioned to her school teacher that I was thinking of getting her tested, and her teacher said she had also begun to wonder about Kayla's language difficulties. Because she pays attention and listens in the classroom, a lot of her work is done from memory. Not every child is academic and I'm ok with that, but she's diligent and yet doesn't quite get the results she should. And I'm not even comparing her with her siblings. I know all three children are different.

She was not on the radar screen of the teachers because apart from being a bit flighty and messy, she didn't have any behavioural issues. Nothing out of the ordinary, so she didn't capture the attention of the teachers. Even at DAS, she went in at a higher level than most kids when they started.

Thankfully, her school has accepted the recommendation that she be allowed extra time during the exams. She also receives single-sided exam papers. Her assessment allows her to be exempted from doing mother tongue, but our application to MOE was rejected.

So, we're going to try for round two. I think this is probably because some parents do take advantage of the assessments to get their children exempted. For example, there was the mum whose son was getting 70 marks, and she had tried twice to get an exemption. She's Malay and the son was doing Malay for mother tongue. So, I thought that's a good thing, right? But she grumbled that it was a lot of effort.

In our case, because I'm Eurasian and my husband is Chinese/Sinhalese, none of the mother tongue choices fit us. So all my children have done Chinese. Kayla has been getting Chinese tuition since K2 because I was trying to prepare her. Her overall average right now is about 30! So I don't think it's fair to make her continue. Of course, if she didn't have this learning difference, I wouldn't even try to get exemption. But dyslexia is a language-based disability.

Also, it affects her confidence. She's going for tuition (and she realises it's not cheap) and she goes for remedial, but she's still not improving, so there has to be some basis for exemption. I do understand that there are abuses by some parents, but MOE should take a case-by-case approach. I don't think it's fair to those who really need it.

She enjoys the classes at DAS because they're slightly different, and she's happy to go. We've not done these things before, so I think they have helped. Her English and math have improved slightly, but her science improved much more. So she's quite happy with herself. As far as I'm concerned, little improvements are good enough, as long as you do your best.

My challenge was telling her about it, because I

didn't want her to use her diagnosis as an excuse for not trying. I just tell her that she has some learning difficulties. So far, she's not had anyone saying nasty things to or about her. She's a very people person, bubbly and chatty (unlike her two siblings). She'll order her food by herself and sometimes even do it for her sister who is older. So she's had no problems socially.

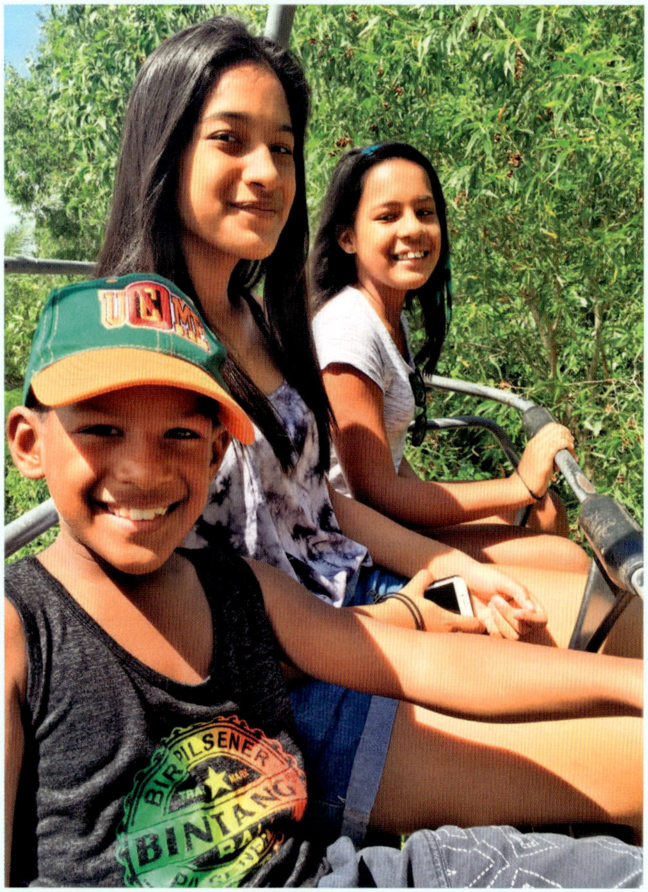

Kayla and her siblings Kiara and Tyler.

I didn't realise that, for her reading, she stumbles and skips a few words. Yet she's not shy about reading aloud in class. She wants to do it. In fact, at my cousin's wedding, she wanted to do a reading. So I asked my cousin to provide in advance what she would read so we could practise. She did an awesome job. She did miss a few words, but the pronunciation was all there. So, during the mid-year Meet-the-Parents session, her form teacher said Kayla paid attention and a lot of it was absorbed, but her teacher didn't think Kayla went home to process it. So, whenever she does her work, it is based on her memory.

I did ask her about what she'd read in her books and what she saw. This is because her cousin says the letters jump when he reads words. In his case, if the word ends with an "e", multiple e's will show. But she said, no, they didn't move. She even got an award as a reading ambassador. At one point, she was teaching the P1s. Hopefully they were simple words and she didn't teach the wrong thing! Now I feel a little bad about scolding her so much before.

I'm hoping that going to DAS will give her coping skills that she can adopt to see her through school, work, and life.

She does have some problems with the concepts in math, but her main difficulty is with problem sums. She did improve somewhat for her English written paper, but for composition (which she generally does OK), she unfortunately went off the point this time; it was long, but totally irrelevant. Her DAS teacher did say that she can write, but can't put it in a flow, and tends to be all over the place. She needs to learn to arrange her thoughts.

Kayla is creative, likes music, and is fashion-conscious. Like many other dyslexic kids, she is chatty. I think that here in Singapore, academic achievements are overly emphasised, and dyslexics get penalised. I recognise that academics are important, but there is more to life. As long as Kayla tries her best, it doesn't have to be all As. For this particular term, I can see a visible boost in her now that she knows she has a learning difference. She'll sit and study without my having to nag. Homework is handed in on time (although sometimes she still slips up).

It has made a difference for her to understand her learning differences, and that has been a blessing. There's always a silver lining to every cloud."

Mrs Desiree Ann Morton
Mother of Kayla

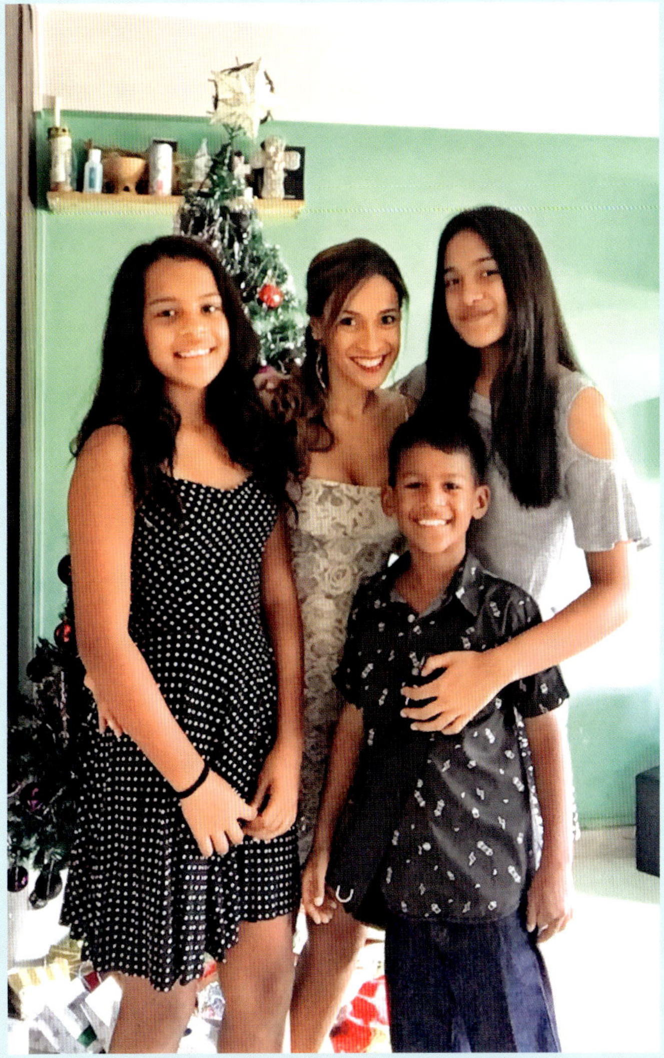

Kayla, Desiree Ann Morton, Tyler and Kiara

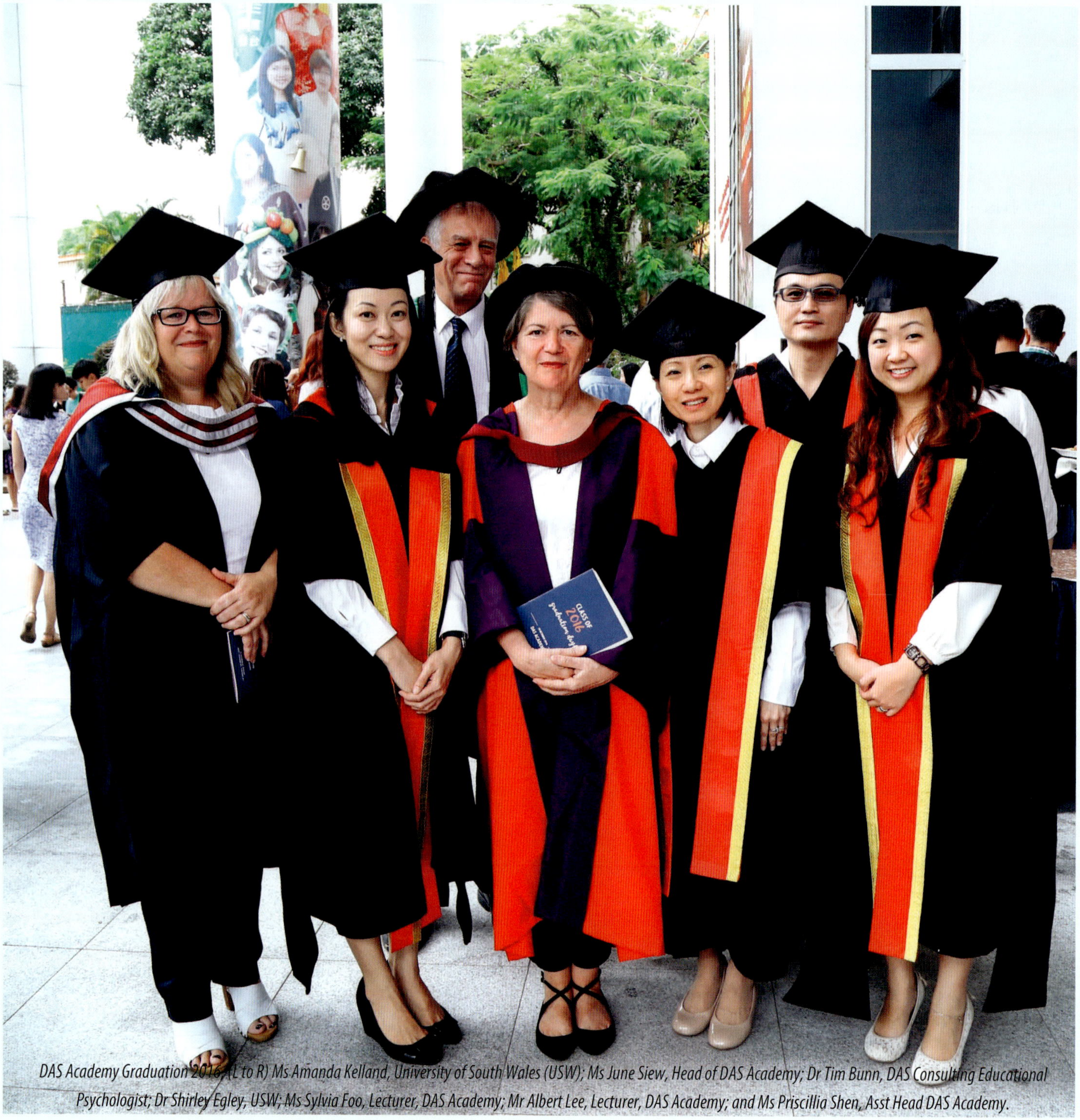

DAS Academy Graduation 2016: (L to R) Ms Amanda Kelland, University of South Wales (USW); Ms June Siew, Head of DAS Academy; Dr Tim Bunn, DAS Consulting Educational Psychologist; Dr Shirley Egley, USW; Ms Sylvia Foo, Lecturer, DAS Academy; Mr Albert Lee, Lecturer, DAS Academy; and Ms Priscillia Shen, Asst Head DAS Academy.

5

CATALYSTS AND MENTORS

Keep me away from the wisdom which does not cry, the philosophy which does not laugh and the greatness which does not bow before children.

Khalil Gibran

H.E.A.R.T.

Everything about the DAS faculty screams h.e.a.r.t. — holistic education and restorative therapy. From the early days—when there was only one teacher with 12 students—to the present cohort of over 3,500 MOE-aided DAS Literacy Programme (MAP) students, one thing has been consistent, DAS exists to help their students overcome dyslexia and be all that they can be.

The heartware is not just obvious from the caring professionalism of the teachers. DAS, as an organisation, also commits a large percentage of its budget to providing bursaries to those who need remediation but cannot afford to do so with their own financial resources.

DAS 25 Anniversary Logo designed by Matthew Tang, aged 12. Matthew described his logo design; "The logo is heart-shaped because it shows the love DAS has for dyslexic kids, patiently helping them, developing them, so that they can cope despite their learning difficulties."

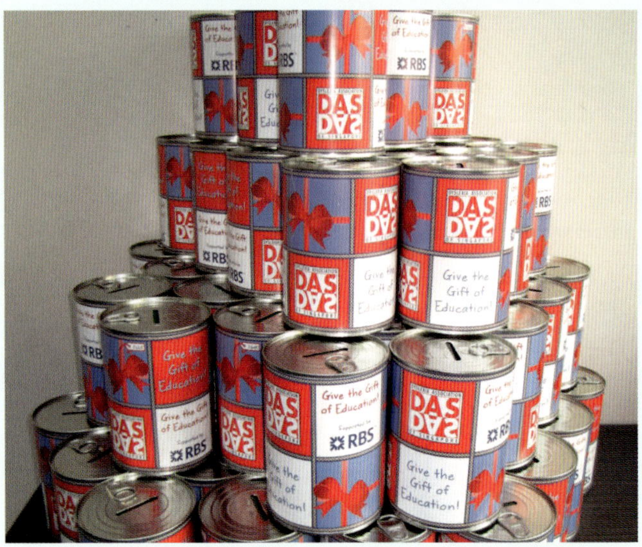

Fundraising at DAS helps to provide bursaries for low-income families.

DAS believes that no child should be left behind because he or she cannot afford the cost of DAS services.

WWW.DAS.ORG.SG/DONATE-TO-DAS

REMEDIATION AND RESOURCEFULNESS

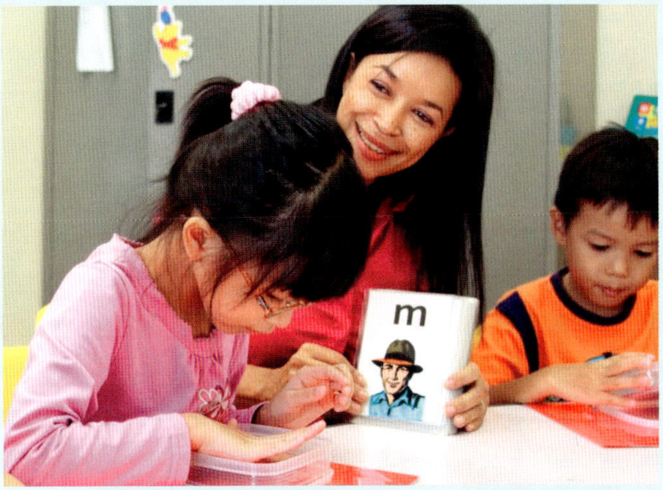

It has been very encouraging to see how MAP has adapted and morphed as DAS grew in its understanding of the varied profiles of its students. In its current iteration, the Integrated MAP Curriculum (IMC) ensures that students progress smoothly in a cumulative and sequential manner, building on their strengths while working on their weaknesses. By developing students into independent learners with the ability to function in a diversity of contexts, the IMC aims to enable students to cope with the curriculum demands they will encounter in school.

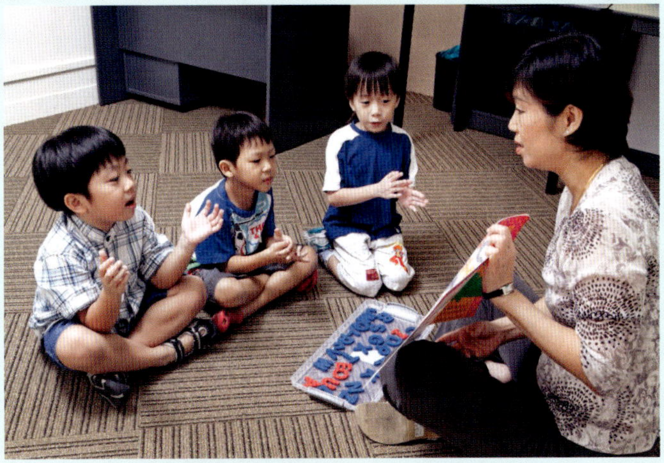

Another division of DAS, the Specialised Educational Services, looks into helping students unlock their potential in more specific areas — Early Intervention, Chinese Language, Mathematics, English Exam Skills, Specialist Tutoring, and Speech and Drama Arts. From the many personal stories that have been recounted by their students, it's clear to see that a sizeable number have been endowed with creative talents that far outstrip their "normal" counterparts in mainstream schools. Nurturing Specific Learning Differences (SpLD) students to overcome their specific weaknesses and to uncover their individual talents has been particularly rewarding.

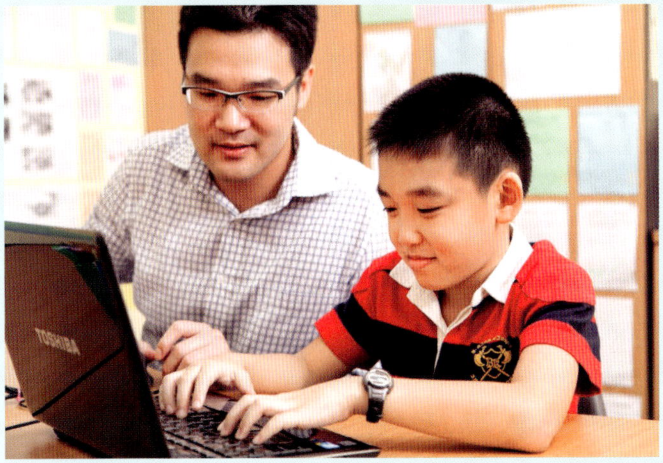

DEVELOPING A POOL OF EXPERTISE IN SPLD

The DAS Academy operates in this niche, but captive market. It is a key provider of Specific Learning Differences (SpLD) training in mainstream, international and specialist schools. Currently, the DAS Academy offers a wide range of courses. Practical workshops provide quick strategies, specialist diplomas provide a comprehensive blend of theory and practice, and academic postgraduate masters aim to transform seasoned practitioners into domain experts. For a decade, the DAS Academy has been tasked by the Ministry of Education to deliver the Diploma in Special Education (Dyslexia) to their Allied Educators. The Master of Arts in Special Educational Needs (MA SEN), offered by DAS Academy in collaboration with the University of South Wales, is a platform for seasoned educators to develop themselves as domain experts in this sector.

Through support from funding bodies, the DAS Academy strives to make its courses more accessible to community partners and stakeholders who will benefit from SpLD training. With course objectives and outcomes aligned to the core competency roadmap outlined by the Social Services Institute (SSI), some of its certificate courses have received support for funding. Voluntary Welfare Organisations (VWOs) working with clients with SpLD can also benefit from the DAS Academy's training by tapping on the VWO-Charities Capability Fund (VCF). This will enhance partnership between VWOs and create a collaborative approach towards caregiving. Additionally, the Caregivers Training Grant (CTG) administered by the Agency for Integrated Care (AIC) has made the DAS Academy's parent workshops more attainable for caregivers who need to build capabilities to better support their children with SpLD at home.

Led by a multi-disciplinary team that has extensive experience in providing direct support to people with SpLD, the lecturers are able to use their skills and expertise in the design and delivery of the programmes offered by the DAS Academy. These programmes provide an academic pathway in the field of SpLD from foundation to postgraduate levels.

Over the past few years, the DAS Academy has developed an academic structure that would be the pride of any university throughout the world. They have designed a rich programme of instruction, partnered with rigorous administrative procedures that ensure equity and reliability in their deliberations, overseen by an examinations board that monitors outcomes, led by Emeritus Professor Angela Fawcett, research advisor to the DAS. Angela supervised the Masters degrees of the key staff, Head of Academy, Ms June Siew, and Assistant Head of Academy, Ms Priscillia Shen, who both achieved outstanding results in their studies. The quality of their teaching is reflected in the solid achievements of their students.

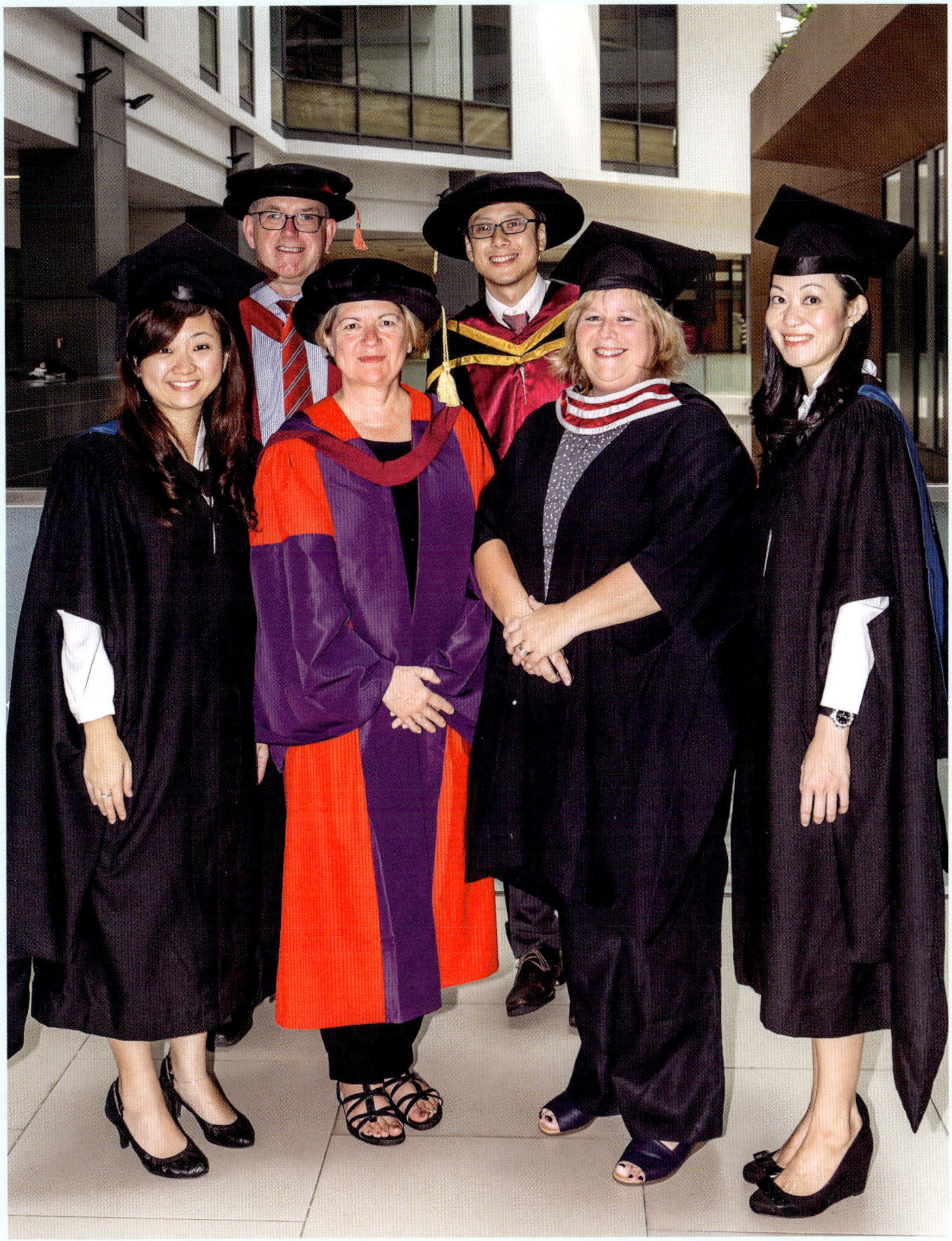

At the 2015 DAS Academy Graduation, (L to R) Ms Priscillia Shen, Asst. Head of DAS Academy; Dr Carl Peters, Deputy Dean, Faculty of Life Sciences and Education, University of South Wales (USW); Dr Shirley Egley, USW; Dr Oei Adam, Lecturer, DAS Academy; Ms Amanda Kelland, USW; and Ms June Siew, Head of DAS Academy.

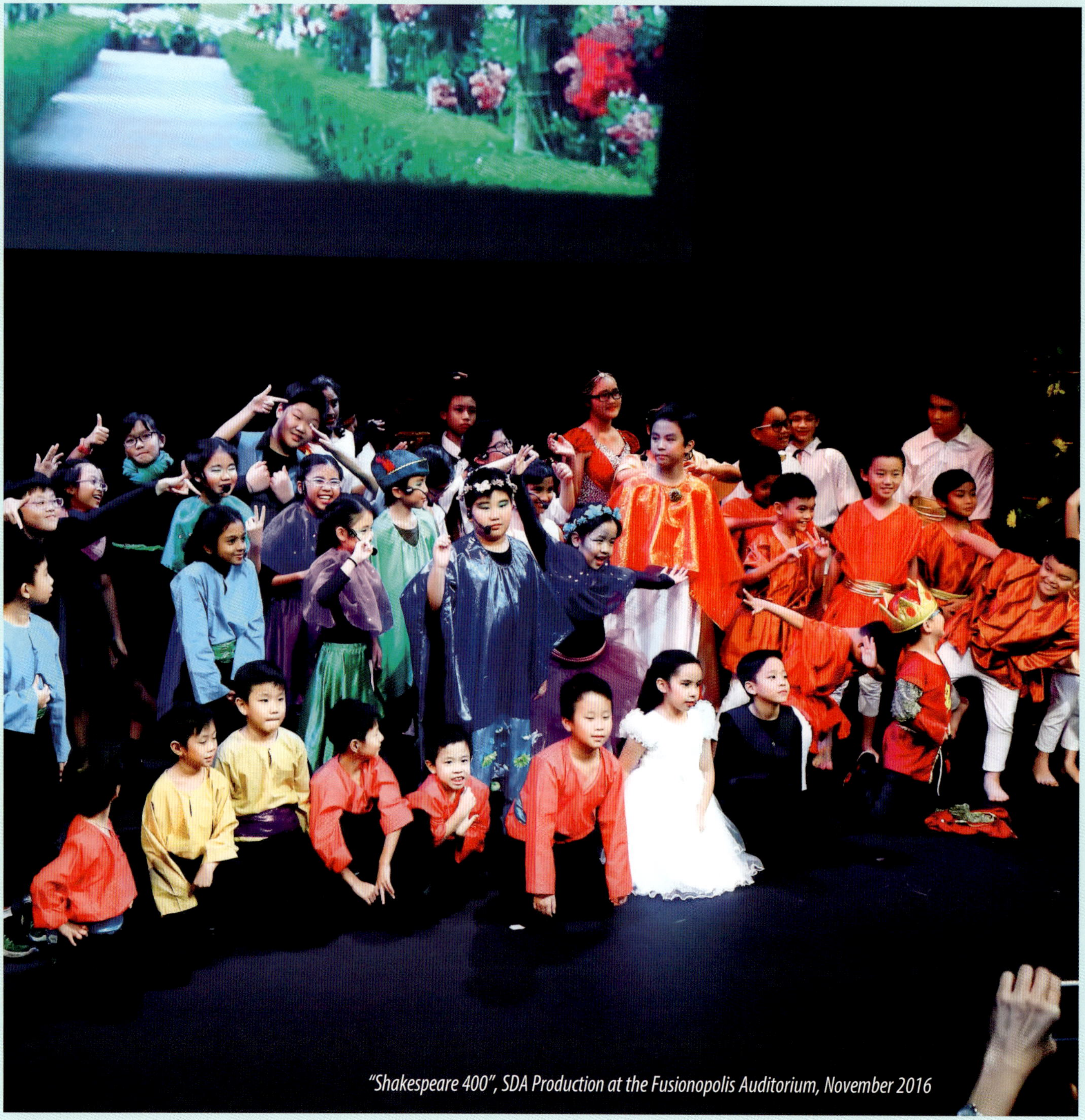

"Shakespeare 400", SDA Production at the Fusionopolis Auditorium, November 2016

SPEECH AND DRAMA ARTS PROGRAMME

SHAKESPEARE 400

The aim of the Speech and Drama Arts Programme is to develop literacy, communication and presentation skills, as well as boost the self-esteem of learners with dyslexia. Drama can be that powerful tool to help increase the confidence of students with learning differences. Using drama activities, students are given opportunities to enhance their persuasiveness and confidence in communication. The Speech and Drama Arts Programme also provides the opportunity for students to perform in a year-end production to showcase their skills.

In 2015, SDA staged a performance on Singapore's history with a cast of 35 students at the MDIS Auditorium in celebration of SG50. In 2016, 46 SDA students presented three Shakespeare play adaptions at the Fusionopolis Auditorium in front of a packed audience of friends and family.

Why Shakespeare? 2016 marked the 400th anniversary of his death and SDA wanted to celebrate the legacy of the world's greatest playwright. Many countries all over the world celebrate Shakespeare and we also wanted our students to appreciate his work, as well as give them the opportunity to be exposed to his plays at a young age, using performance-based methods. Shortened and simplified versions of several plays were introduced to the students via suitable drama activities to scaffold the stories. This has been highly beneficial to the students' understanding of the great poet and playwright's work.

The children performed adaptions of *Midsummer Night's Dream, The Merchant of Venice* and *King Lear*. Each play was a 40-minute presentation, giving SDA drama students a chance to be on stage.

Although it was an ambitious effort by the team, it would not have been possible without the support of the DAS Executive Committee and the General Management Team.

Presentations such as these require mammoth effort and encouragement from the entire DAS community. The SDA team, a group that is defined by its strength and dedication, worked tirelessly to make the production a success. The parents of students gave their full attention and dedication, as well, throughout the entire preparation period. Their support, and especially their trust, gave the SDA team the encouragement to take our students to new heights and it gave their children the confidence to shine on stage.

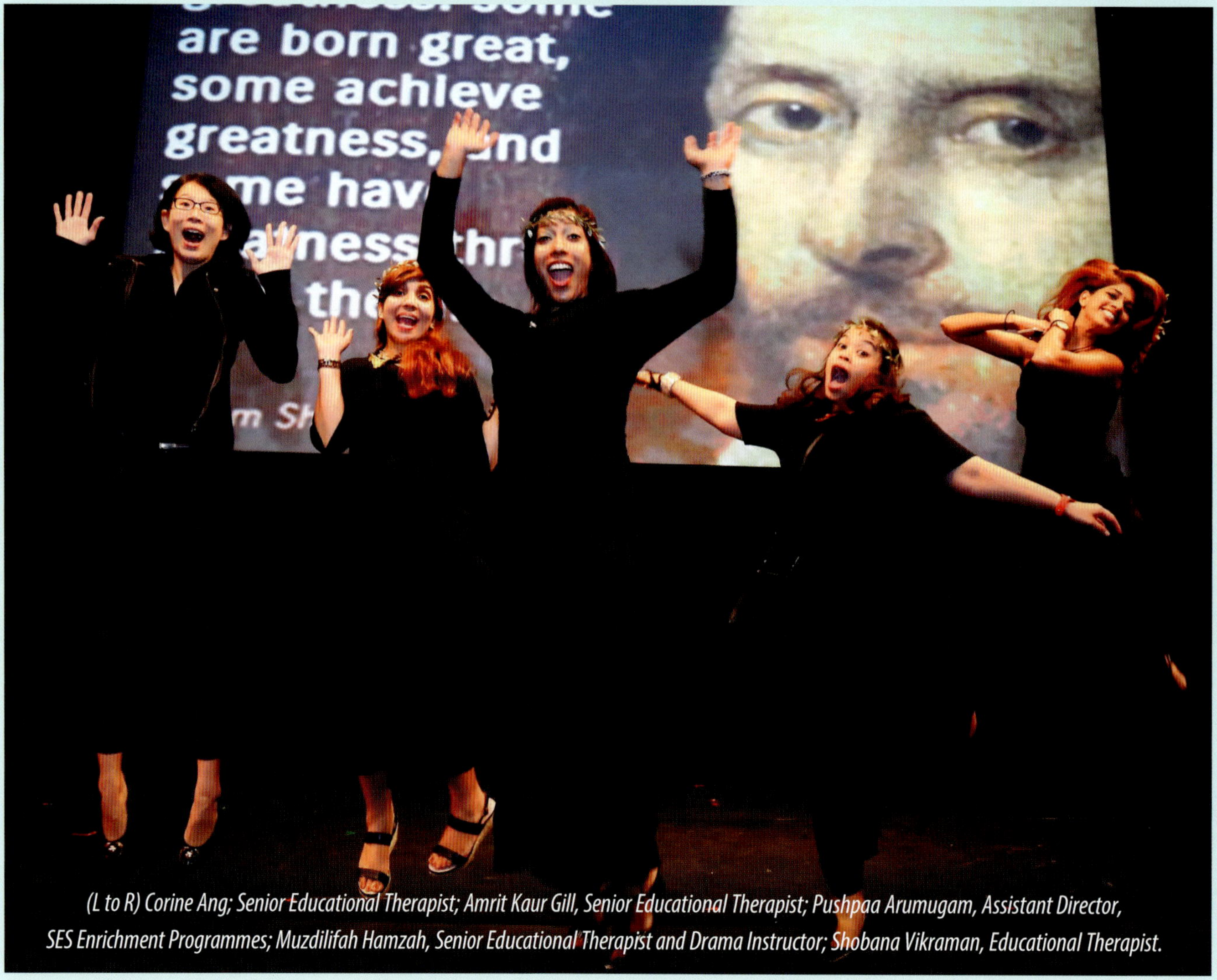

(L to R) Corine Ang; Senior Educational Therapist; Amrit Kaur Gill, Senior Educational Therapist; Pushpaa Arumugam, Assistant Director, SES Enrichment Programmes; Muzdilifah Hamzah, Senior Educational Therapist and Drama Instructor; Shobana Vikraman, Educational Therapist.

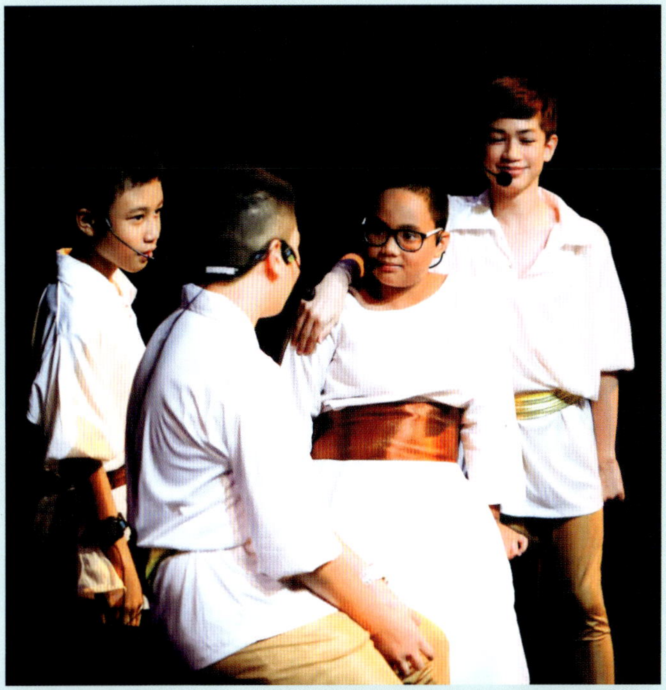

Our dearest students have worked extremely hard to display their hidden talents and potential each week, despite the challenges they are facing. Every student at DAS has the potential to reach greater heights with consistent hard work and immense effort like our 46 students in this Shakespeare production.

Ms Pushpaa Arumugam
Assistant Director of SES Enrichment Programmes

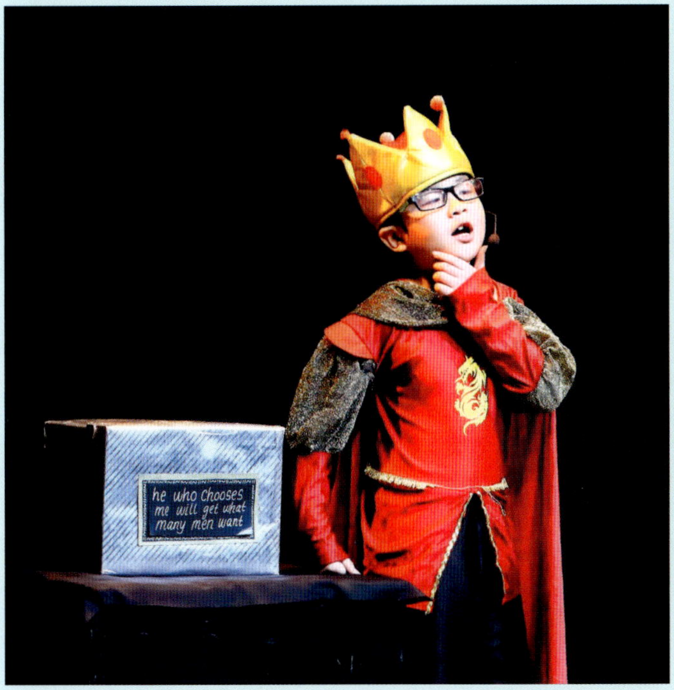
he who chooses
me will get what
many men want

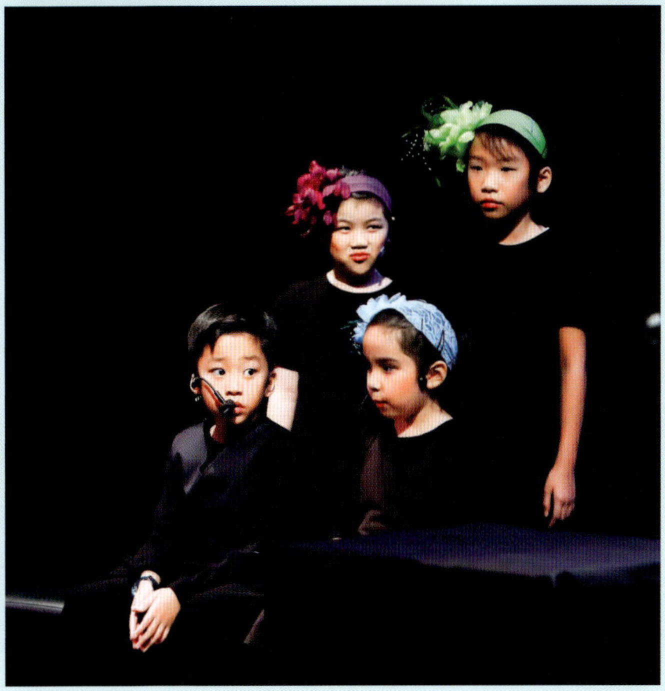

"Guiding the students through this amazing journey has indeed been incredible! The students have not only been dedicated to their role in the play but also motivated and selflessly helped each other during rehearsals. I am extremely pleased to have guided these amazing children!"

Ms Shobana Vikraman
Educational Therapist

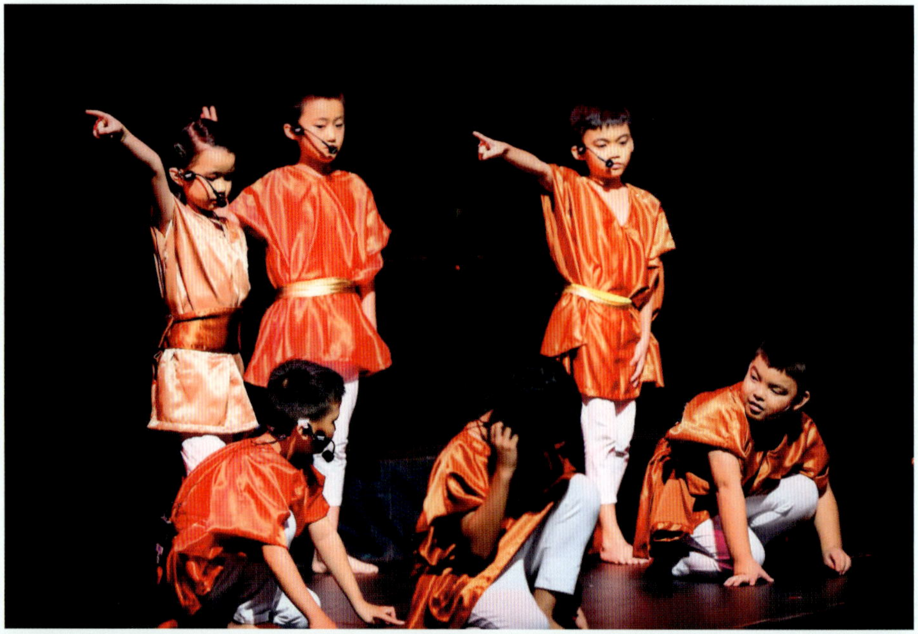

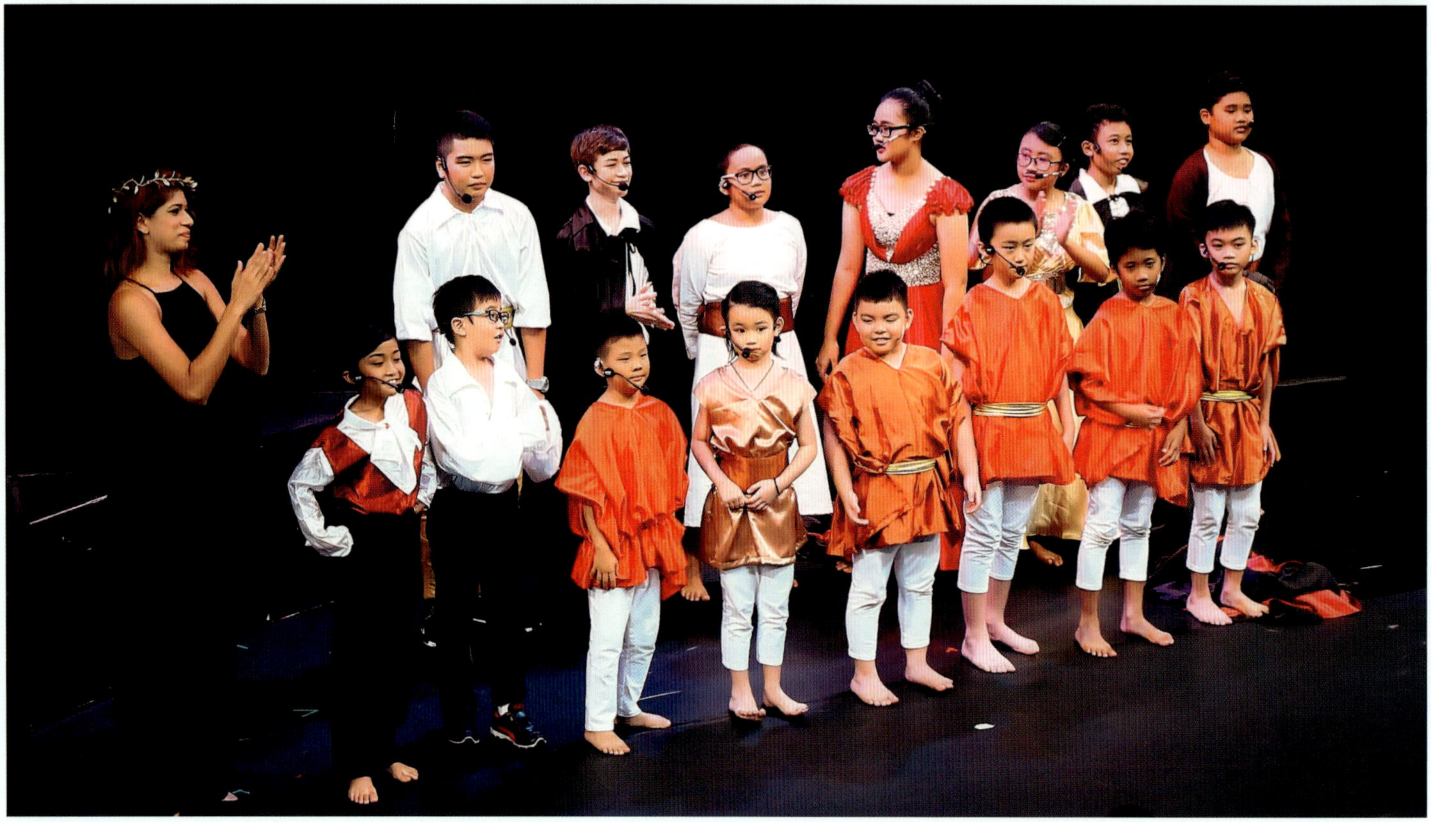

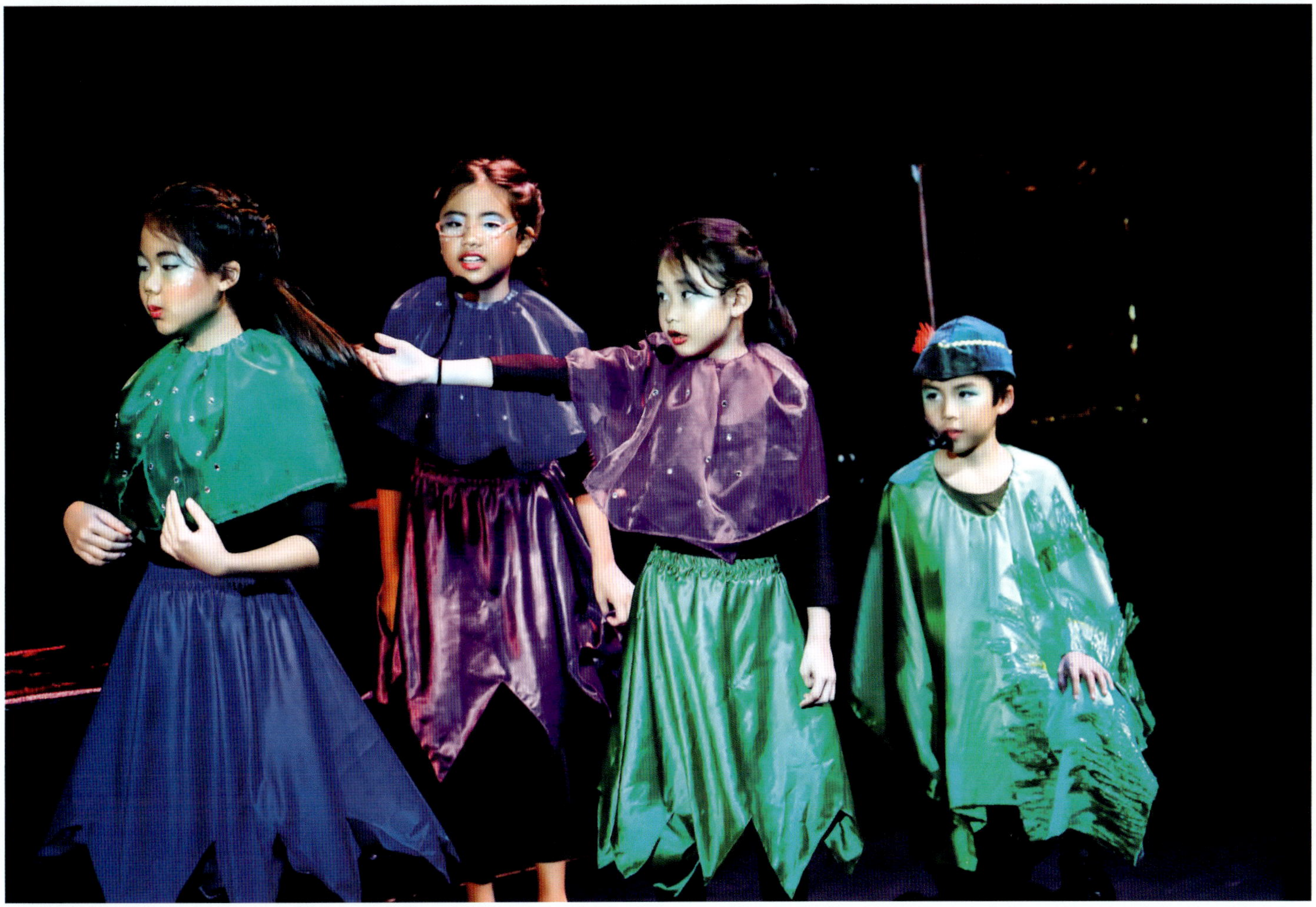

"I am truly amazed by the commitment shown by our students for this play to materialise. They accepted the responsibility of learning their lines and actions from the beginning and persevered throughout until the actual day of the performance. They were able to maintain a positive attitude when dealing with challenges and constantly looked out for each other during rehearsals. I hope this camaraderie builds their self-esteem and gives them a sense of achievement in this journey."

Ms Muzdalifah Hamzah

Senior Educational Therapist and Drama Teacher

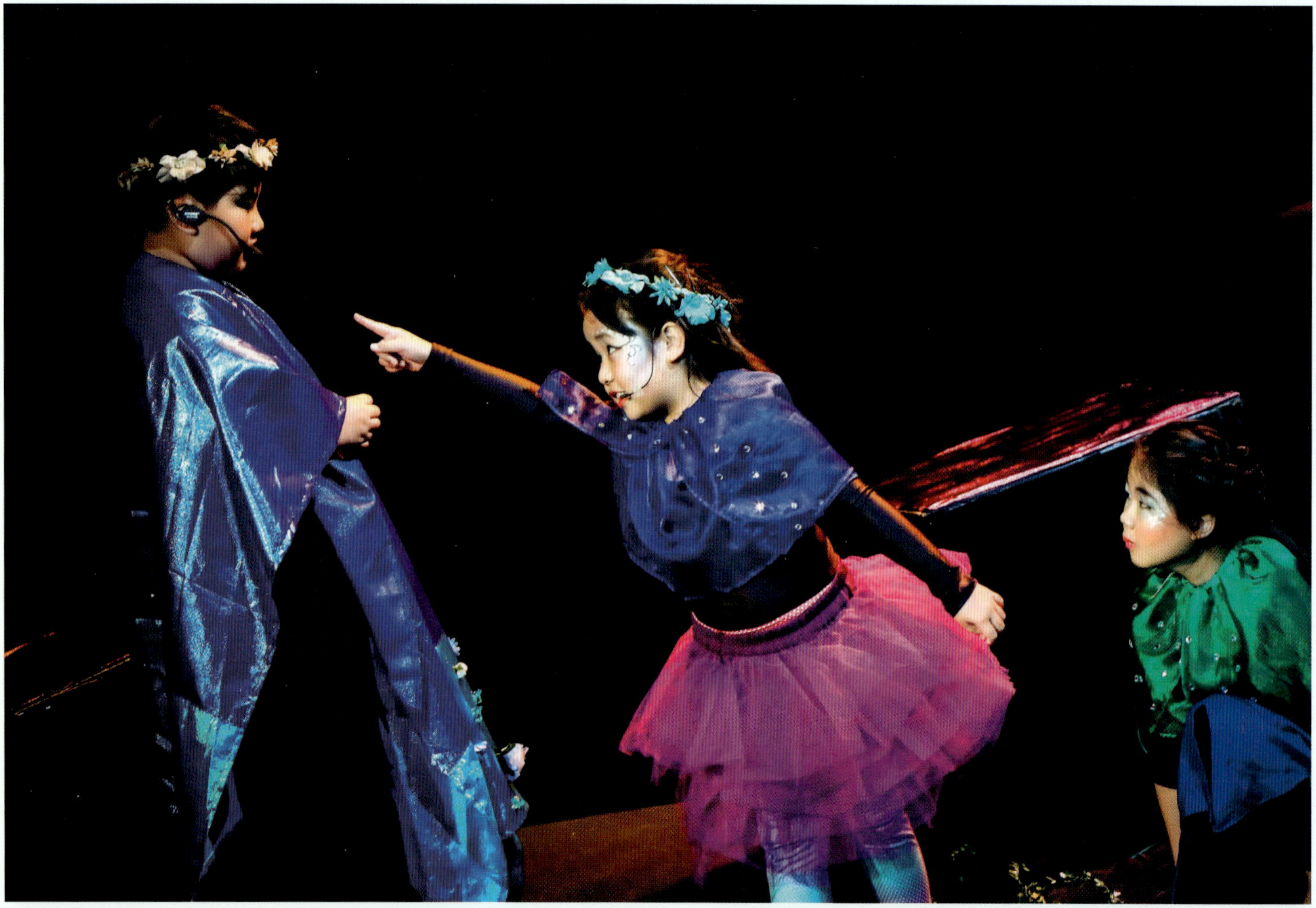

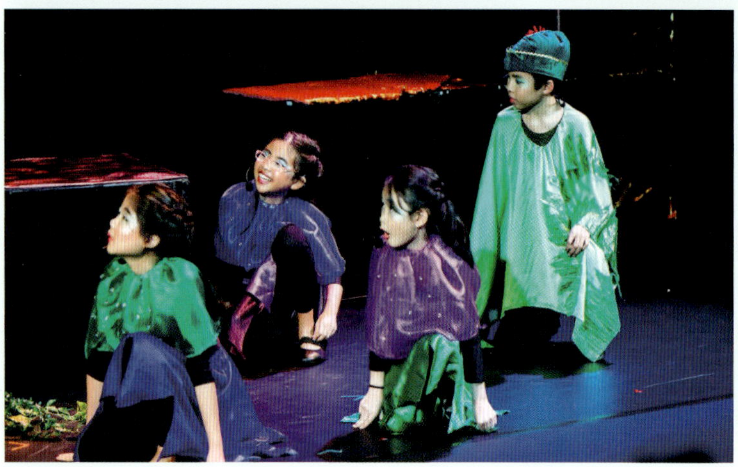

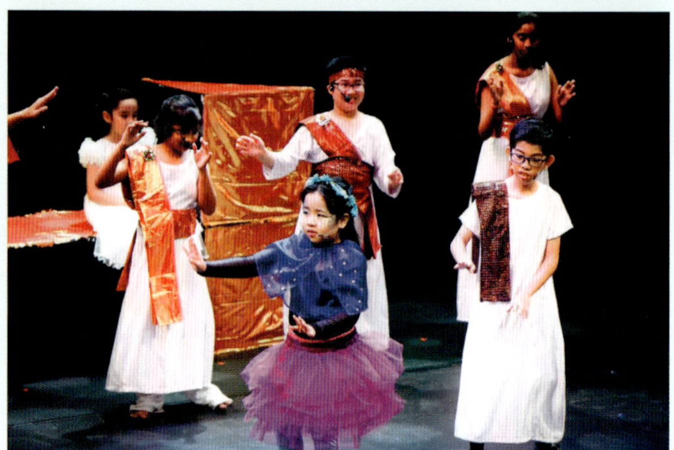

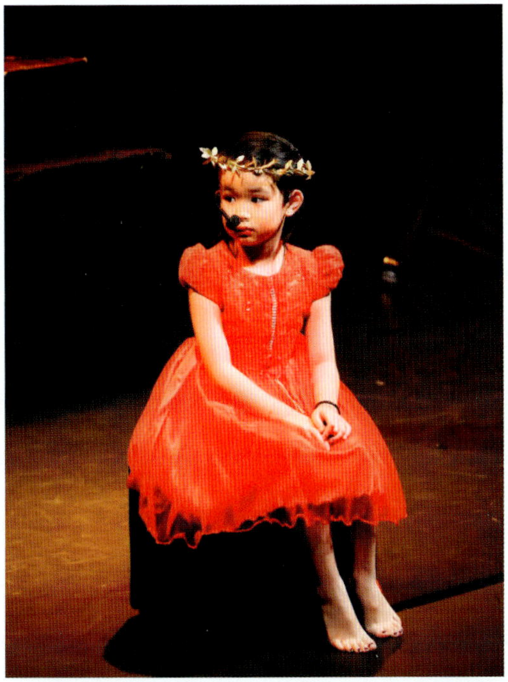

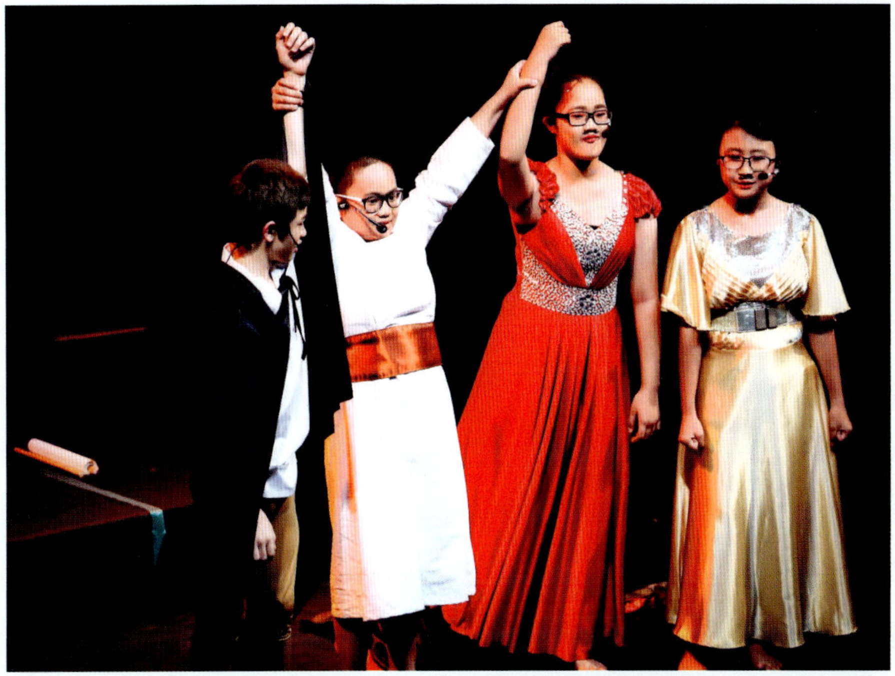

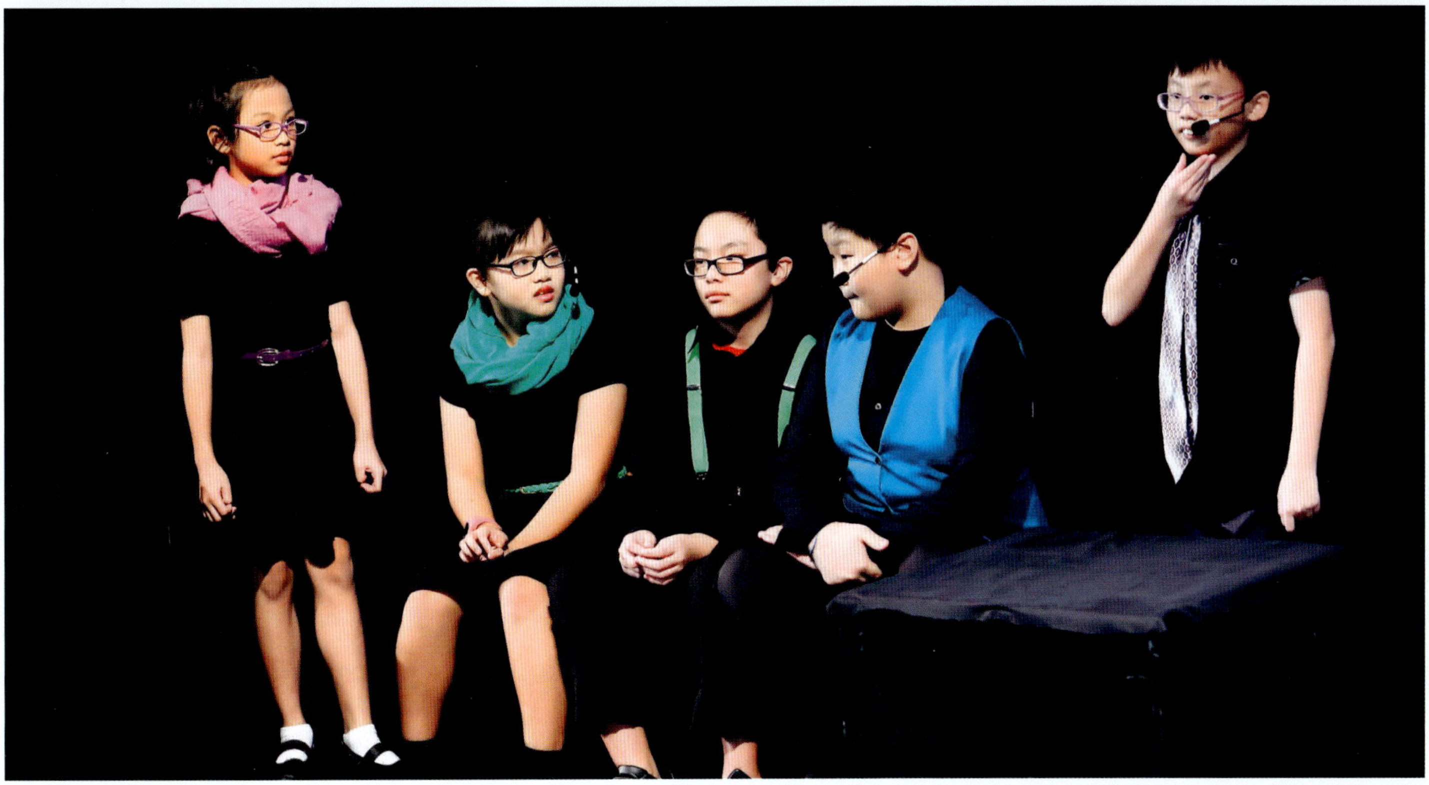

TURNING THE ORDINARY INTO THE EXTRAORDINARY

The ethos of an organisation, when well articulated, will permeate all that it does and unite its members. DAS's educators, psychologists, therapists, and administrators are totally sold on the organisation's mission of "Helping Dyslexic People Achieve". Many are at DAS because they feel their own experiences can inspire students to achieve their dreams.

"I've always been interested in teaching, and that's exactly what I've always been doing. Even when I was in school, I was giving tuition – teaching in one form or another. But although I planned on a career in teaching, things didn't go as planned. While it was easier to give up, and I certainly indulged in such thoughts for a while, I decided to pursue my Masters instead. The people around me, including my family and friends urged me on and I enrolled in NUS to pursue a Masters degree in Literary Studies.

I was about to graduate when I saw the DAS advert and realised that they provided teacher training - there was my chance to regain my dream. I started to read up to find out about dyslexia. And what struck me—and I vividly recall saying this during my job interview as well—was that I felt that I could relate with dyslexic children because of the setbacks I faced in pursuing my dream. I felt that I would be an empathetic teacher and channel that determination back into the classroom, by modelling the message to my students, "If you don't succeed now, don't give up because we can create opportunities for ourselves. So today, thirteen years later, I hope to continue to help our children to become self-advocates and to embrace their dyslexia and the strengths that come with it."

Ms Geetha Shantha Ram
Director of MOE-aided DAS Literacy Programme (MAP) and Staff Professional Development

"I was seeking career opportunities to work with children within the social services as I found the work there to be meaningful. I realised that I could actually relate quite well with kids and enjoyed working with them.

So when I saw the DAS ad offering a position as an educational therapist, I jumped at the opportunity. They offered training, quite comprehensive ones, and when I listened to the description of dyslexia, I felt that some of it mirrored my own learning journey. I could empathise with the struggles that dyslexics go through because I had faced similar struggles, particularly in the areas of focus and attention back in school.

On top of that, I could never understand how some my friends who seemingly didn't need to study were passing with A's while I needed to struggle to get the grade which I desired. I became curious and that curiosity blossomed into a commitment to find out what the ingredients of success were. I remembered thinking to myself that if I could find out what these ingredients were and turn it into a formula, I would be able to replicate the process and help other students succeed as well. That set me on a mission, a mission that I am still on today."

Mr Nor Ashraf Bin Samsudin
Director of Specialised Educational Services (SES)

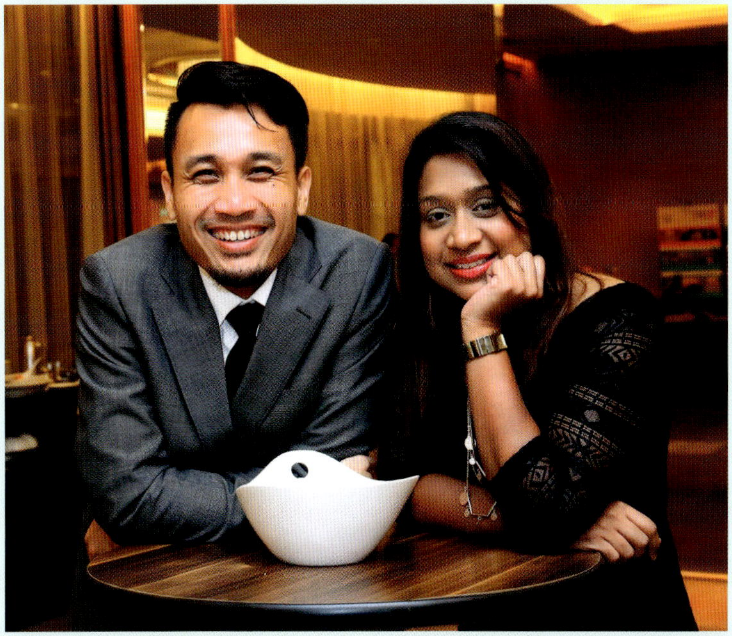

Mr Nor Ashraf Bin Samsudin and Ms Geetha Shantha Ram at the 25th Anniversary Dinner 2016

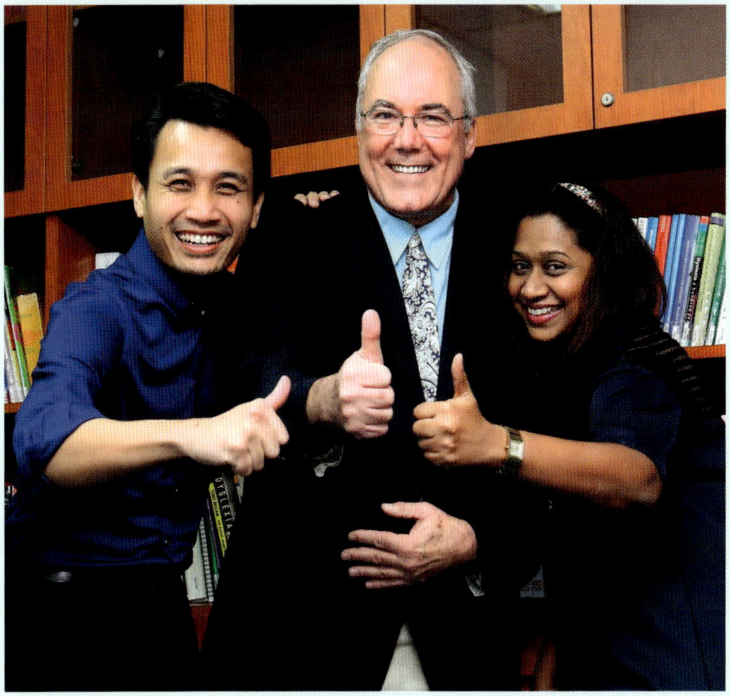

Mr Nor Ashraf Bin Samsudin, Dr Charles Haynes, and Ms Geetha Shantha Ram

RECEIVING AS MUCH AS THEY GIVE

While DAS acknowledges that their educators, psychologists and therapists have played and continue to play a key role in being catalysts and mentors to their young charges, it must also be said that the relationship is a two-way street. More often than not, even as they are giving to their students, the educators themselves are on the receiving end.

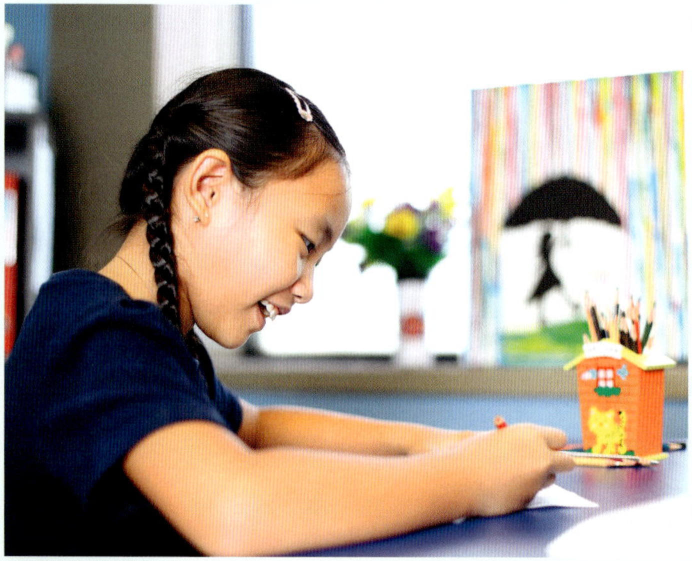

"I recall this one child I used to teach. she would fall sick exactly a week before any exam. It was like clockwork; she would fall sick, and she would have a high fever. The same child would be performing fine in my classroom but if you put her on the spot and asked her a question, which she wasn't confident in answering, she would start to cry. No warning. And as the teacher, you think about her just being nine years old and having to go through such emotional challenges everyday, but still she does it – goes to school, struggles to do what many of her classmates appear to have no difficulties doing and you realise the impact of her experiences. The strength and courage that child showed is something that I admire and think we could all learn from. As adults, we encounter a lot of difficult situations, and we complain and whine and cry. But the courage our students show, is a reminder that we just have to keep at it."

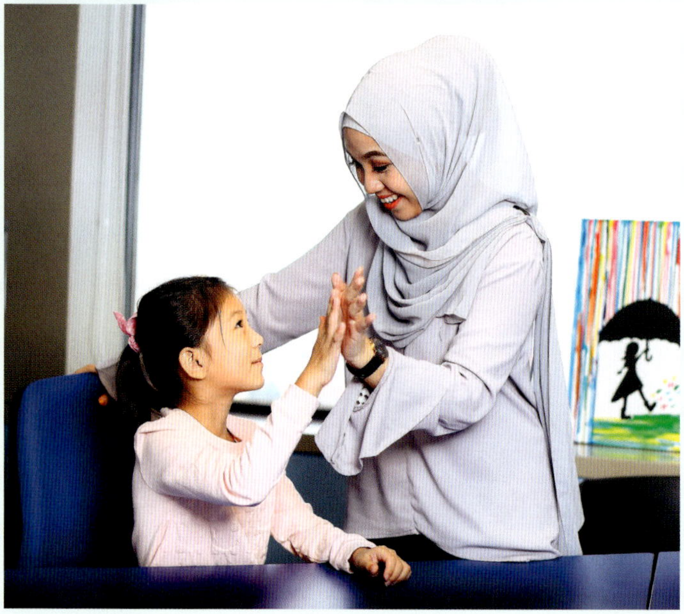

Ms Geetha Shantha Ram

KUDOS FROM PARENTS AND STUDENTS

What happens in DAS classrooms is "no state secret", as they often say. The educators apply sound teaching methodology to help their students overcome the challenges they face. What the onlooking public is less privy to, however, is the encouragement that the students give to their teachers. The DAS's litmus test for the learning experience in their classrooms is simply, "Will the students come running back for more?"

It is not uncommon for teachers to encounter scenarios like: "Student X was given medical leave, but he argued with his parents to send him for DAS classes."

And there is no greater joy than to receive positive feedback from both parents and students.

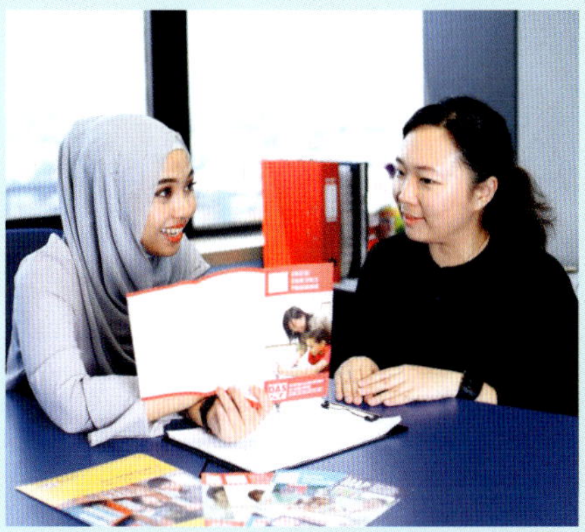

"My daughter's PSLE result is 239. She got A's for all 4 subjects. She said she promised to let you know."

"I am very happy that Ken passed his English for PSLE. He has never passed English before."

"Our son was awarded Best in Progress in English Language in his cohort at school. He would not have achieved this without the help from his teacher at DAS. We celebrate his humble success. Thank you."

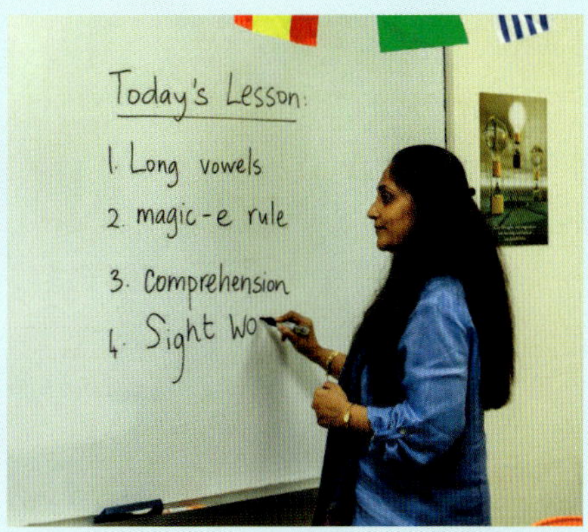
Today's Lesson:
1. Long vowels
2. magic-e rule
3. Comprehension
4. Sight Wo

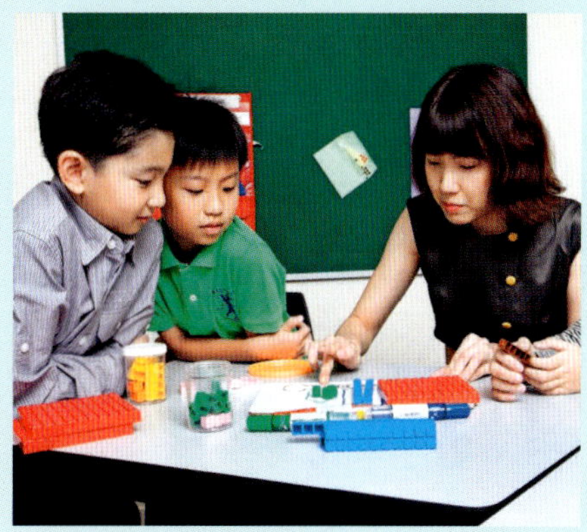

"Thank you very much for helping my daughter in her 1st and only year of Primary School Maths class tuition. She has never passed her maths before and I am very thankful for DAS to have maths tuition for a child like her."

"My child enjoys coming for classes and even though I wanted him to stop Chinese classes at the DAS, he wanted to continue. He is motivated to attend the Chinese class, is interested to learn Chinese, and now does his homework without reminders."

"Hello teacher. I got my PSLE results already. Thank you so much. I can get into Secondary School!"

"I am very happy that my son has passed his English for PSLE. He has never passed his English before!"

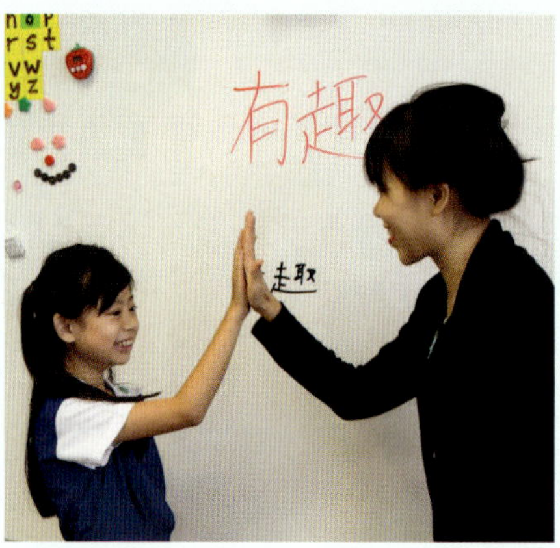

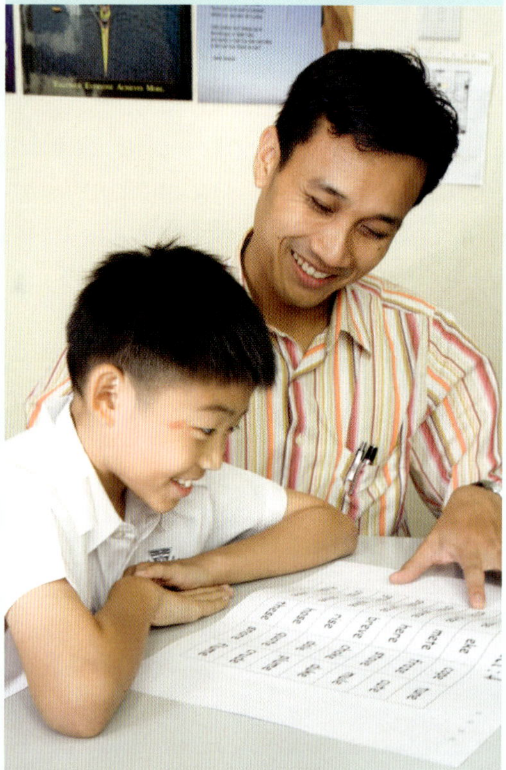

"I am impressed with my son's English Exam results, he has improved from a low C during his prelims to achieving a B in PSLE. His comprehension has shown great improvement. I hope he will continue to apply the skills throughout his learning journey, Thank you DAS!"

"I love DAS Maths because my teacher uses interesting and creative games for us to understand Maths better. She also helps me to improve my maths to a higher grade."

"Interestingly, since my son started your Drama programme, his school teacher noticed the positive change in his attitude; he is more cheerful and he is happy to learn. He has since improved extensively in his overall result this year and he will be receiving the Edusave Good Progress Award this year. Thank you very much for all the encouragement and positive notes given to him."

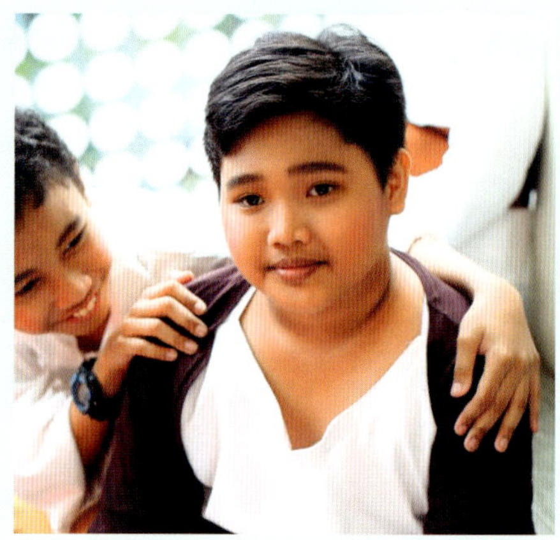

"Two mornings a week my daughter looks forward to coming to DAS for her specialist tutoring lessons. On these two days my daughter jumps out of bed and is joyfully ready to go. As a matter of fact, I would say she is impatient for these classes. She walks out of them feeling confident in herself and her abilities to be successful at her school. Boosting her self-esteem is not a small feat either since she just cannot seem to catch up with her peers at school.

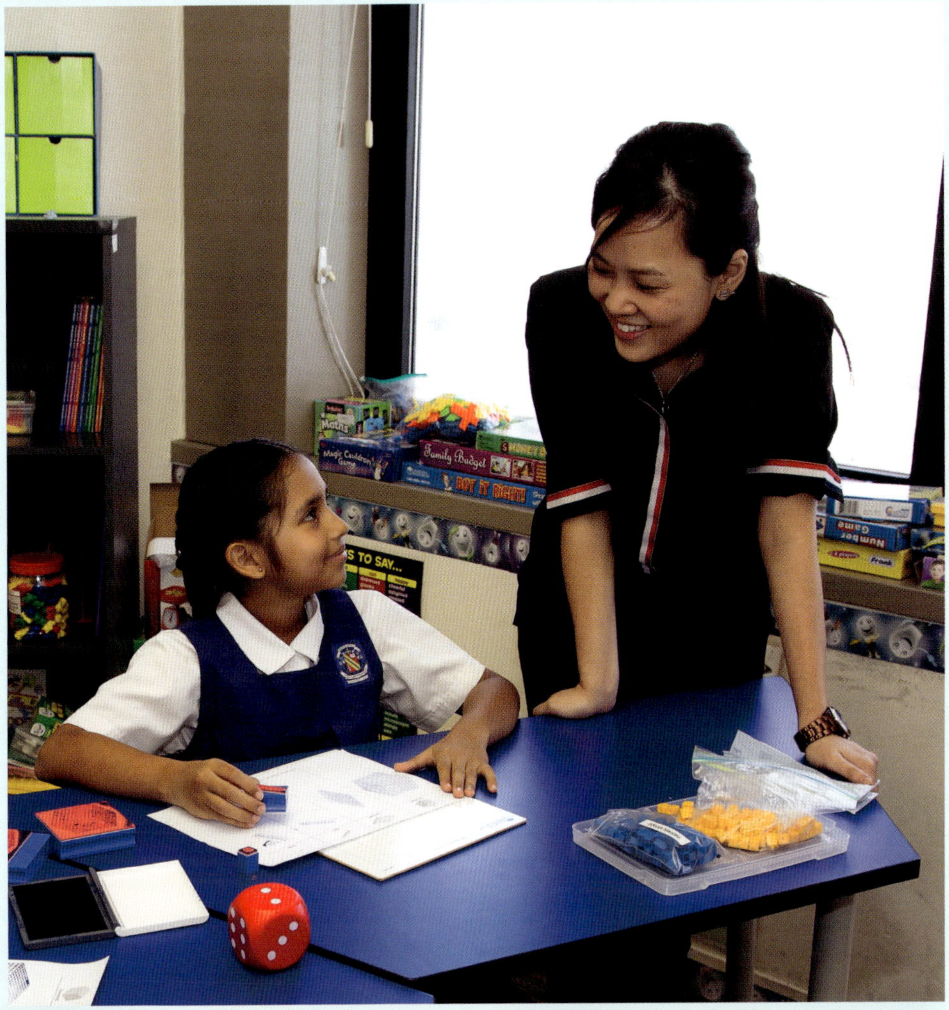

I felt utter despair for her academic future, even though there are countless numbers of successful dyslexics. The despair came from the fact that I did not know how to help her or even where to begin finding help. Now my initial panic has subsided and it has been replaced with hope. If my daughter was lucky enough to find one excellent teacher, then maybe she will find more along her academic journey."

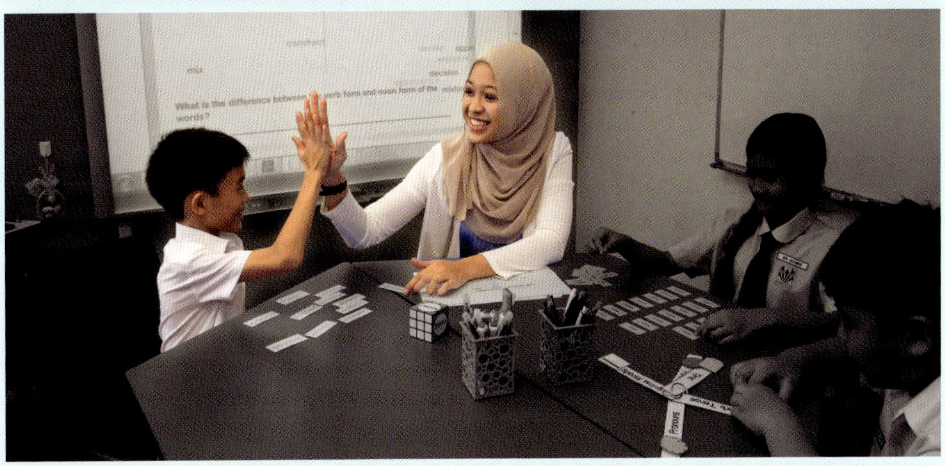

STUDENT GRADUATION AND AWARDS CEREMONY

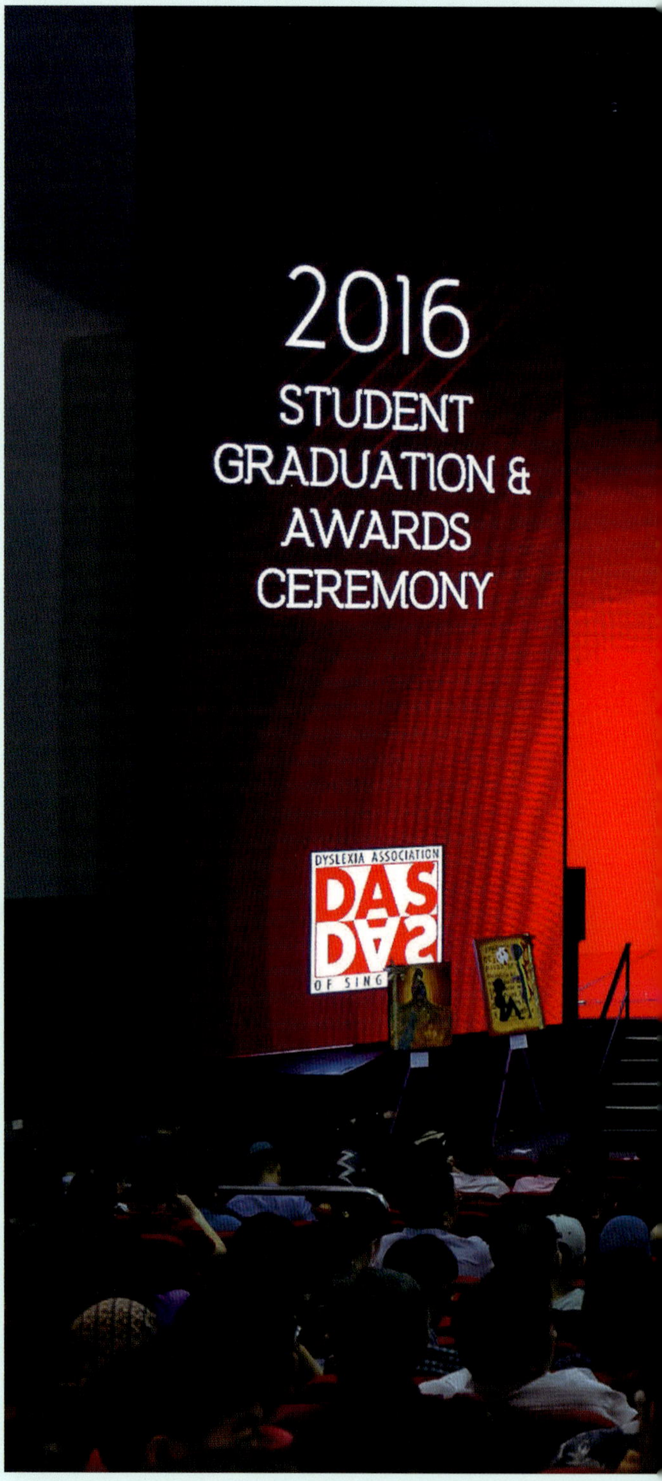

The annual DAS Student Graduation and Awards Ceremony is a celebration. It highlights the successes and achievements of DAS's students not only in their academic performance but also their strength and resilience to improve and overcome their learning difference.

The graduation held in DAS's 25th Anniversary year was the largest to date with 216 graduating students from the MOE-aided DAS Literacy Programme (MAP) having attained a competency in literacy that will facilitate their success in school and their overall learning journey. Together with the graduating students, other students received the DAS Special Achievement Awards. These were the ones who had demonstrated exceptionally high levels of commitment and determination in their pursuit of success in Sport, Arts or simply All Round Excellence.

At Student Graduation, DAS also celebrated the success and achievements of their alumni; past students who have continued to excel. The hope is that these outstanding young people will be an inspiration and role-models to the current students.

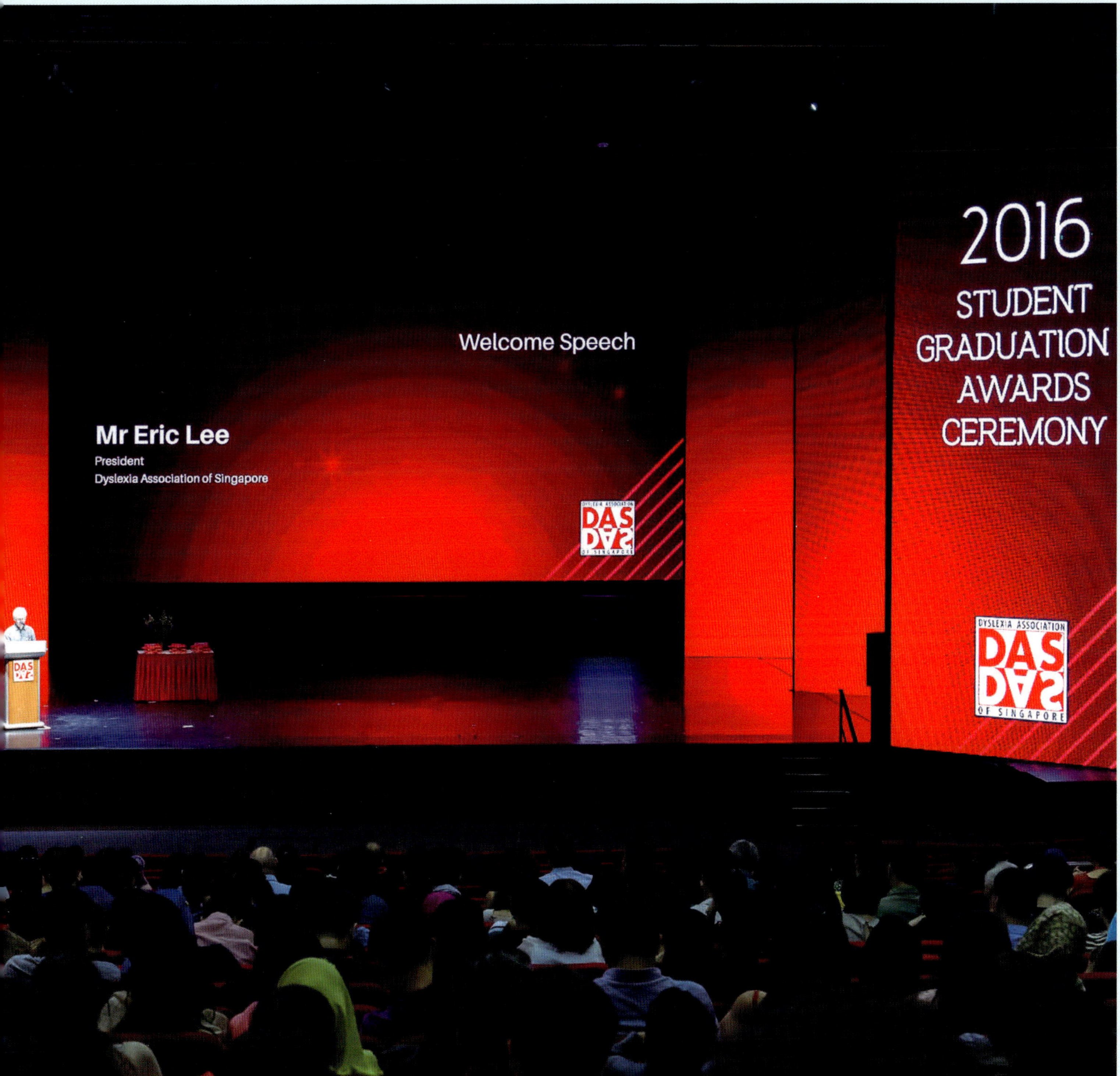
Welcome Speech
Mr Eric Lee
President
Dyslexia Association of Singapore
2016
STUDENT
GRADUATION
AWARDS
CEREMONY
DYSLEXIA ASSOCIATION
DAS
OF SINGAPORE

Graduation also sees the presentation of awards to students who have made outstanding progress while on programmes delivered by the DAS Specialised Educational Services (SES) division. SES saw its enrolment cross 1,100 students in 2016.

This was led by the Preschool and Maths programmes with almost 300 student each. The English Exam Skills and Chinese programmes also saw enrolment of more than 100 students. This is an indication of the varied challenges children with dyslexia face across age groups, languages and school subjects and the importance of providing a wide range of programmes for them.

While the achievements of the students are applauded, there was also an acknowledgement of the DAS Educational Therapists (EdT) who work ceaselessly in support of their students. As part of the ceremony, the MAP EdT of the Year Award was presented to acknowledge the incredible work EdTs do in the classrooms. In 2016, three DAS EdTs received this award; Mr Roslan Sa'ad, Ms Phoebe Goh Huimei and Ms Winnie Wee Poh Hua.

The MOE-aided DAS Literacy Programme now has an enrolment of almost 3,100 primary and secondary school students. MAP compliments the Ministry of Education's School Dyslexia Remediation Programme which is now available in all primary schools. These developments reflect the significant number of school-age children whom DAS still needs to identify and help. The corresponding need for more

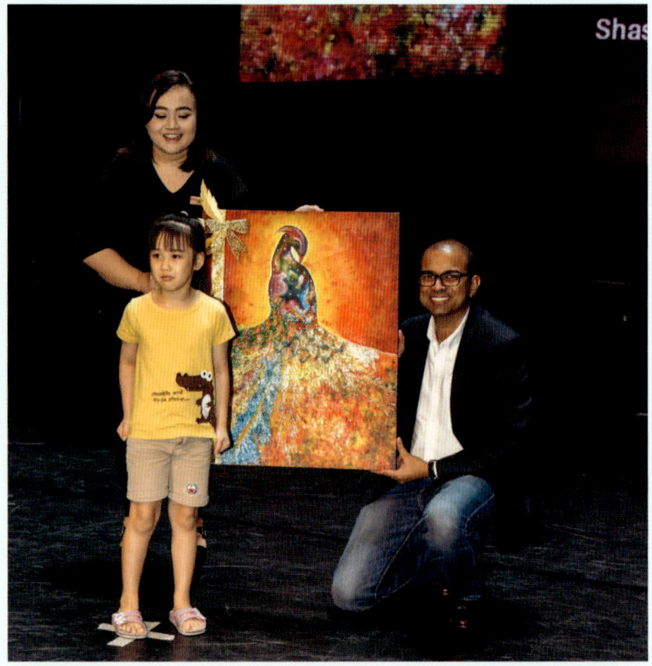

Artwork by DAS Students are presented to Dr Janil Puthucheary, Minister of State, Ministry of Education, and Mrs Goh Chok Tong, DAS Patron.

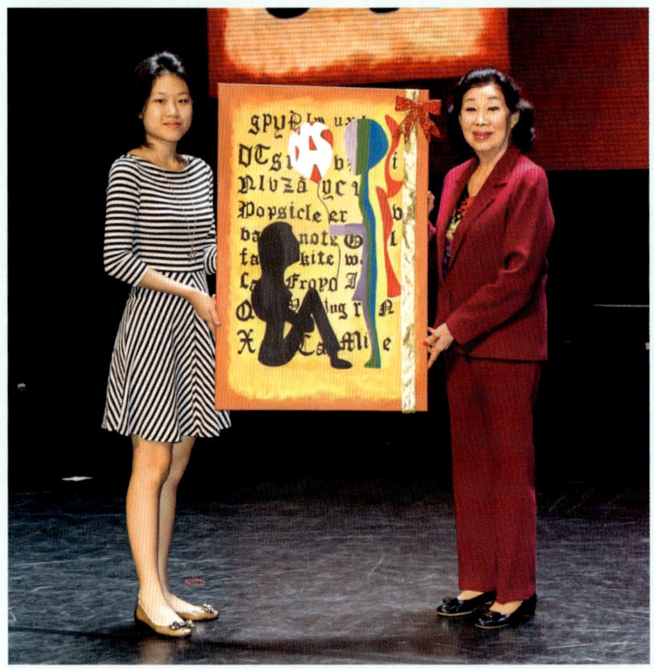

dedicated and well-trained EdTs is also paramount.

The event was graced by DAS Patron, Mrs Goh Chok Tong, who presented the MAP EdT Award of the Year. The Guest of Honour was Dr Janil Puthucheary, Minister of State, Ministry of Education, who in his speech on the day paid tribute to all the graduating students and to the founding DAS President, Dr Jimmy Daruwalla. He said, "I had the pleasure of meeting Dr Daruwalla and was touched by his concern for children with dyslexia and commitment to expanding and improving the work of DAS. He championed the cause of dyslexia and sought to create awareness about the condition. Dr Daruwalla's passion to provide the best possible support for students with dyslexia has resulted in the growth of DAS into the organisation we see today. For his dedication and contributions to dyslexic children of Singapore, Dr Daruwalla was awarded the *Tabla!* Community Champion award in 2011. His contributions to the dyslexia community in Singapore will be acknowledged and I am sure DAS will continue his legacy by bringing its programmes and services to the next level."

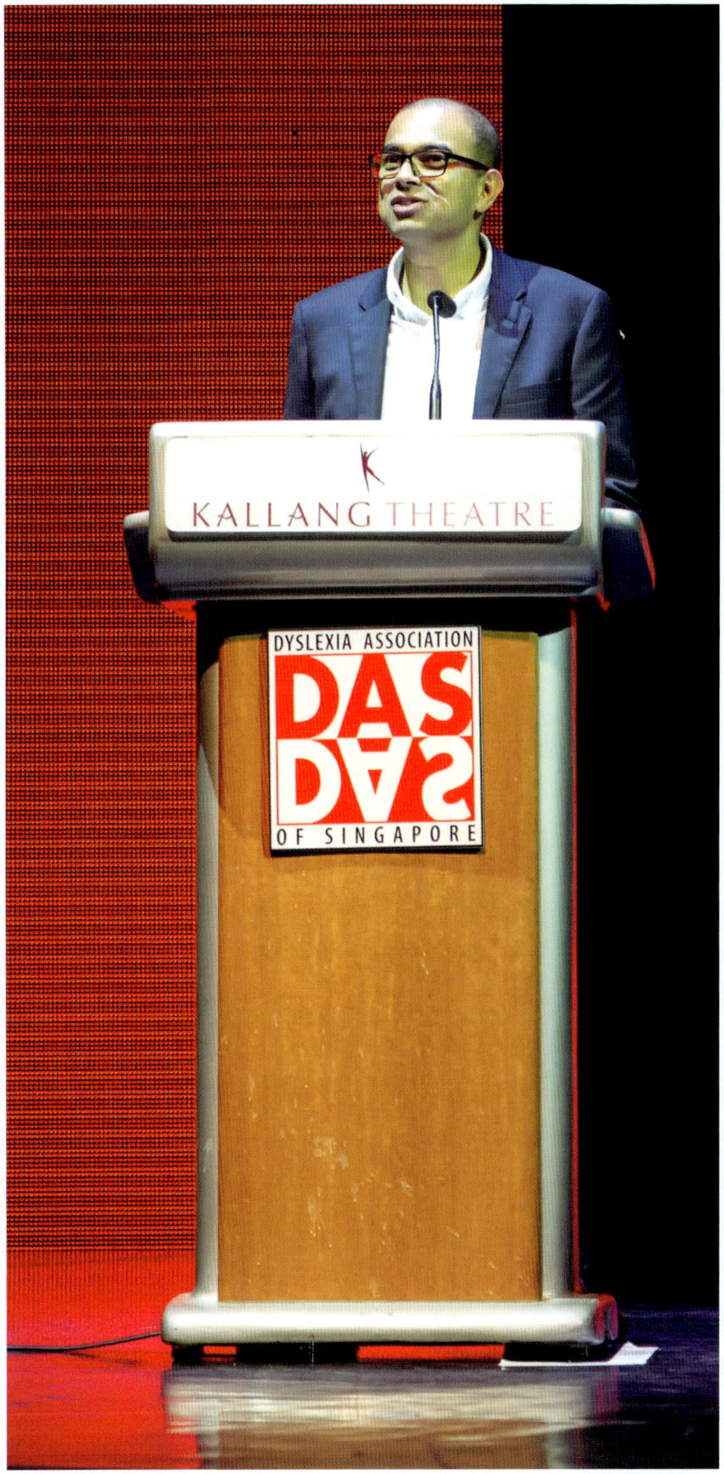

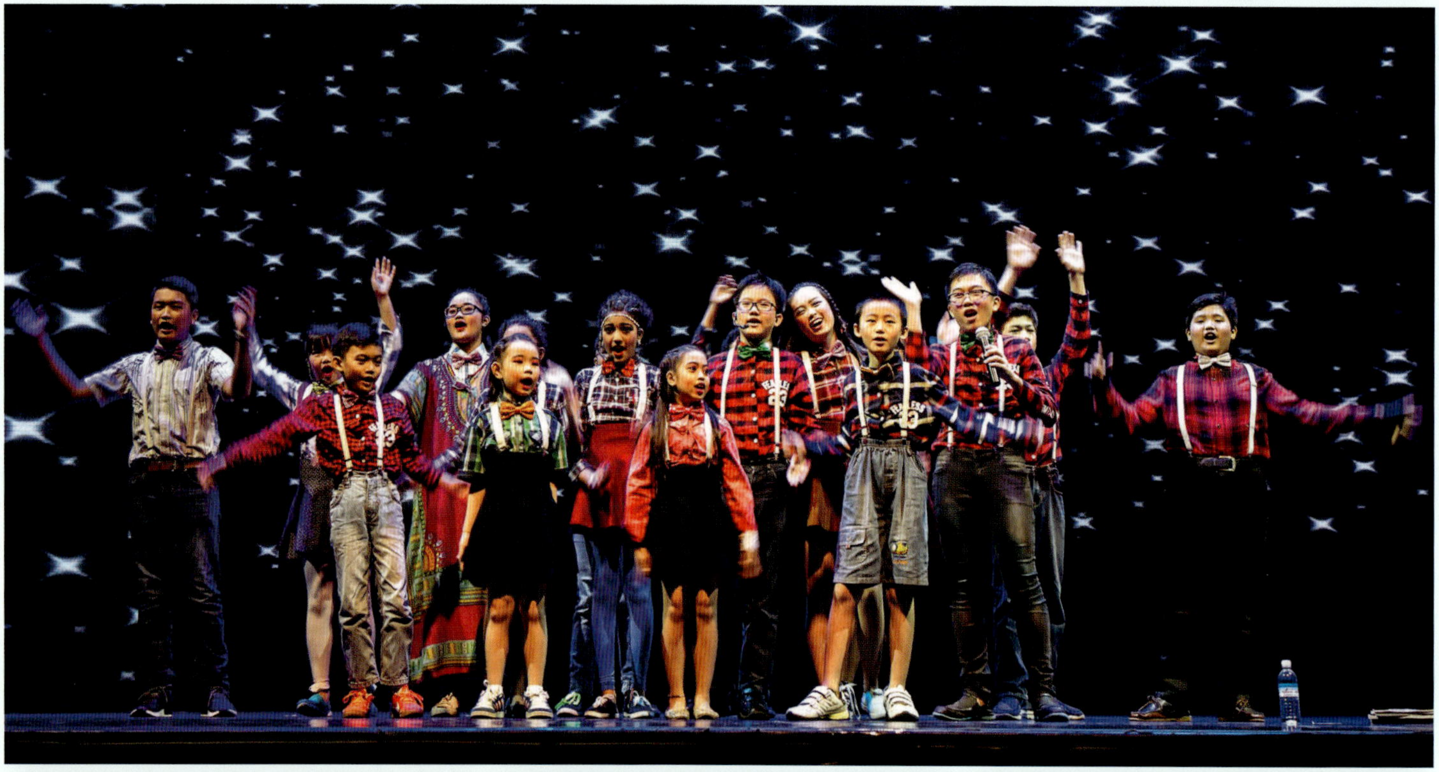

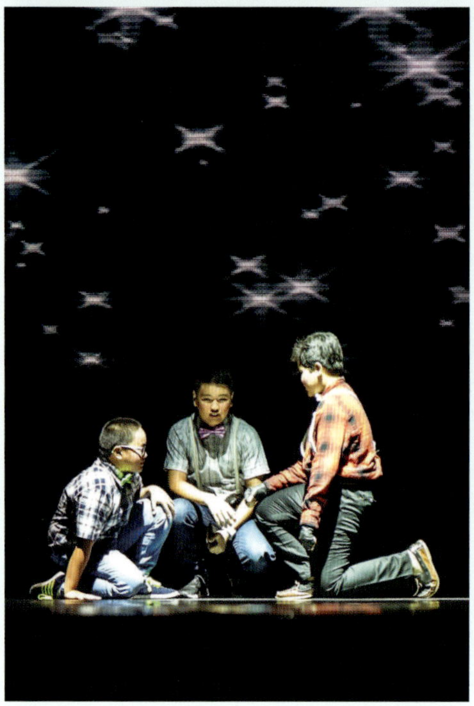

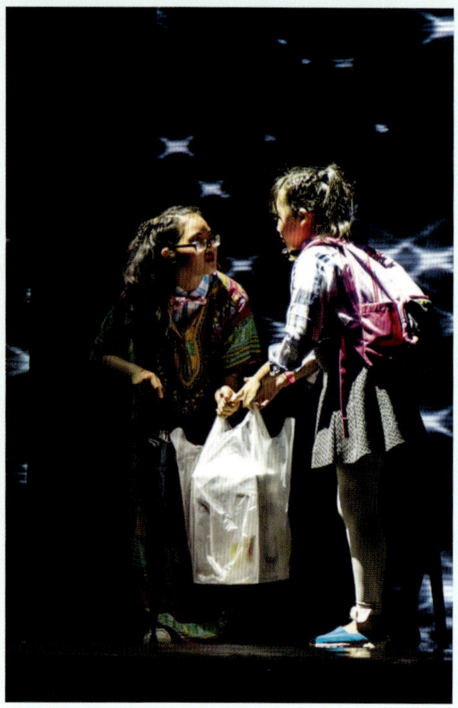

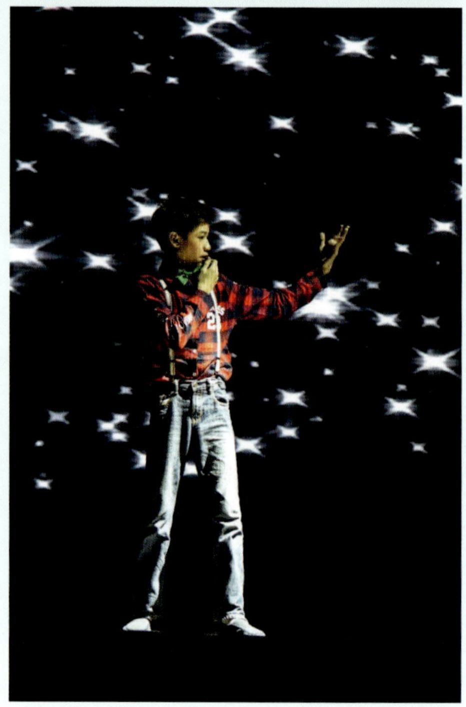

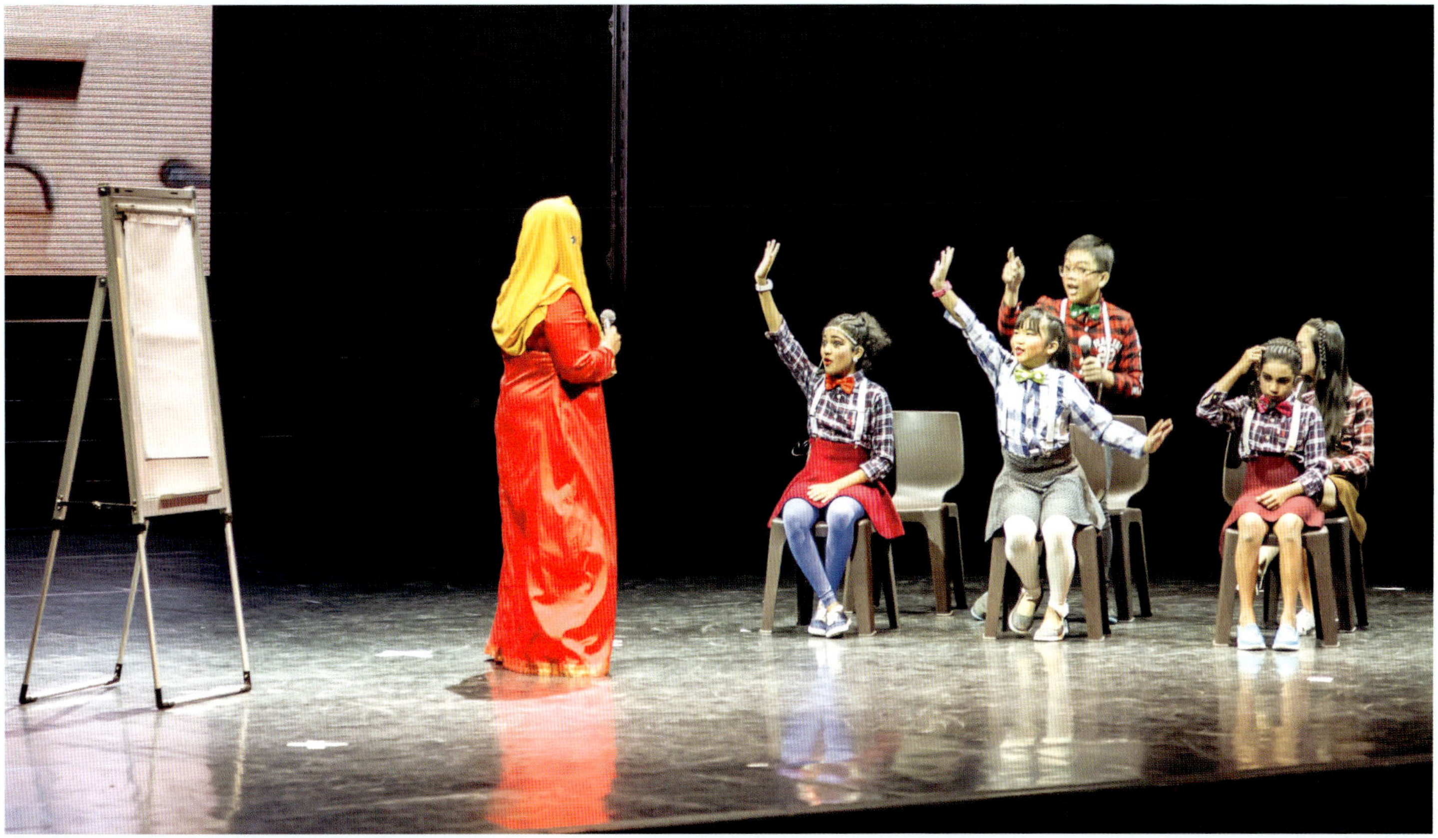

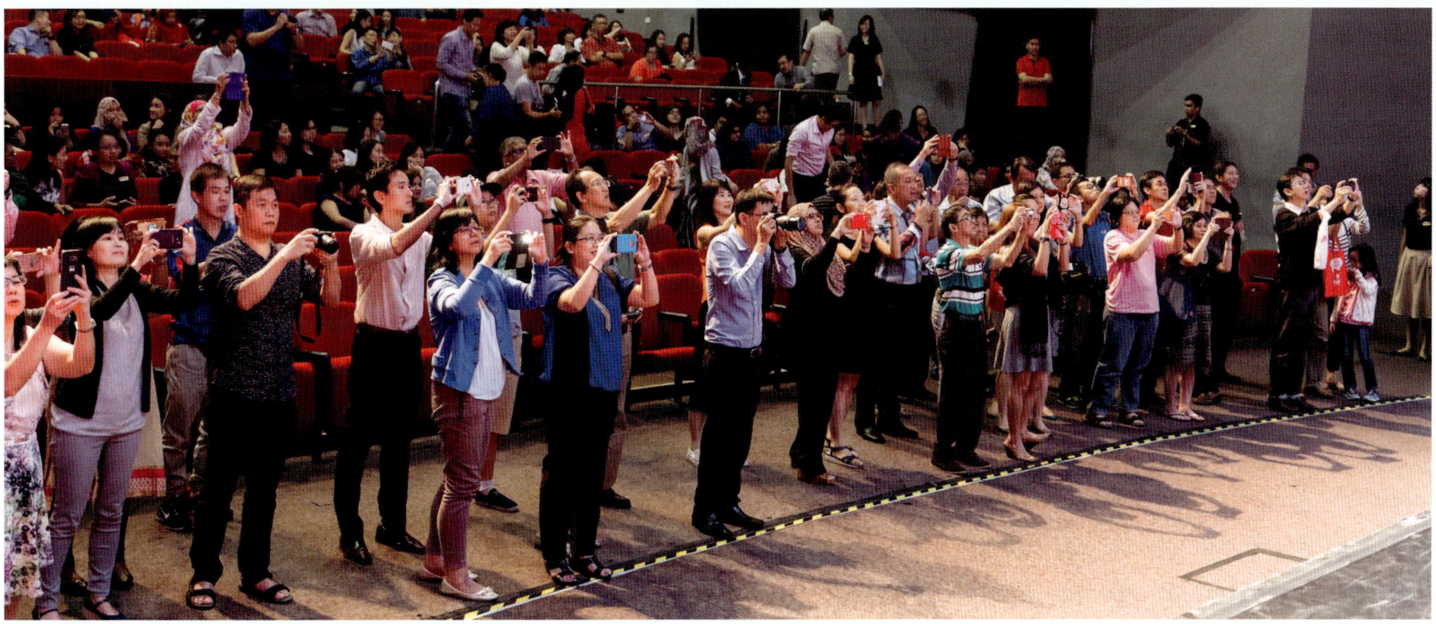

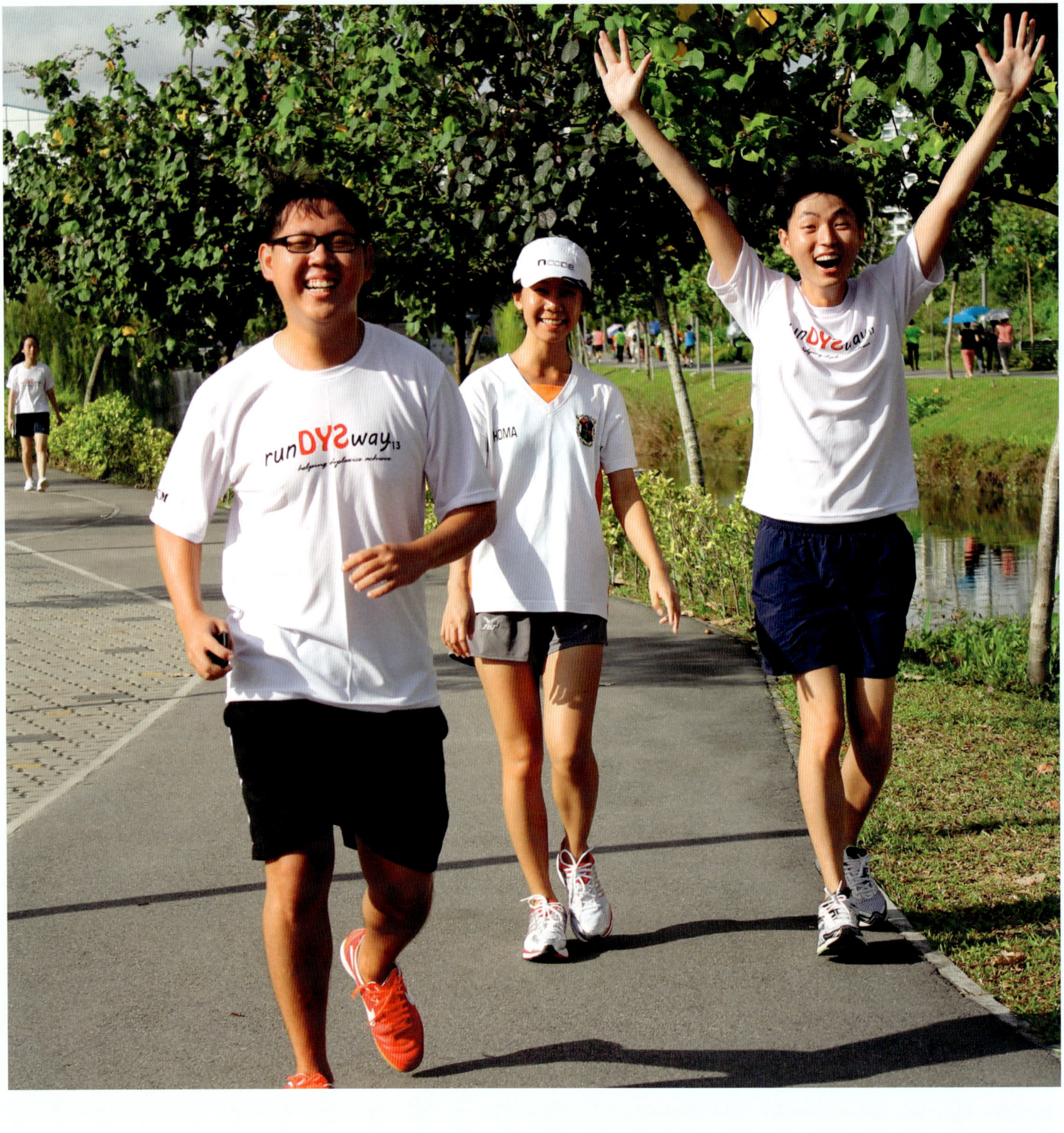
runDYSway'13

6

SIGNIFICANT OTHERS IN THE MAINSTREAM SCHOOLS

A single act of kindness throws out roots in all directions, and the roots spring up and make new trees.

Amelia Earhart

AWARENESS AND OUTREACH

In the 25 years that DAS has been in existence, it has achieved much in helping those who fall within the dyslexic spectrum. Because remediation for those struggling with learning differences has been so urgent, the priority has naturally been given to helping the dyslexic community.

Perhaps, the time has now come to look beyond DAS's immediate sphere of influence to provide more public education. While directly helping dyslexics continues to be the focus, educating the general public will enhance the benefits for both dyslexics and the wider society in the longer term.

It has been encouraging to see reports in the newspapers about achievements by dyslexic students who have surmounted the odds to do well in their studies. This has fleshed out the challenges that are faced by dyslexics and has gone some way to helping the general public understand and appreciate what dyslexics go through. DAS CEO Mr Lee Siang has, through his letters to the press, continued to keep dyslexia in the public eye. That both mainstream media and social media have reported on dyslexia and DAS extensively reflects the media's acknowledgment that there is an important story worth telling about people with dyslexia.

In 2015, DAS also conducted more than 60 activities which have helped to increase awareness of the needs and strengths of people with dyslexia. These efforts have included awareness talks in schools, free mass computerised screenings, and open-house events. Every year, letters are sent out to all schools to offer awareness talks, with an average of at least 60 schools taking up the offer.

TEACHERS WHO CARE

According to figures from the Ministry of Education, there were 18,000 students with special needs in mainstream schools in 2015, compared with 11,000 in 2012. It has been a slow and hard road, but DAS has doggedly done its part on behalf of dyslexic students these past 25 years, to be their advocate in an education system whose focus on meritocracy and achievement has seen many fall by the wayside for lack of a helping hand. The higher rate of identification in schools today is the result of the inclusive approach of MOE towards students with special needs.

It is heartening for DAS that its labour is not in vain. In March 2016, for instance, Mrs Chitra Devi Guna alerted her student's family to the fact that he was severely dyslexic. Sri John Albert David was already in Primary 6 and preparing for his Primary School Leaving Examination. But he had so much difficulty with English and Mathematics, Mrs Chitra realised that he needed help. So she convinced his grandparents (who are his guardians) that he should downgrade to the foundational stream. With the help of specialised teaching, revision support from a group of friends, and having the exam questions read to him, Sri John overcame his difficulties and did well enough to qualify for both Normal (Academic) and (Technical) streams. All this, in no small measure, because his teacher was sensitive to the needs of her dyslexic student.

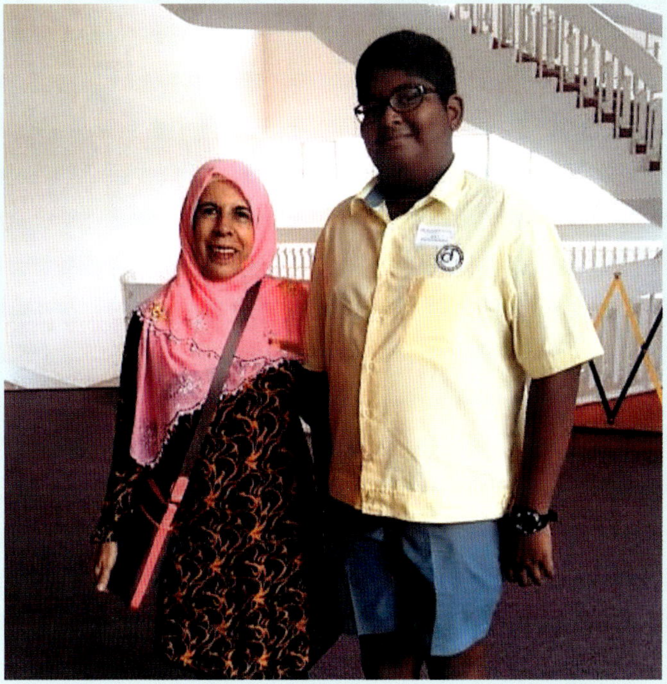

Above: At the 2016 Student Graduation and Awards Ceremony, Sri John S/O Albert David received a Maths improvement award. He is here with his DAS Maths Teacher Ms Aishah Abdullah, known as Ms Albel.
Below: Sri John is with his very proud grandparents. He obtained a Grade 1 for Maths and Science in his PSLE and Grade 2 for English and Tamil.

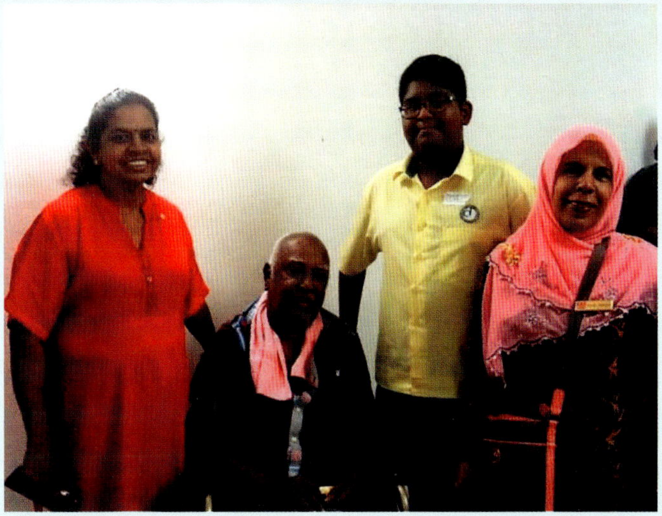

COMMUNITY AWARENESS

At a macro societal level, DAS's efforts to create greater awareness has also placed dyslexia on the radar screen of organisations and other educational institutions. In partnership with institutional sponsors and mainstream schools, DAS has also benefited from Community Involvement Programmes (CIP) and Character and Citizenship Education (CCE) projects run by local schools. In return, DAS has begun to make an impact on the lives of countless young people by imbuing in them a propensity for kindness and doing social good.

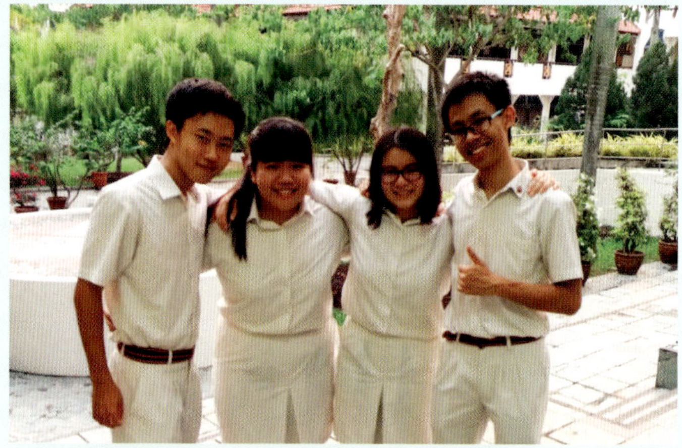

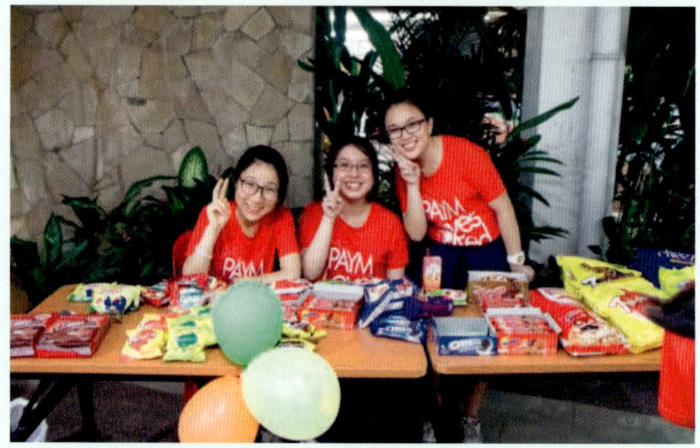

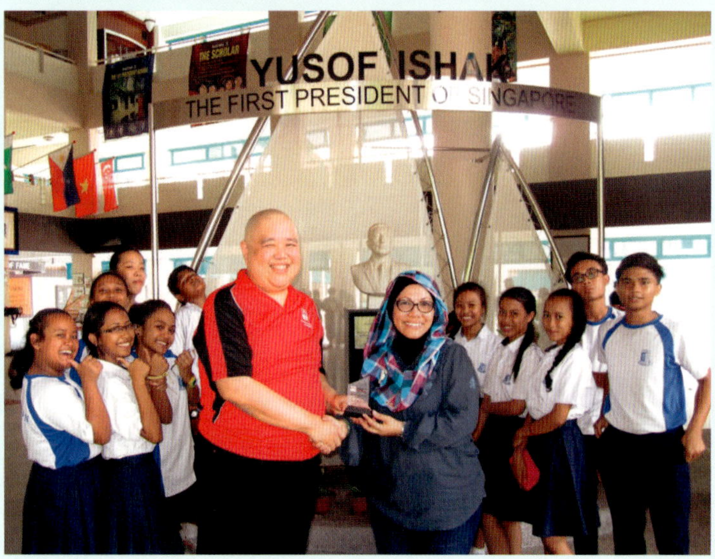

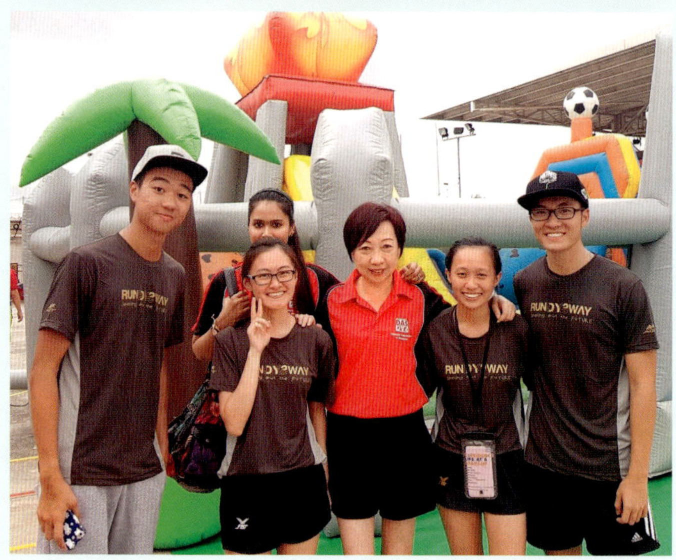

CITI-YMCA YOUTH FOR CAUSES

One of the institutional catalysts for fundraising and awareness-raising has been the Citi-YMCA Youth For Causes (YFC). This is a community initiative started by Citibank and the YMCA of Singapore in 2003. Funded by Citi Foundation, the programme helps to promote social entrepreneurship and community leadership development among Singapore youths. It provides youths aged 15 to 25 with a platform which includes seed funding, training and volunteer mentorship for executing self-initiated projects to raise public awareness, funds and mobilise volunteers for Voluntary Welfare Organisations (VWOs) of their choice.

EMPOWERING YOUTHS TO PUT THEIR VALUES INTO ACTION

YFC complements the "Values in Action" (VIA) programme that is a part of the Ministry of Education's Character and Citizenship Education. The youths, in teams of four, seek to demonstrate values such as harmony, respect and responsibility as they champion their social causes.

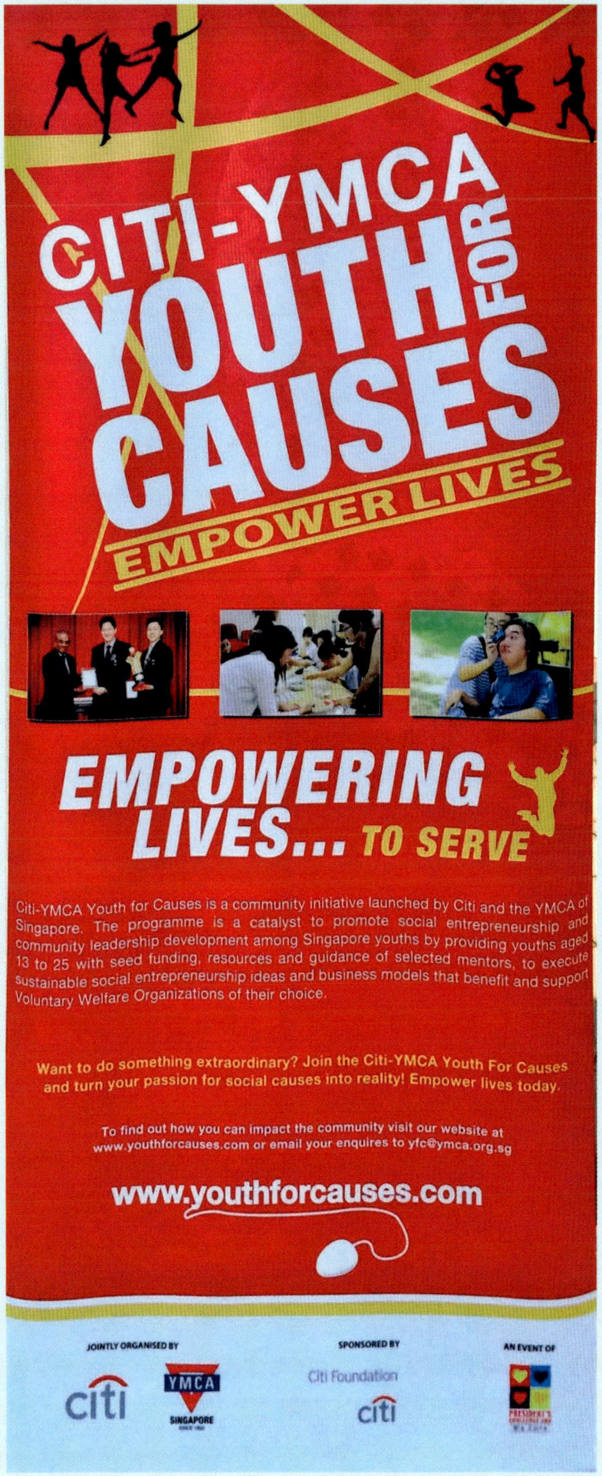

Left: Ms Jacqueline Song, DAS Head of Fundraising with the Run-Dys-Way Team.

IMPACTING OUR COMMUNITY

The YFC programme empowers participants to be the masters of their own project, working closely with VWOs in Singapore, and gaining first-hand experience in organising events to champion a social cause. Students get to learn lessons outside of the classrooms to spark their entrepreneurial spirit, and be developed into socially responsible community leaders.

NATIONAL YOUTH COUNCIL GRANTS

The Young ChangeMakers (YCM) grant, administered by the National Youth Council (NYC), provides seed-funding for youths to implement projects for the community.

Young ChangeMakers aims to build platforms where young people can congregate, connect and collaborate with like-minded individuals to make a difference to the community. Youths who are looking at organising community projects or starting ground-up initiatives can come together for monthly YCM Open Mic sessions to kick-start their ideas and work on solutions for community needs. Successful applicants can receive YCM seed-funding of $3,000 or up to 80% of total allowable project cost, whichever is lower. Projects that demonstrate exceeding merits in terms of project scale and impact will be awarded up to $5,000 or up to 80% of total allowable project cost, whichever is lower.

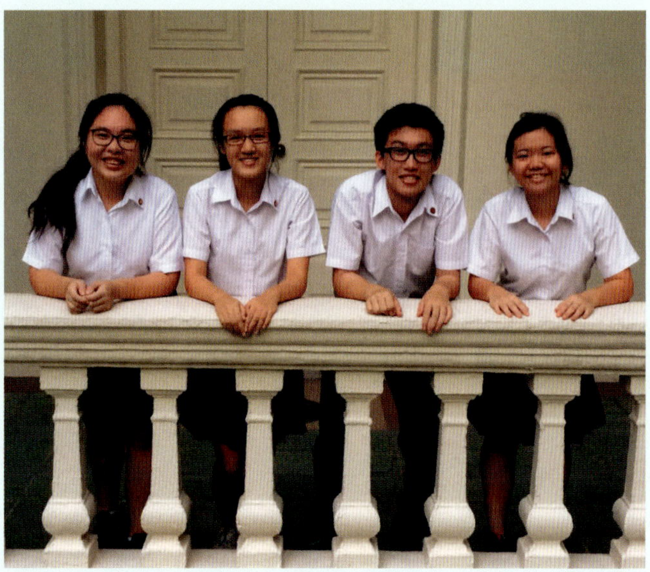

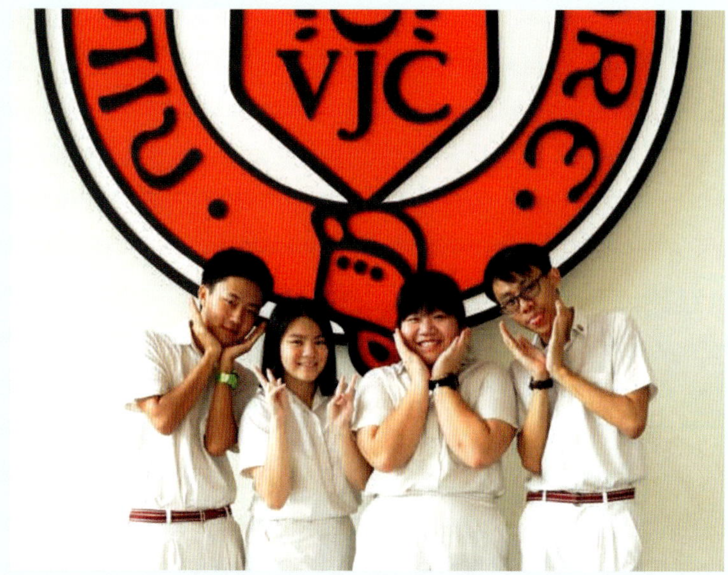

TEAM D'SLEXIA

WHAT WE DID

In 2013, when we were still studying in Dunman High School, we applied for the Citi-YMCA grant under Youth for Causes. This provided us with seed money to carry out a charity project in partnership with our chosen VWO.

After looking through the list, we chose DAS because we deliberately wanted to leave out VWOs who already had a higher profile. We realised that there was very little awareness of Dyslexia in society. People know how to say Cancer and Dementia in Chinese, but not Dyslexia.

In fact, most of the people we spoke to would ask, "What is Dyslexia?" So we thought it would be good to raise awareness and give DAS the support that they needed. Parents often misunderstand the condition and think that their children are stupid or slow.

There were only two teams that had nominated DAS that year. In the case of Team D'Slexia, we carried out street sales, did busking (Take Dys Step), organised a run (Run Dys Way), and had our own internal school sales of keychains we had designed and DAS merchandise.

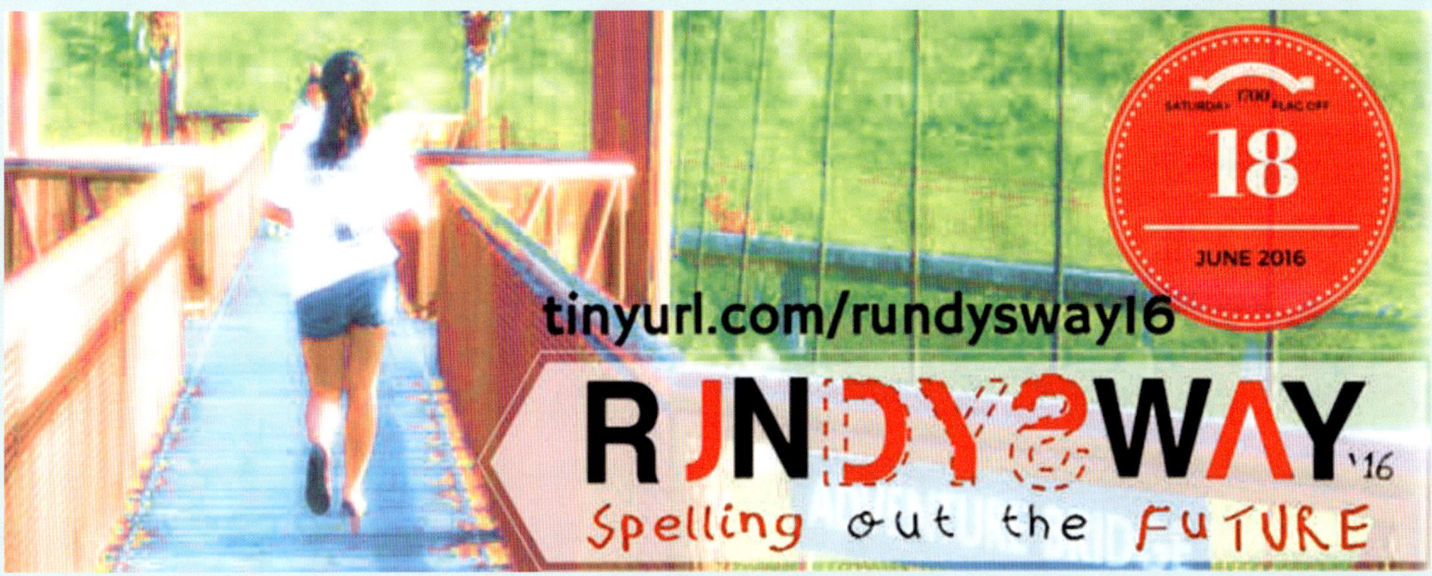

WHAT WE ACHIEVED

By the end of our activities in 2013, we had raised $16,000 for DAS. More importantly, dyslexia was better known and understood that year at Dunman High.

At the beginning, we didn't think about the sustainability of the whole project. But the good thing was, we were able to pass on the project to our juniors (Team D'Code) the next year. They also received the Citi-YMCA grant.

Continuity

In 2016, it was good to organise another Run-Dys-Way because it provided continuity and involved people in a way that showed our involvement wasn't just a one-off. So we reached out again to our Dunman High community.

Although awareness of dyslexia still lags behind illnesses like cancer and heart disease, we think that we have made slow and steady progressive steps in the right direction. It has to start somewhere, so this year, together with Team D'Code, we collaborated with Punggol 21 Community Club as a third-party fundraiser for DAS. As a result, we were able to reach out to a greater public beyond the school. Just by publicising the event, many more were made aware of dyslexia.

Participants of Run-Dys-Way had to pay for a ticket to run. Additional donations were also accepted on the day itself. We capped the total number of runners at 200. We also managed to get sponsors for the goody bags. There were more public runners this time round and the Punggol 21 CC organised a carnival alongside the run.

In 2013, our project was simply to show support for dyslexia by creating better awareness. The event in 2016 went beyond that to include raising funds for DAS.

Spreading the Word

We feel that more should be done to spread the word to parents and educators. One of our friends only found out he is dyslexic during his pre-enlistment army medical check-up. Apart from him, we don't even know anyone who is dyslexic.

During the period when we were carrying out our DAS project, we were hoping to meet and interact with some dyslexics so that we can better understand the challenges they go through on a daily basis. But because of our tight school schedules, it was difficult to arrange for the team to meet them.

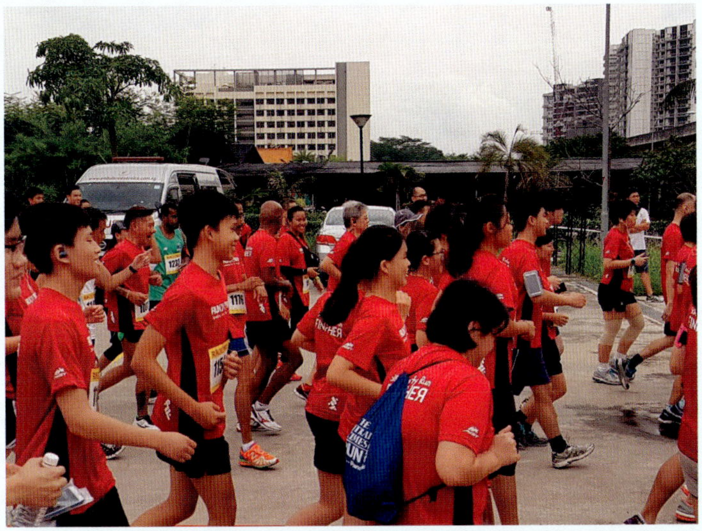

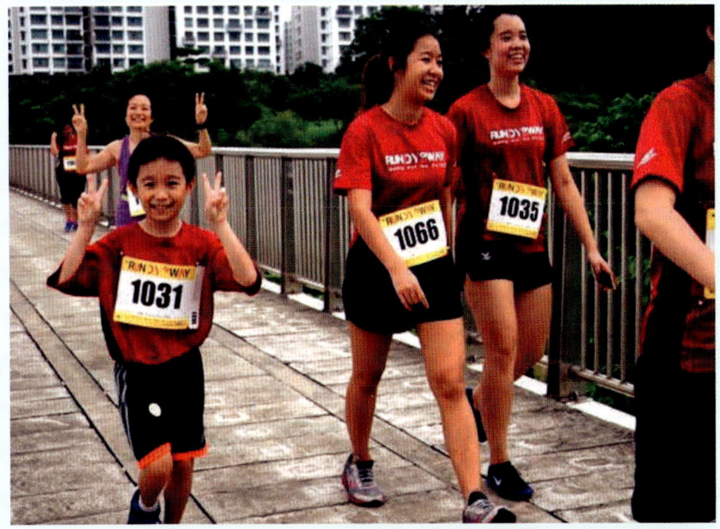

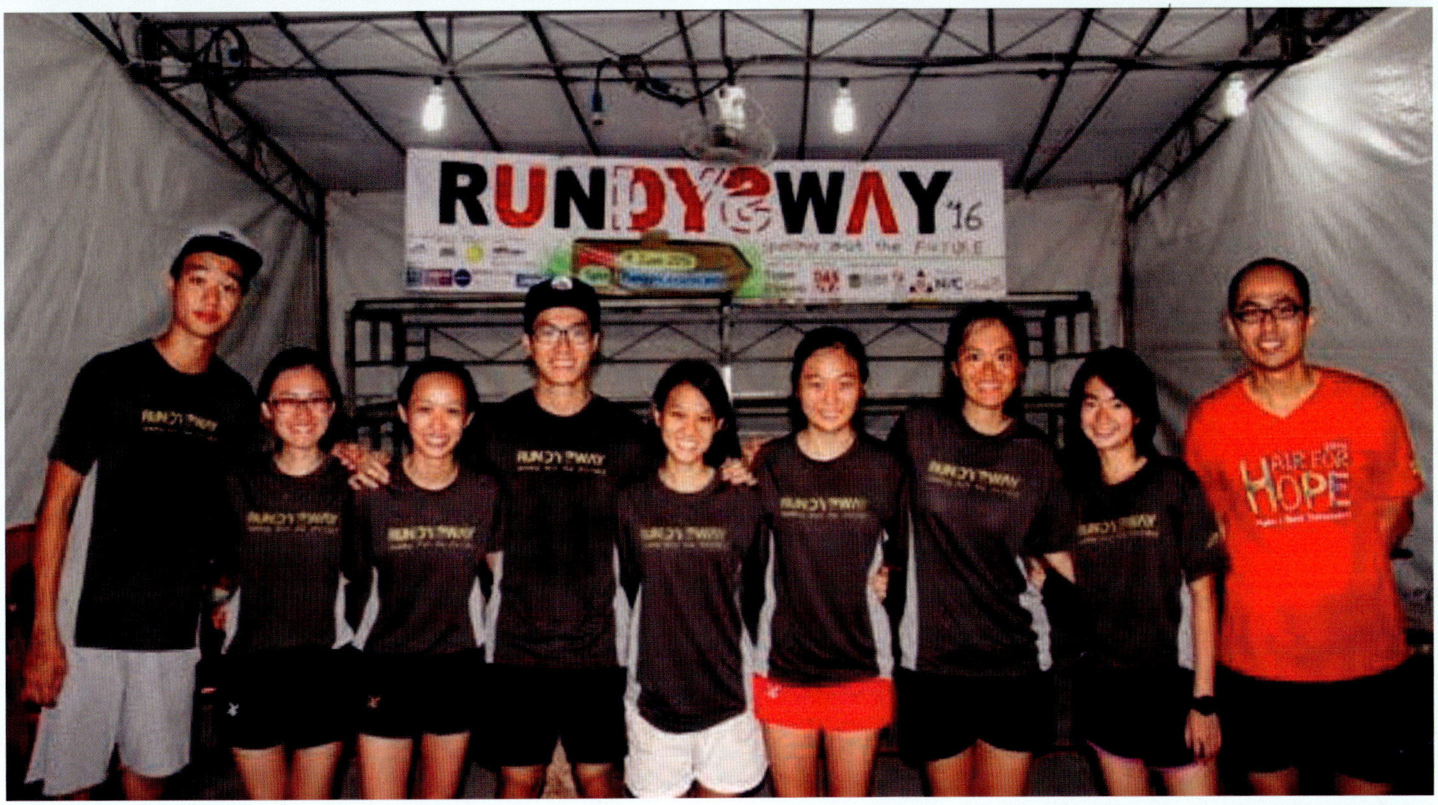

Run-Dys-Way 2016, Runners and organisers of this successful event and great support for DAS

Personal Growth

There were many facets to our project and we learnt organisational skills, self-motivation, and how to contribute to the community. All this added a different dimension to our lives.

I don't think any of us would ever have imagined doing this. It was only after embarking on it that we realised we were quite passionate about the project.

In 2013, we only had about one to two months to organise the run. We enjoyed having control over our own project.

We had done other CIPs in the past, but most of the time, we didn't fully know what we were doing. This time, we had control and were therefore more self-driven. We had to organise the event, liaise with companies — pitch the reasons for doing this and explain why we should receive help, and how we can contribute to the company as well.

Understanding people and handling them with a smile even when they rejected us (interpersonal skills) was something else we learned. In the final analysis, we felt that we received more than we gave to DAS in doing this project.

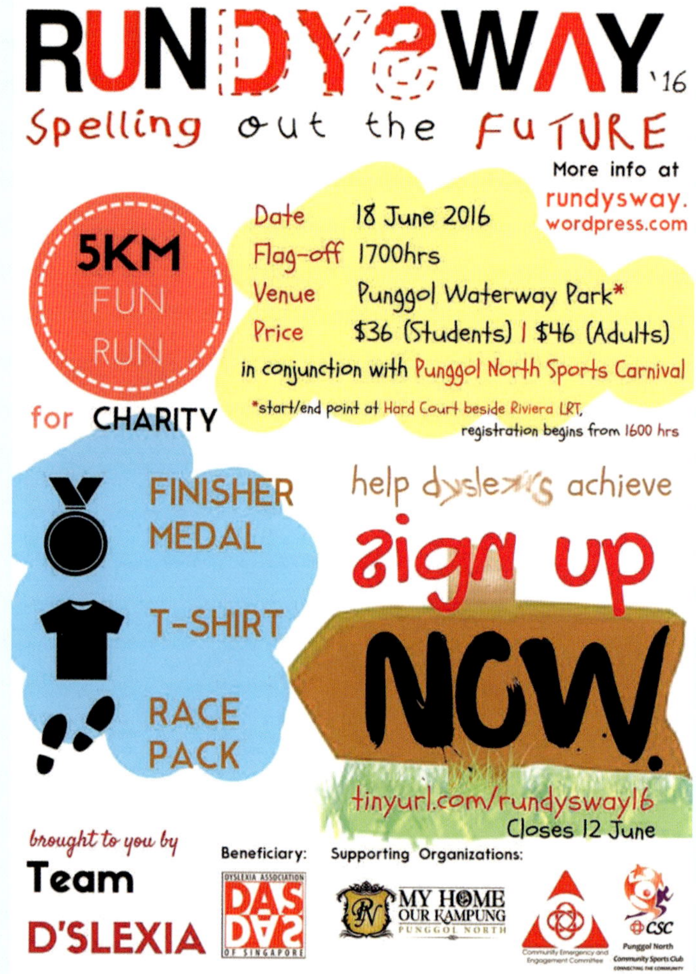
RUNDYSWAY '16
Spelling out the FUTURE
More info at
rundysway.wordpress.com
5KM FUN RUN
for CHARITY
Date 18 June 2016
Flag-off 1700hrs
Venue Punggol Waterway Park*
Price $36 (Students) | $46 (Adults)
in conjunction with Punggol North Sports Carnival
*start/end point at Hard Court beside Riviera LRT,
registration begins from 1600 hrs
FINISHER MEDAL
T-SHIRT
RACE PACK
sign up
NOW.
tinyurl.com/rundysway16
Closes 12 June
brought to you by
Team D'SLEXIA
Beneficiary:
DYSLEXIA ASSOCIATION
DAS
OF SINGAPORE
Supporting Organizations:
MY HOME OUR KAMPUNG
PUNGGOL NORTH
CSC
Punggol North Community Sports Club

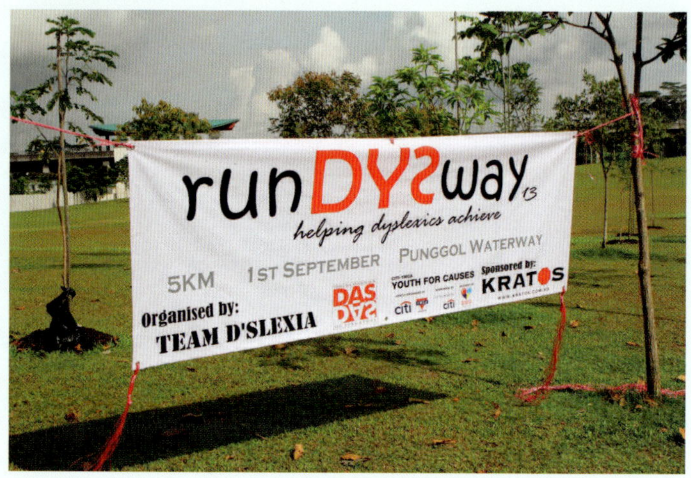
runDYSway13
helping dyslexics achieve
5KM
1ST SEPTEMBER
PUNGGOL WATERWAY
Organised by:
TEAM D'SLEXIA
YOUTH FOR CAUSES
Sponsored by:
KRATOS

TEAM VON

WHY DAS?

We are a team of 16 students from Nan Chiau High School who embarked on our Service-Learning Project in partnership with DAS last year under the mentorship of our teacher, Mr Tan Jia Hao.

After contacting DAS and getting to know more about dyslexia, we strongly felt that there was a need to spread awareness among Singaporeans about this special-needs community.

We specially chose "Von", the Icelandic word for "hope", as our team name. Hope represented a central theme of our project as we sought to encourage dyslexics with the thought that there is indeed hope of a brighter future ahead.

With our vision in mind, we applied for a grant under the National Youth Council's Young Changemaker (YCM) programme and were successful in kickstarting our project.

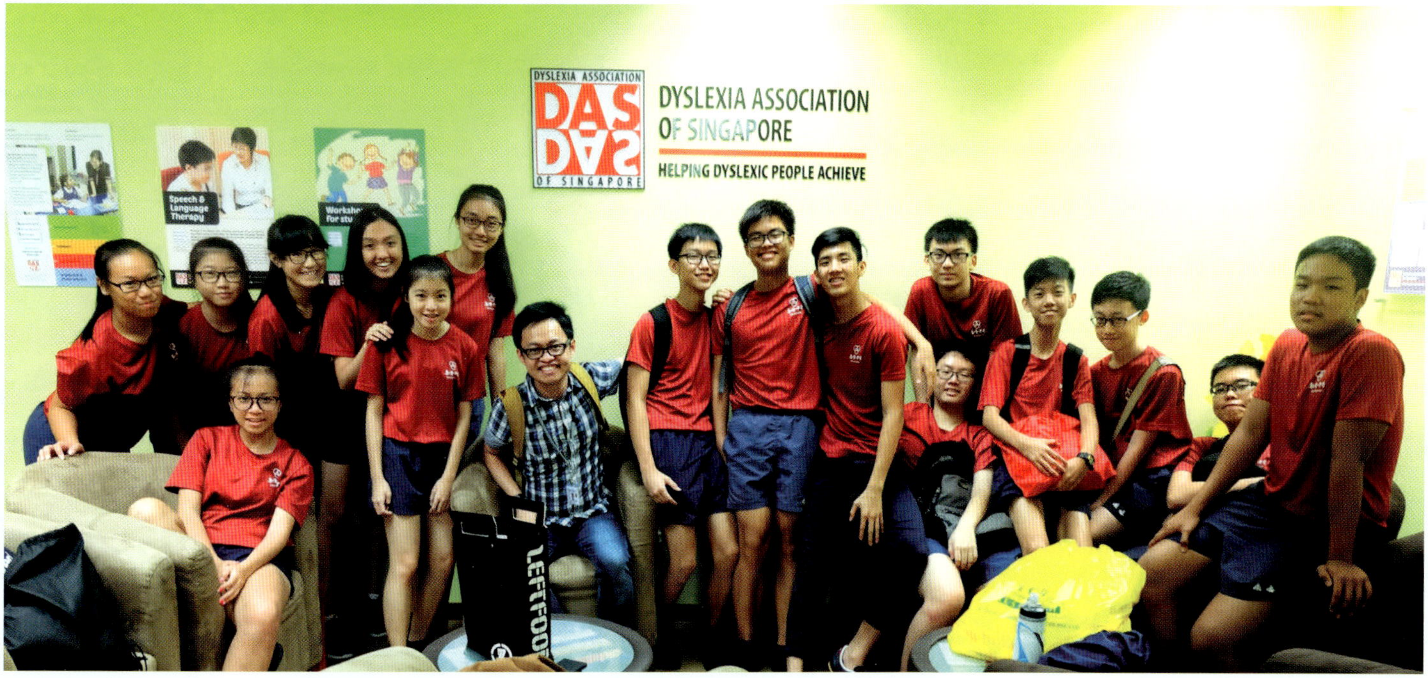

WHAT WE DID

Since the main needs of the DAS revolve around the raising of awareness of dyslexia within the community, as well as the raising of funds to support their programmes and operations, we designed our activities to target these areas.

As part of our fundraising initiatives, we conducted door-to-door sales in the neighbourhood. This presented us with an opportunity to share about DAS with the people we spoke to.

In addition, during school events such as our combined sports meet, movie screening event, as well as our annual carnival, we sold merchandise and took this opportunity to publicise the work of DAS. Eventually, the publicity took off and more volunteers from our school and the public joined our cause. Partners such as Ben & Jerry's also came on board to sponsor ice cream for our fundraising efforts.

By the end of the project, a net sum of $11,000 was raised. Despite the heavy commitments balancing schoolwork, CCAs and Service Learning, this proved to be indeed a very satisfying experience as we had achieved more than our projected target.

Throughout the journey, we also learned valuable project management skills such as planning, team collaboration, and time management. Through it all, we learned to be more thankful.

PERSONAL GROWTH

Trevor (One of the team leaders)

I found that not many people are aware of the problems dyslexics face. We took the opportunity to share their problems and to enlist the help of others. I learnt to be a better person because I learnt to care for people with dyslexia. In my role as a team leader, I realised that I needed to be more proactive in planning, for example in applying for street sales licences. We learned marketing skills and also found ways to reduce the cost of our goods by using recycled materials.

Through this project, I have gained a better understanding of the struggles that people with dyslexia have in coping with their studies. I'm impressed by their perseverance even in the face of difficulties.

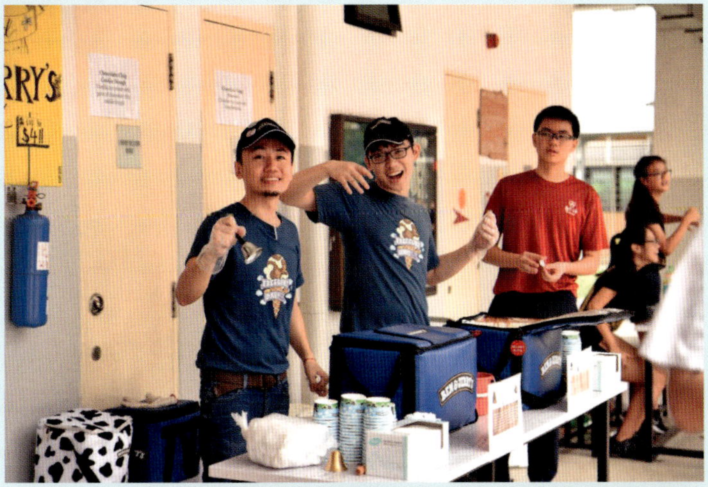

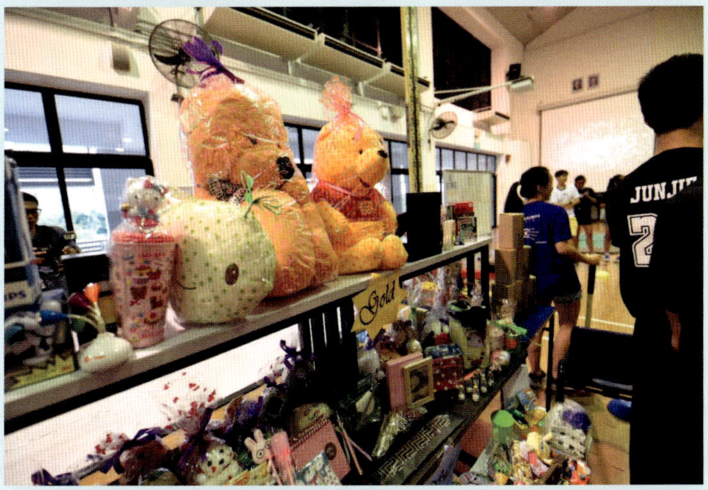

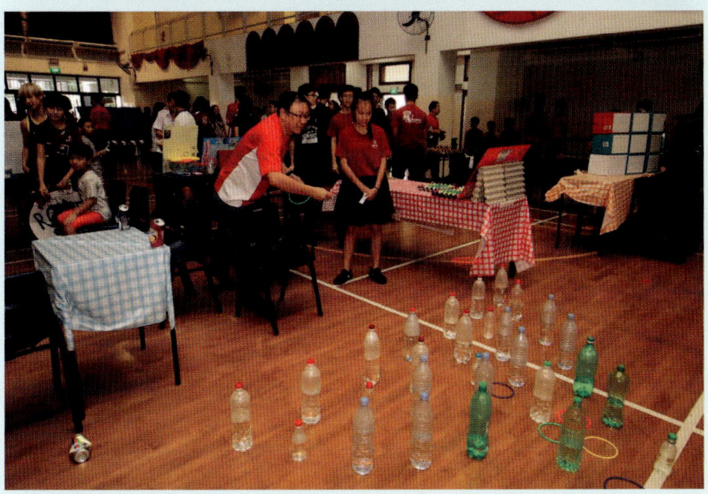

It has been a steep learning curve for me. I learned new skills that enabled me to carry out my role in the team, including being able to reach out to strangers for donations. I am also thankful for the encouragement from the other leaders, and the members who have worked very hard together with me.

Yun Xin (Overall leader)

Through this project I have learned to delegate work and lead a team. Initially, my members were easily dejected and demoralised by the poor takings during our street sales. I had to keep encouraging them to keep going and not give up.

Although the group members were shy, they still stepped up to do their part. At one point, two of our members had to collect 30 donation tins from the DAS office and bring all of them by public transport back to our school. And because the trains and buses were quite packed, they sometimes had to get off to make way for others who were alighting, and then get back on again to continue their journey. All these had to be done while they were carrying 15 tins each!

For direct service, we went down to Rex House to help with the laminating of their books. We were given a briefing about dyslexia and also given codes to decode so that we would have a better understanding of what dyslexics experience when they read.

It was very rewarding to set a goal which we exceeded in terms of fundraising. I was very shocked by this because throughout the process many team members weren't cooperative, and there were many hurdles we had to overcome.

But we were very thankful for DAS's support and also the connection to Ben & Jerry's. This came at a time when we were very dejected because all our suggestions for games during the school funfair had been rejected. It gave us the strength to push on. I even asked my mother to bake cookies for sale.

Zhi Qian (Internal fundraising)

I was the only person overseeing this, so I had to make sure that everything ran smoothly. My family wasn't very supportive when I first told them about our project because they were afraid that it would interfere with my studies. My mother relented and said that as long as I could cope with the extra work, I could go ahead. As a result, I learned the skill of juggling my studies, CCA and service learning.

As a team, we also learned to tap on each other's strengths and support each other through our weaknesses.

Being the highest-grossing team, we received a lot of mention at the end of the project. We were delighted as each time our achievements were highlighted, the DAS also received more publicity.

Jia Yew (Another team leader)

I learned about being resilient in tough times. Our mentor, Mr Tan, also deserves mention as he was there for us throughout the duration of the project. In our team, we went from being strangers to becoming friends. We gained better insights into one another and we made use of our strengths to help each other work through with our weaknesses.

Our appreciation and admiration for our teacher-mentor, Mr Tan, grew considerably during the time he worked alongside us. Among the 18 teams, we were probably the most difficult to control, but he stood by us all the way. He came for every single street sale and cheered and encouraged us.

FROM A TEACHER'S PERSPECTIVE

Mr Tan Jia Hao

We started planning in early February. I had to guide them in their planning and also manage their expectations. The students were the ones who chose DAS. It was quite a good collaboration and we're happy we had a chance to help DAS.

It was quite tiring for the students because they were doing this in addition to their regular school workload.

I told them that they have to remember that this is charitable work, so they need to adopt a positive mindset as they came out the work. It has no direct bearing on their studies, but is a part of the Character and Citizenship Education (CCE) module in school. Nan Chiau focuses on CCE to enable students to learn to contribute to the society. I am very pleased that Team Von pulled together and learned precious life lessons along the way.

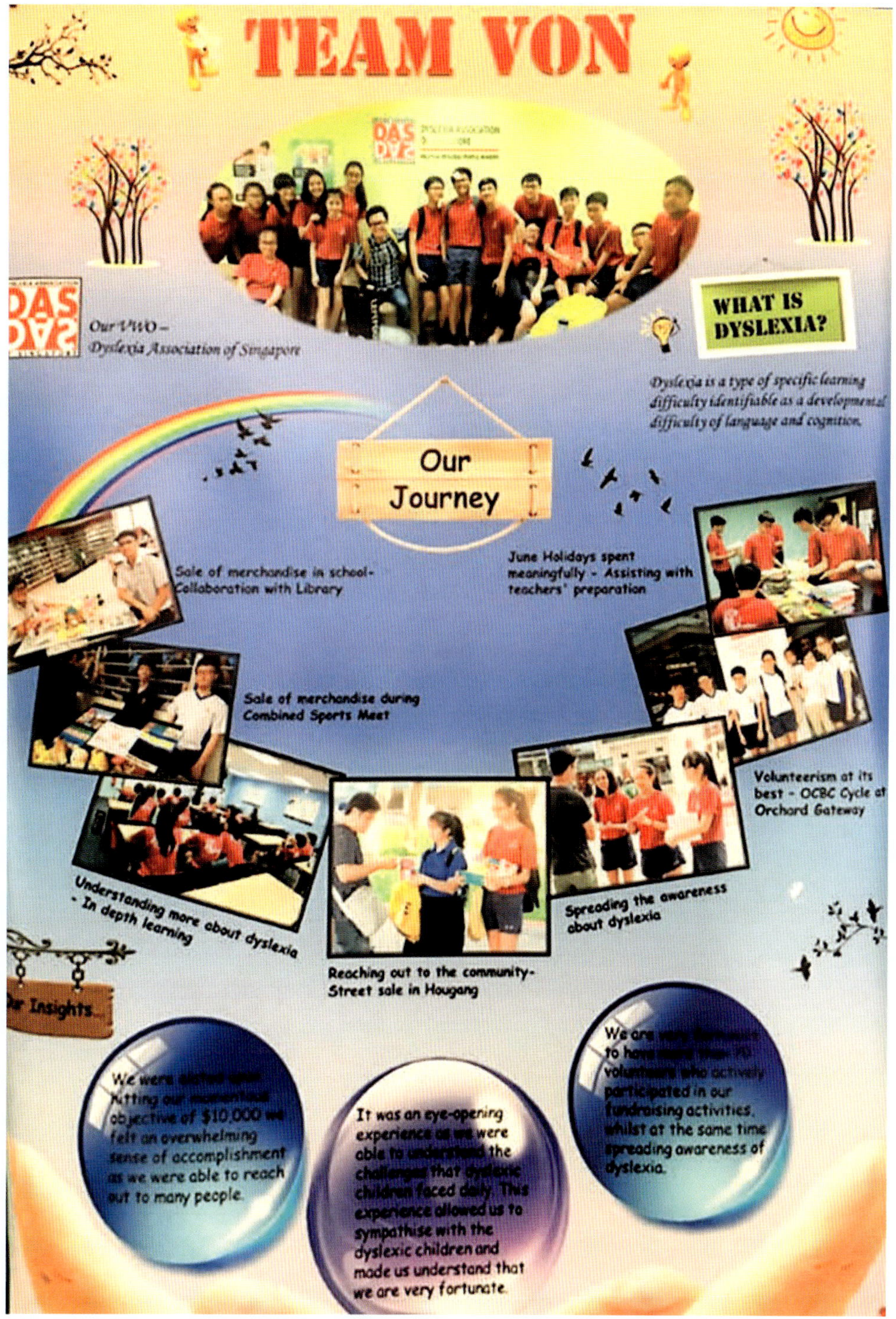

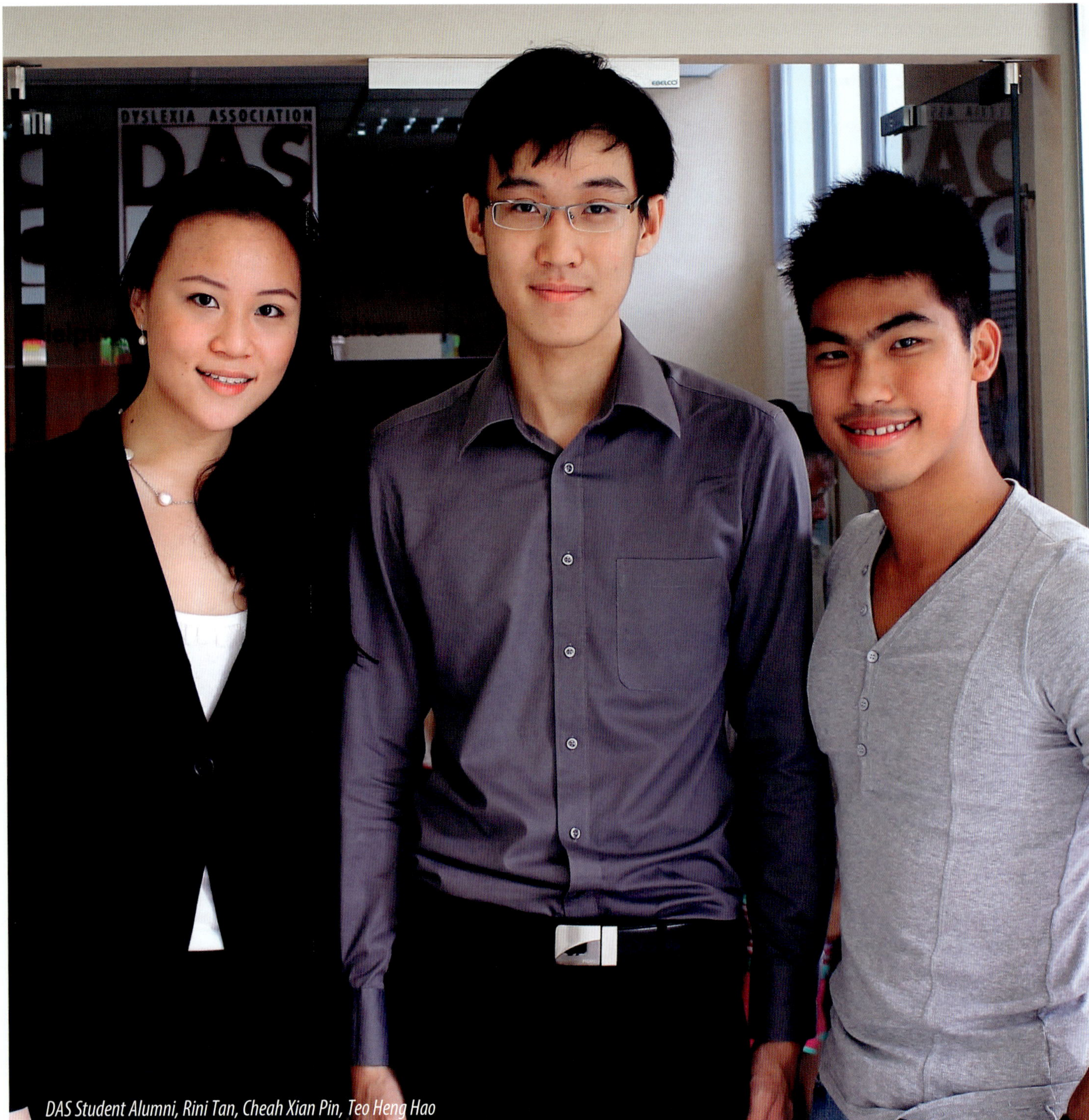

DAS Student Alumni, Rini Tan, Cheah Xian Pin, Teo Heng Hao

7

LIVING TOGETHER, WORKING TOGETHER

Being dyslexic can actually help in the outside world. I see some things clearer than other people do because I have to simplify things to help me and that has helped others.

Richard Branson

AWARENESS AND OUTREACH

The good thing about turning 25 is that an organisation has the opportunity to see the fruition of its plans and the growth of those it has helped. In a speech that the late Dr Jimmy Daruwalla made to share his Embrace Dyslexia vision in 2014, he said:

> *"They [dyslexics] have the ability to see the big picture, without being bogged down in the details. They have the drive and determination to succeed where others would give up having faced failure frequently in their earlier days and have developed creative solutions to deal with it.*
>
> *While reading may slow them down, they do learn to read people and are good at choosing people who they can delegate these responsibilities to, be it a parent, sibling, co-worker, etc.... They have mastered the art of verbal communication, which is so important in doing business — and in employee relations it was found that the turnover rate is lower in businesses run by dyslexics."*
>
> *Dr Jimmy Daruwalla, 2014*

DAS has seen many of its alumni entering the workforce and making an impact in society. It would be simplistic to paint a happily-ever-after picture of their lives because most of them have to make considerable adjustments to a working world that can often be less than accepting of learning differences. But Dr Daruwalla's comment about dyslexics' drive and determination to succeed has been borne out time and again by the life stories that have been shared. Employers also have a key role to play in understanding the challenges of their dyslexic staff, and creating solutions that can help them flourish.

DAS STUDENT ALUMNI

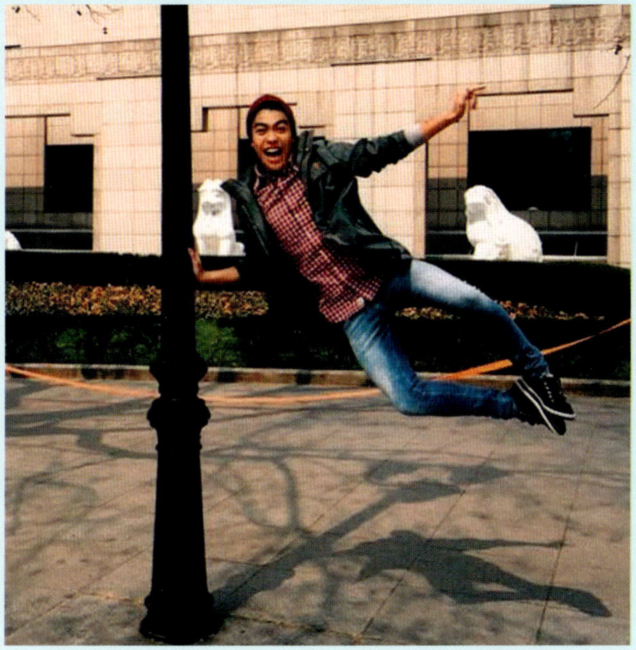

TEO HENG SOON

"Being a dyslexic was a problem then and it still is. I think the basic fact is that a dyslexic has to study three times more than their peers to do slightly better or just to be on par with them. I am no exception to that. I cannot say I have overcome dyslexia and I don't think I will ever overcome it. I would say what is more important is to understand it and not fight it, as it is part of me, trying to push it aside would not help.

Understanding it taught me that there were indeed lessons to learn from this learning difficulty. It helped me to be disciplined and focused. When my friends would play, I would have the discipline to keep on studying. This has helped me be very patient with myself especially when it comes to exploring and developing the talent or interest for karate, dancing and cinematography. Through this, I am convinced that hard work is highly important to get somewhere in life. Dyslexia has really given me the drive to do my best to be an all-rounder in studies, social interactions and in my interests."

DAS STUDENT ALUMNI

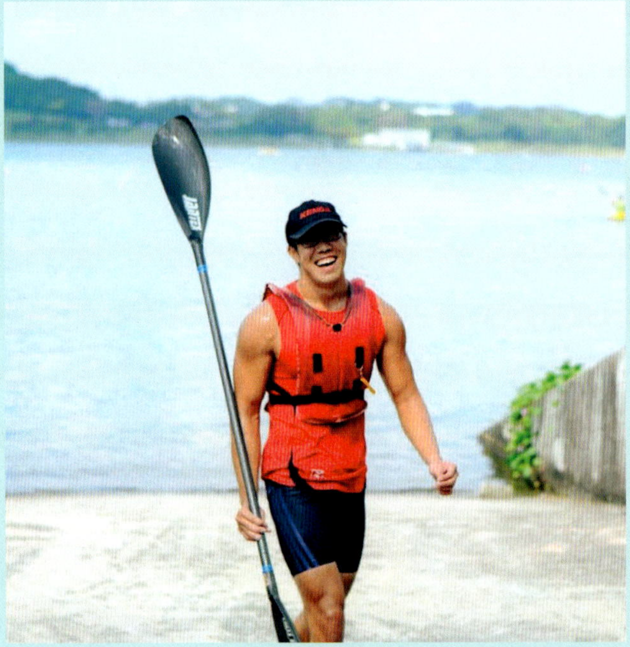

HENG YI ZEN

"Sometimes I felt that dyslexia made me inferior to the rest. It vexed me, and what made it worse was when my classmates wished they had dyslexia too, so that they could get extra time during examinations. Although they were kidding, it did hit a raw nerve. I understood that the extra time granted to us was to enable us to compete on an equal footing with the rest of our friends. I made sure that I did my best and never blamed any of my problems on dyslexia.

Dyslexia has helped me to discover myself more, and it taught me that if I really want to achieve anything all I needed to do was work hard for it. Everything has a price tag on it; the question is whether you are willing to commit the time and effort. When the going gets tough sometimes all you need to do is look behind, see how far you have already travelled and look at the people who are supporting you. Once you have done that, you would realise that the only one who thinks that you cannot achieve it, is you."

DAS STUDENT ALUMNI

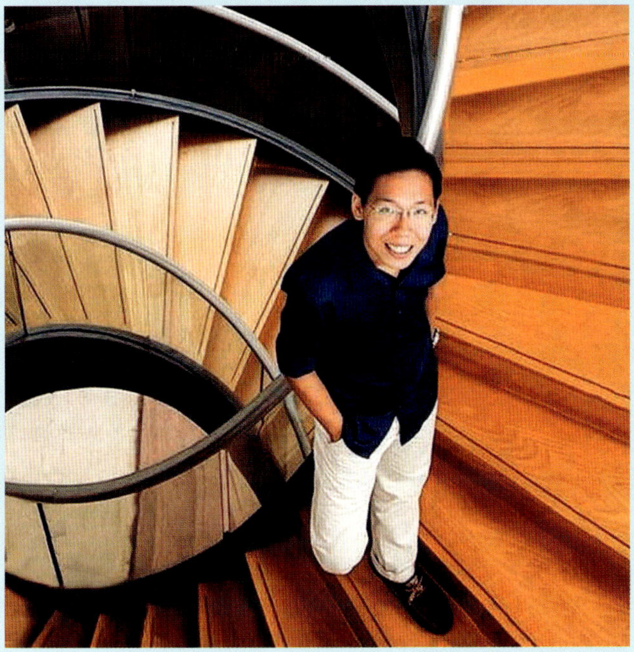

EDWARD YEE

"I never really saw dyslexia as something to overcome but a strength/tool to make use of. Throughout my schooling years, I was able to solve problems differently from others and was never wholly able to solve them the conventional way taught by teachers. Dyslexia also helped me understand that it is okay to fail; but to embrace and learn from mine and others' failures, hence my favourite quote by Sir Isaac Newton, "If I have seen further, it is by standing on the shoulders of giants."

There is an African proverb that says, "If you want to go fast, go alone. If you want to go far, go together." I did not make it to where I am today alone. My family has always supported me throughout and ever since I was young I have been told whenever I failed that I definitely could do well if I just put in the hard work. This has helped me develop a growth mind-set over time. To the other dyslexics, I will borrow the words of Albert Einstein, "Everybody is a genius. But if you judge a fish by its ability to climb a tree, it will live its whole life believing that it is stupid."

DAS STUDENT ALUMNI

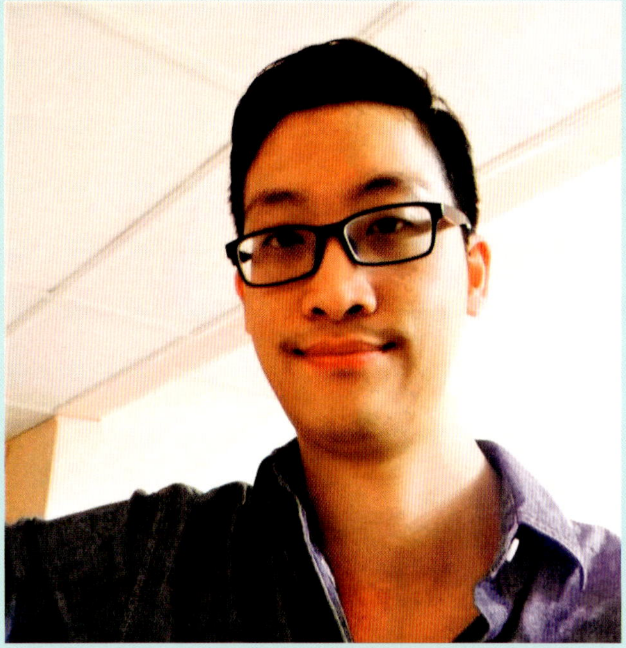

CALVIN YIO

"In those early days, when I first found out that I was dyslexic, there was not much information about dyslexia and there was no internet. All I knew was that I was different from my siblings and felt rather left out. However, with the dedication of my mother I was able to learn to cope with the hurdles that being a dyslexic brought about. I would say that being a dyslexic opened up my views on many areas and how to approach many things. It empowered me to try out and dare to take risks in various areas of my life.

My parting advice to the other dyslexics out there; be confident and do not falter. If you have a dream pursue it and follow your heart, do not let others put you down, do not be afraid to fail and do not be afraid to keep trying. Do what you feel is right and do not be afraid to take risks. This was what I did in order to pursue my passion as it had allowed me to break into the industry in which I was most passionate about. And allowed me to grow my knowledge and desire to understand new things in this current age, time and society."

DAS STUDENT ALUMNI

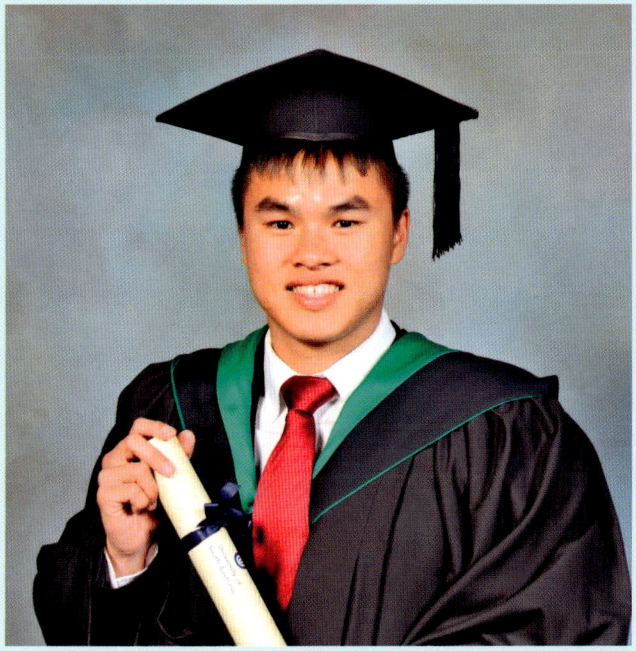

JEREMY LIM

"An American musician B. B. King once said, "the beautiful thing about learning is that no one can take it away from you." As someone with dyslexia, I encourage other dyslexics to continue to strive ahead in your pursuit of knowledge and pace your studies to a level that suits your learning just as I have. I see dyslexia as a gift and a chance to be unique!

I embrace it! I have had a successful educational journey and have graduated with first-class honours from a Civil Engineering Degree and the greatest accomplishment is being gainfully employed and receiving my first month's pay. It is like all the struggles, worries and anxiousness I once had in school disappeared and now I am doing something I am passionate about."

DAS STUDENT ALUMNI

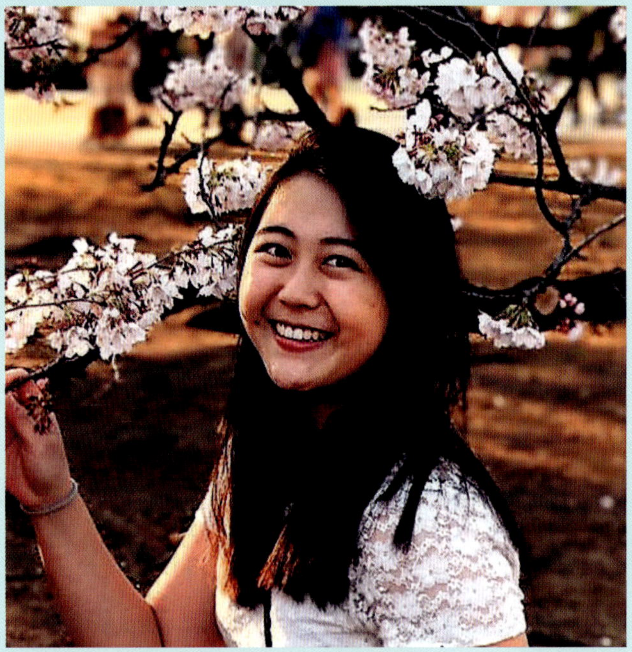

AERIN LIM

"Growing up, I was always a slower learner. Given the same amount of time to complete an exam as everyone else, I constantly found myself only managing to answer half the questions posed. In the past, this made me feel intellectually inferior to my peers. However, dyslexia is not an impairment that cannot be overcome. By putting in more effort and being more meticulous in your learning, you will still be able to excel in your studies. What really helped me was finding a study style that worked for me. It will take some experimenting, but when you manage to work out a system that can help you to effectively memorise the contents and methods of application of whichever subject you are learning, the subject will become much easier to master. Even now, I am still constantly trying to improve on a study style that I can effectively apply to my discipline to allow me to do better. Also, it is very important to believe in yourself and never give up despite how difficult learning may seem to you. A lack of self-confidence will always limit one's potential.

In a nutshell, do not lose confidence or hope despite your struggle with dyslexia as it is a learning difference that can be worked upon. Embrace the fact that you can think differently from others as something that makes you special, and never doubt your own worth or capability. Your potential is probably far greater than you have managed to unleash on your learning journey thus far."

DAS STUDENT ALUMNI

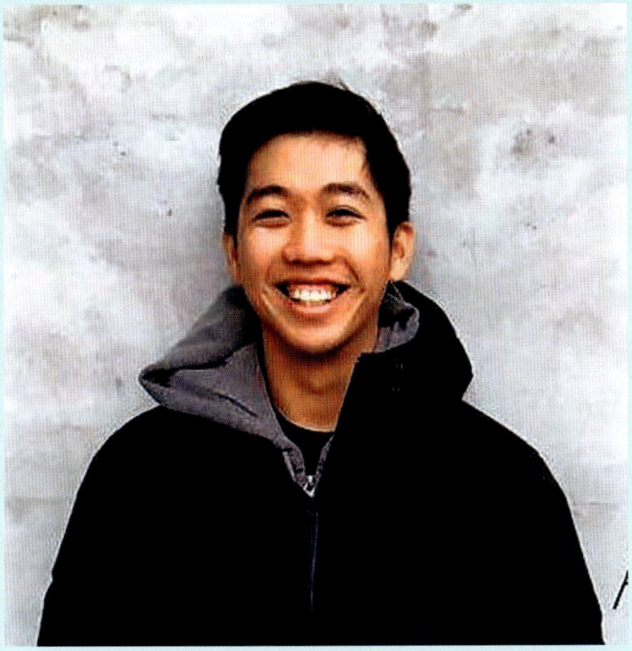

RYAN LIM

"Being dyslexic, I have had to put in much more effort than others at each juncture of my life to overcome my impediments. The first semester of law school was no exception. However, I believe that one has not lived life to its fullest until he has done everything he can to achieve his full potential. To overcome dyslexia I have learnt resilience, developed a strong work ethic, a keen eye for detail and the ability to think out of the box. These are skills I believe are highly sought after in the legal field. I am grateful to the Dyslexia Association for helping me when I was young, and I hope to remain involved in their activities. It is a great source of pride for me to be featured in the dyslexia publications to serve as an inspiration to other dyslexics. Incidentally, the previous SG50 edition featured Mr Lee Kuan Yew, who is one of my biggest heroes, I hope that other dyslexics will draw inspiration from these stories and not view their dyslexia as a disability but instead as a strength. I cannot thank the Dyslexia Association of Singapore enough for their continuing support in my life, without which I would not be who I am today. I have no doubt that the association will continue to greatly benefit and support younger dyslexics in the many years to come."

LIFELONG LEARNER JENNY KHNG

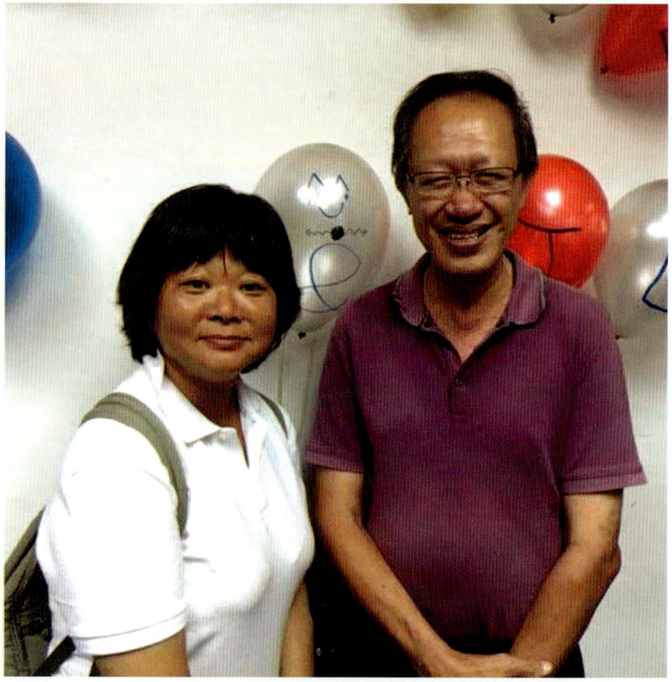

Ms Jenny Khng and Mr Tan

The advent of technology has unfolded a myriad of possibilities for Ms Jenny Khng, a dyslexic who is mother to three dyslexic children. Heavily reliant on her iPhone, Jenny proclaimed it is her best friend. She uses voice recordings during meetings so that she can review them when she's home. The automated voice-controlled personal digital assistant, Siri, as well as the text-to-speech feature are life-savers for Jenny. She dictates messages to her phone and triple-checks the correct spelling before sending it out.

Aside from her phone, her former boss and now business partner, Mr Tan, has been a tremendous help in her life. She first met him when she applied for a position in a waste management company. He recognised her difficulty with administrative tasks and volunteered to help her with them.

One of her main duties was bag collection; she had to drive around and pick up filled trash bags left on roadsides by the cleaners. The job was not as easy as it appeared, and there was a need to come up with a plan to do her job effectively and efficiently.

Already having trouble with recognising directions and road signs because of her dyslexia, she also had to pick up the bags by a specified time. Mr Tan came to her rescue by helping her to calculate distances and planning out a feasible route with her. He helped by summarising large chunks of information into bite-sized pieces that she could digest.

Although Mr Tan encouraged her to upgrade herself by attending courses, she balked at the thought of subsequently being promoted to an administrative position where she would have to write reports. After a 10-year stint at that company, Jenny decided to venture into a recycling business with Mr Tan. Combining her passion for a clean and green Singapore with the desire to acquire new skills, she started the business so that she

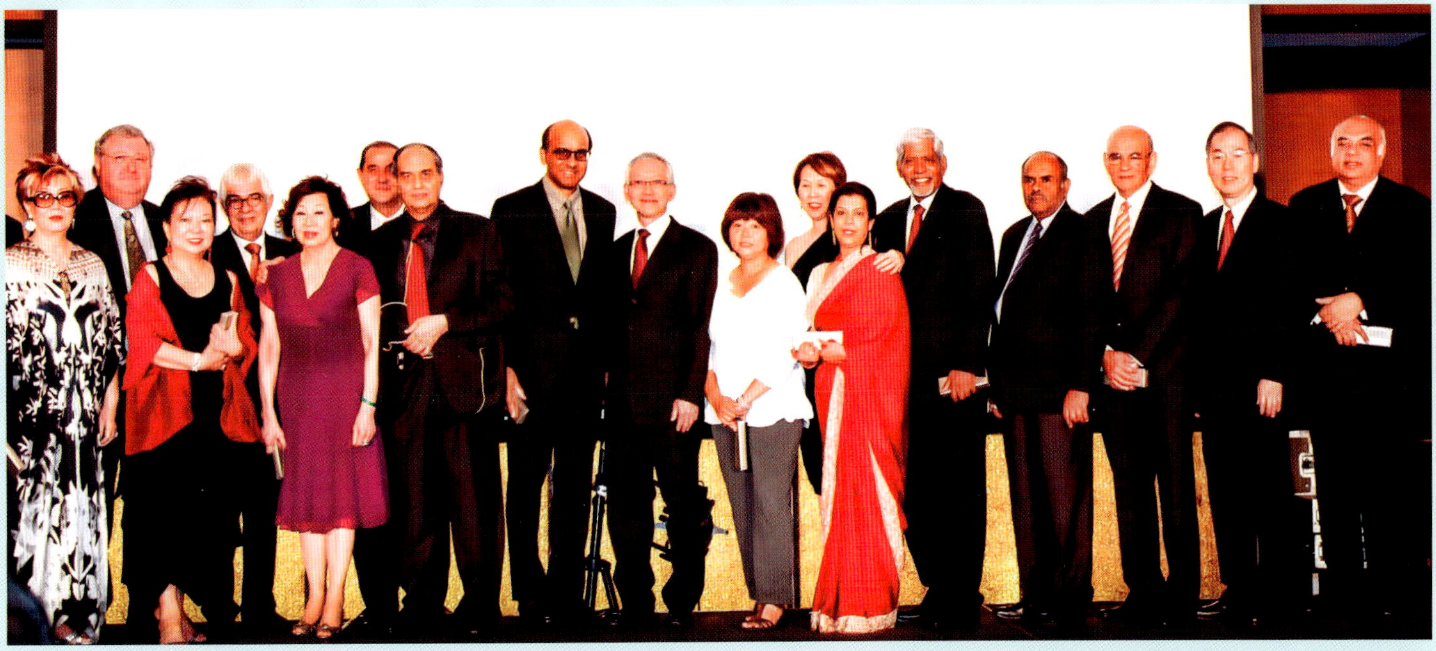

Above: Jenny Khng was recognised for her long-term support of the Dyslexia Association of Singapore along with other current and ex-members of the DAS Executive Committee at the 21st Anniversary Gala Dinner in 2012. Jenny is in the white blouse in the centre of the picture
Below: Mr Tan is reading Jenny's story in the Embrace a Different Kind of Mind *at the book's launch in 2015.*

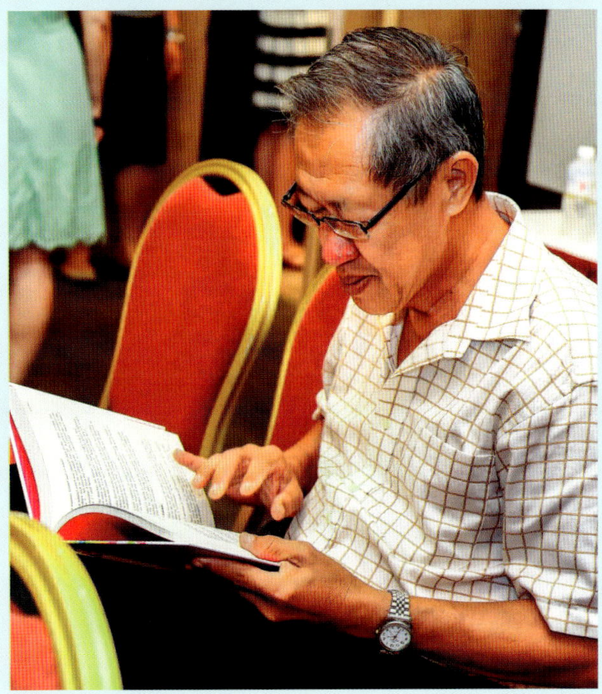

would not have to go for interviews. And, fortunately, Mr Tan could help with the paperwork and free Jenny to focus on the other aspects of the work.

Mr Tan handles all the administrative aspects of their business and patiently continues to try to teach Jenny in spite of her lack of interest in and aptitude for writing reports and financial statements.

Jenny's word to younger dyslexics, "It is better to learn slowly than never to learn at all."

"WHEN I LOOK BACK, I CRY…"

KYDZ International is now in its 12th year. The specialist educational toy company was started by Mr Gary Seow as a last-ditch attempt to provide for his wife and three young children. He was in despair after having resigned from yet another job… his 10th.

Gary used to work in sales. Even though he tried to learn to adapt and cope with the demands of his job, he would fail time and again. Sometimes he would be told to resign; other times he would be "shelled" in front of other colleagues. That was his normal. But he continued to record his sales figures wrongly. As a junior member of the staff, his supervisor would scold him for being dishonest and he was accused of overclaiming. After all these years, he is now able to say that they were honest mistakes.

When Gary started KYDZ International, he only had a range of nine toys. All had been bought from distributors. Initially, he said that he had to endure a lot of insults, and had to eat humble pie. After one year, Gary realised that he needed staff to help him process the orders. However, going through the process of explaining things in detail to "normal" people was and still is very torturous for him. He's more interested in the end result. So, for his staff, initially it was a case of "We didn't know he's dyslexic, so we didn't understand what he was trying to say". For him, when he says, "Here's the order", his mind has already processed the whole sequence of events and he's very clear about the end result of having the order fulfilled. The staff, however, needed more instructions on the specifics before they could carry out his instructions. In his words, "My thoughts jump. My sequence would be something like 1,3,7,8,10 when, for other people, it would be 1,2,3,4,5,6,7,8,9,10."

After some years of his business growing in spite of all the frustrations and anger, his wife Carrie decided to step in to help him. It was only nine years ago, at the age of 47, that Gary discovered what had been plaguing him all these years. When he and his wife Carrie made a presentation of their educational toys to Mr Kevin Smith at DAS, Kevin recognised immediately that Gary was dyslexic. With Carrie's corroboration of Gary's symptoms, Kevin confirmed the diagnosis on the spot.

In the early days after the diagnosis, Gary was quite

uncertain about how the general public would view dyslexics. He used to explain to clients that he was "abnormal" because he wasn't sure they'd understand what dyslexia was, and the people would end up reacting negatively. Now, he uses the "D" word quite openly, and Carrie is always there to run interference should the need arise.

Business dealings have become quite formulaic. In the current setup, Gary is the front man who welcomes customers and introduces the products. Carrie is the one who will help each customer to pick out the items they need and will then filter the information to the staff. If Gary has to communicate with the staff, he will often use paper and pen to draw the steps he needs done. With more junior staff, he will just keep things brief and short.

Even speech can be a problem if a person speaks too quickly. "I used to think I was having these difficulties because I was Chinese educated," Gary said. But fortunately, with his wife working alongside him, she's able to discern those parts of a conversation that he would have difficulties understanding and would then "translate" for him. Now things are easier, because he's aware of his problem and will ask for help.

In the days when Gary used to go out to make sales calls or to make purchases, he would end up having a lot of small notes and coins in his pocket by the end of the day. It was just easier for him, when there

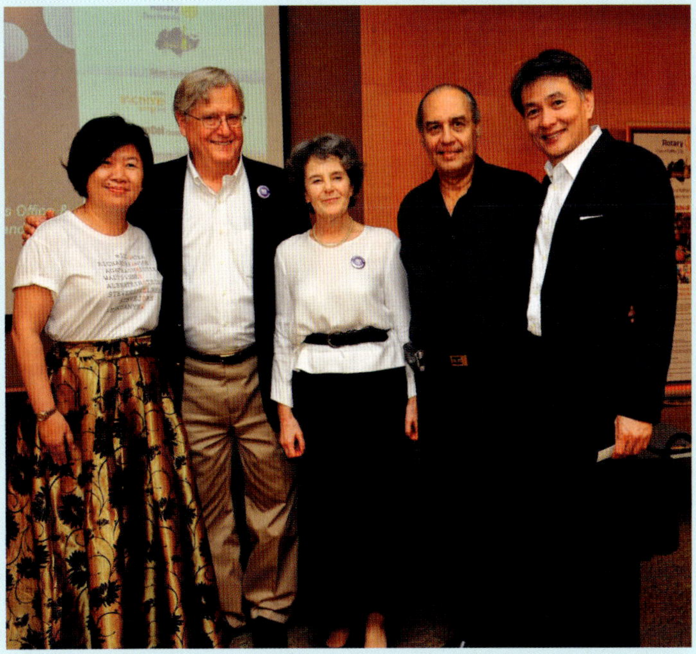

At the Embrace Dyslexia Dinner held in November 2014, pictured above from left to right, Ms Carrie Chan, Mr Thomas G. West, Mrs Margaret West, Dr Jimmy Daruwalla and Mr Gary Seow.

were money transactions, to give a big note and receive change in return, rather than have to count out the right amount because the numbers would stump him and he wouldn't be able to react fast enough. What would take others one second to process or decide would take him ten. This challenge continues to haunt him till this day.

Now KYDZ International has two showrooms and one warehouse that they have fully paid up for. They export to Indonesia, Thailand, Vietnam, and the Philippines. Malaysians tend to just come down south to make their purchases. Gary is also the poster boy for dyslexia in Indonesia and is often invited by the founder of the Dyslexia Association of Indonesia to gives talks. This also gives him an opportunity to sell his products, many of which he now designs and manufactures.

KYDZ International has diversified, in a sense, and now also services the eldercare sector. They recently recognised that many of their educational toys can also help those grappling with the onset of dementia. So they now supply many of the nursing homes and daycare centres for the elderly with games and toys that aid in motor and memory skills. Gary and Carrie are thankful that they can play a meaningful part in the community and are in a position to enjoy the fruits of their labour. Yet, when asked how he felt about having come this far, he covers his face and says, with his voice breaking, "When I look back, I cry".

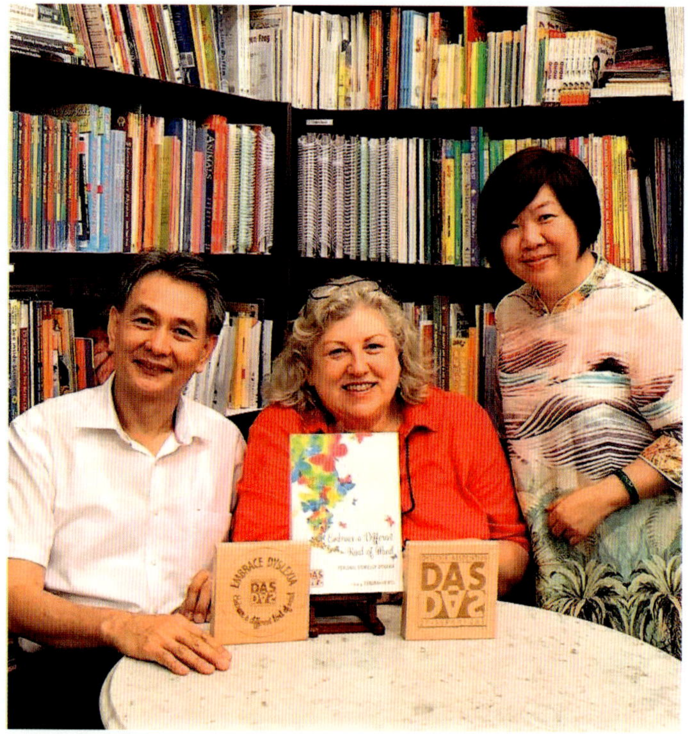

Above: (L to R) Mr Gary Seow; Mrs Deborah Hewes, Editor of Embrace a Different Kind of Mind, *and DAS Head of Publicity and Publications; and Ms Carrie Chan.*

Below: Some of Gary's wood products that he designs and manufactures

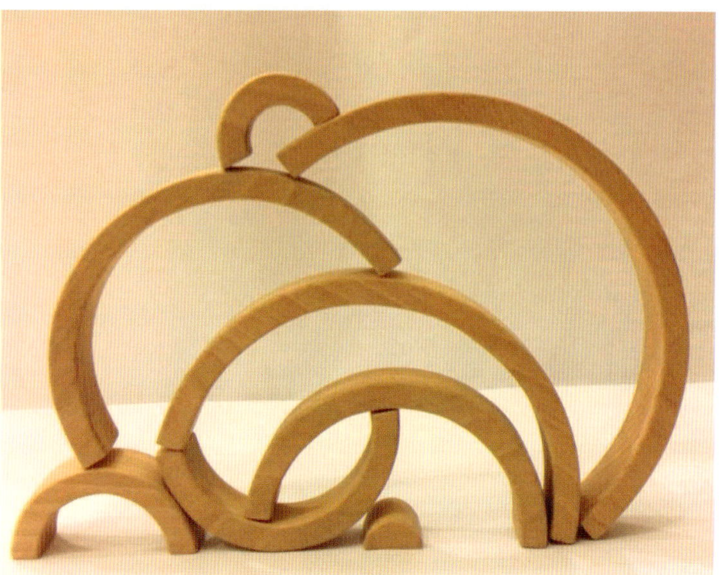

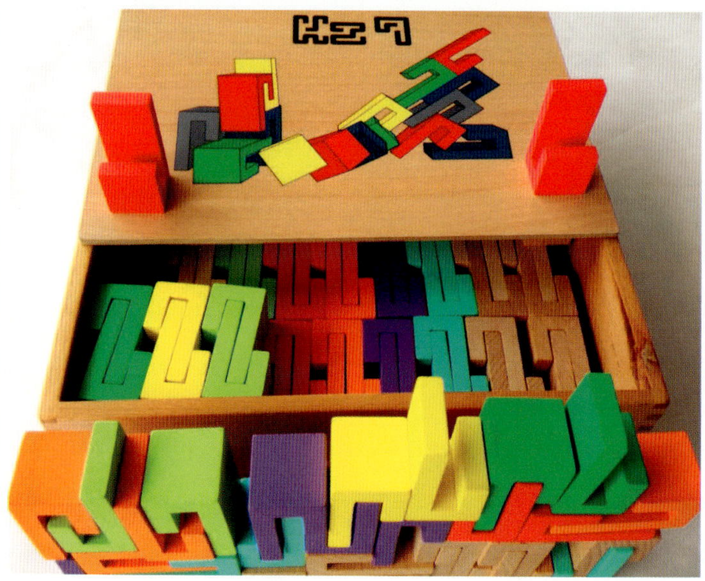

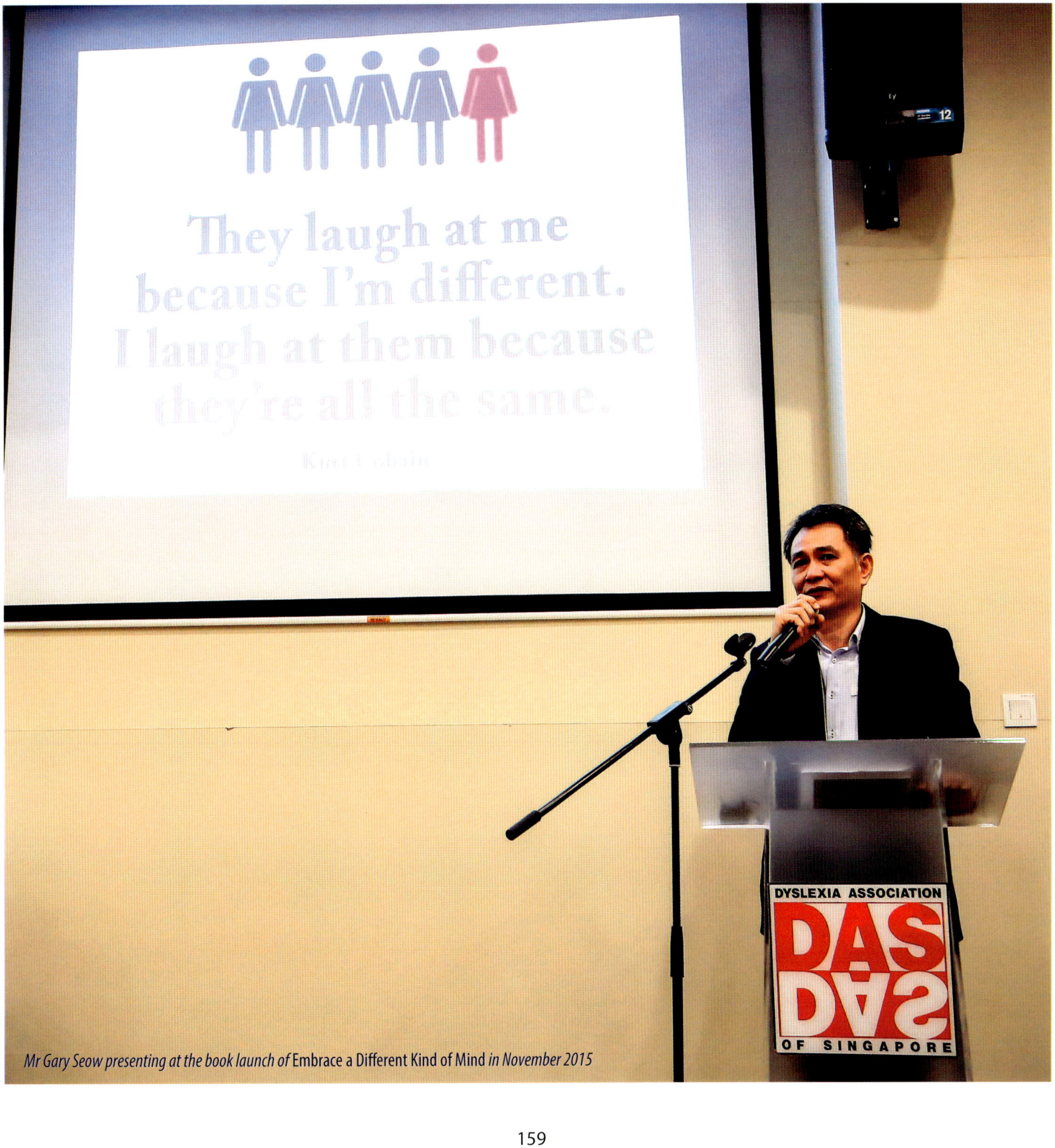

Mr Gary Seow presenting at the book launch of Embrace a Different Kind of Mind *in November 2015*

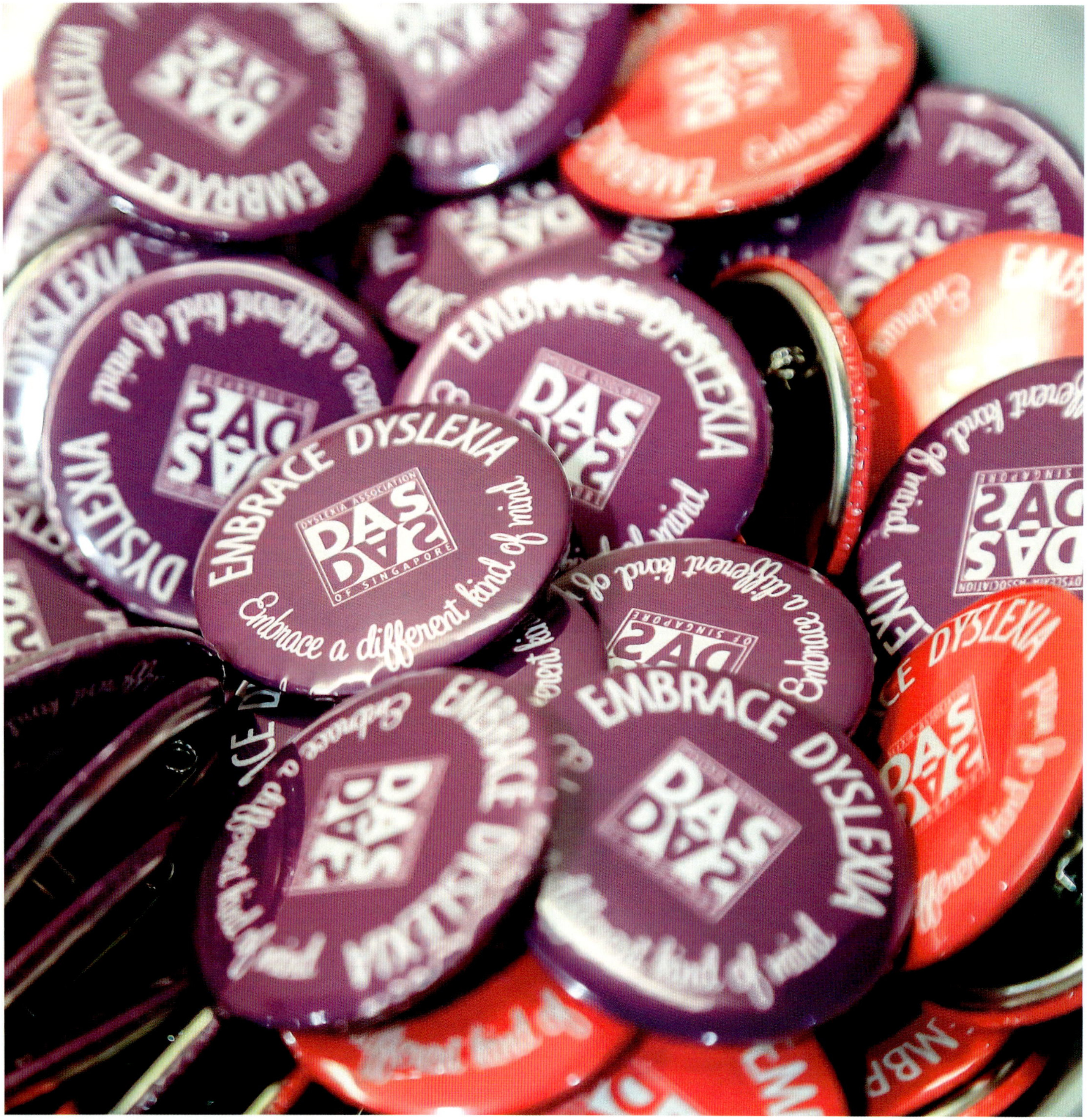
EMBRACE DYSLEXIA
DYSLEXIA ASSOCIATION
DAS
OF SINGAPORE
Embrace a different kind of mind

HOW CAN PEOPLE IN THE WORKPLACE HELP?

Be an Embrace Dyslexia Advocate in your workplace! We are seeking companies who are willing to make their workplace a friendly environment for people with learning differences. What this means is that your company makes a commitment to Embrace Dyslexia in the following ways:

1	**RAISE AWARENESS FOR EMBRACE DYSLEXIA BY:** Sharing information about dyslexia in the workplace; Inviting DAS to conduct Awareness Talks and Including information about dyslexia in the staff handbook.
2	**EXPLORE OPPORTUNITIES TO WORK WITH THE DYSLEXIA ASSOCIATION OF SINGAPORE BY:** Workplace giving or Volunteering initiatives and Mentoring DAS Alumni for internships or work experience.
3	**CHAMPION DYSLEXIC INDIVIDUALS BY:** Recognising their strengths and understanding their weaknesses and Providing appropriate support and encouragement.
4	**DONATE TO DAS PROGRAMMES** To help low-income families with bursaries. www.das.org.sg/donate-to-das
5	**ADVOCATE FOR EMBRACE DYSLEXIA BY SIGNING THE EMBRACE DYSLEXIA COMMITMENT** Please contact us at info@das.org.sg and we will mail you an Embrace Dyslexia Pack.

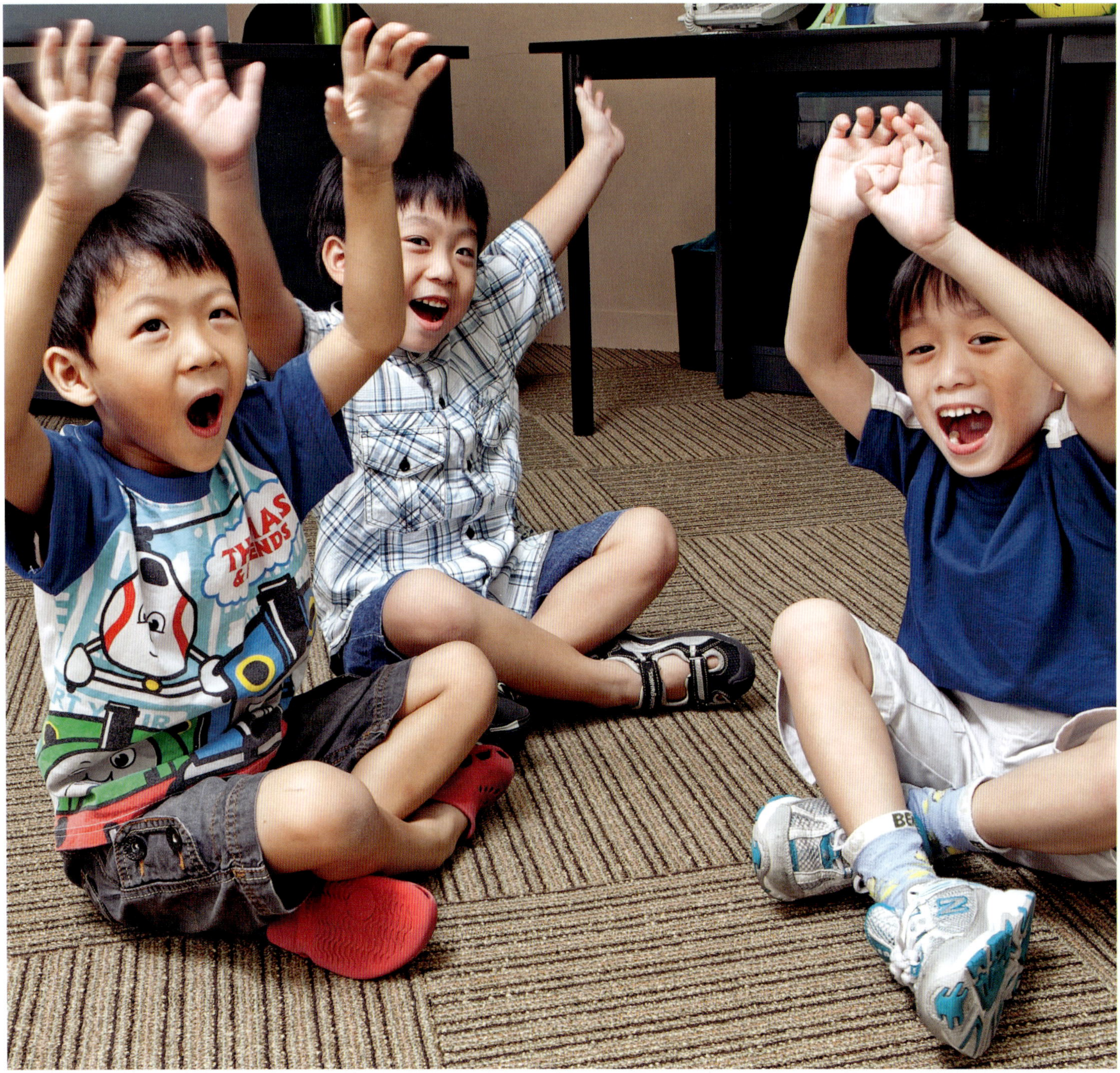

8

TO INFINITY AND BEYOND

We colour the world,
Not with the darkness of our pasts,
But with the rainbow of our hope.

Jenim Dibie
The Calligraphy of God

MUCH MORE TO DO...

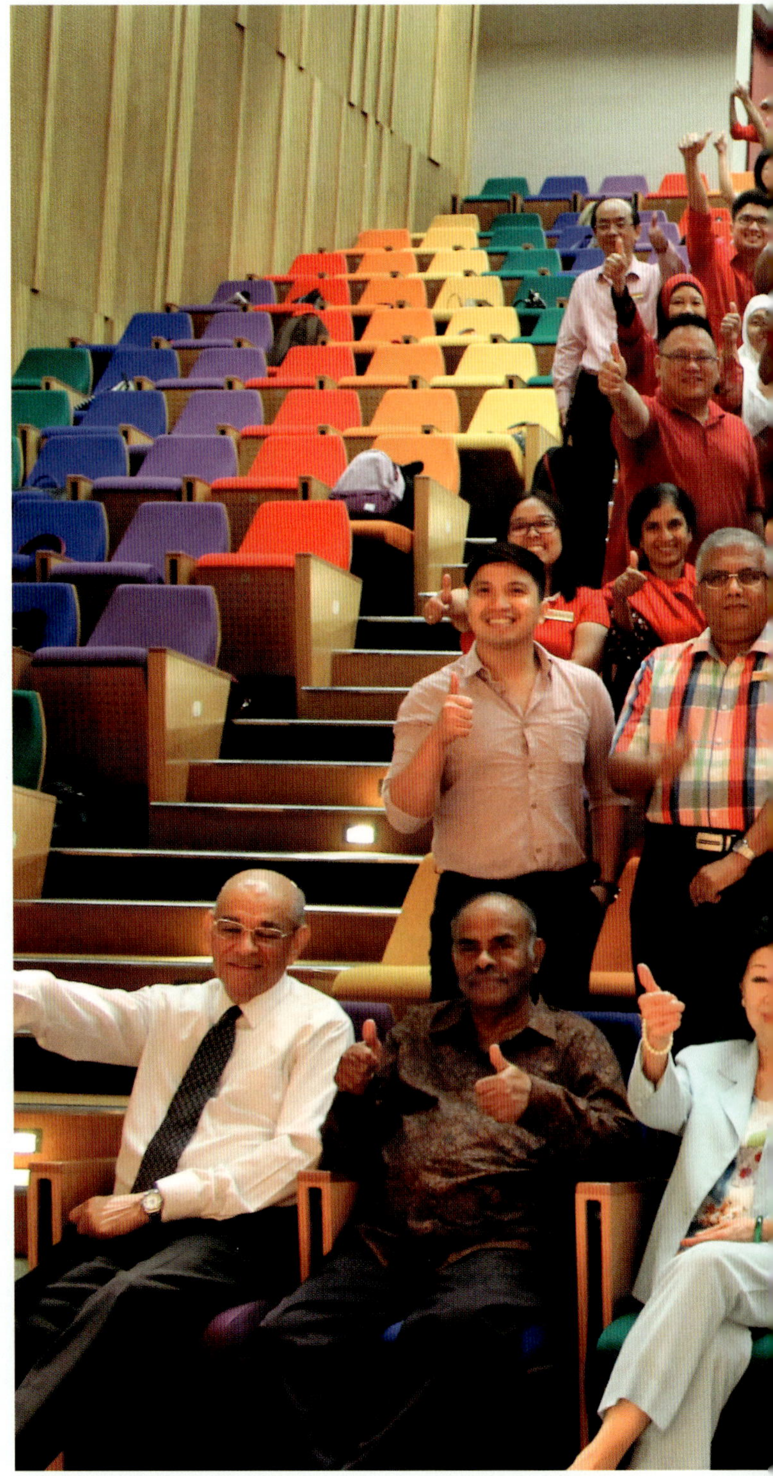

DAS has been given the privilege of helping those whose pasts were shrouded in pain and rejection to reach a place of hope and acceptance. All the stories that you have read in this book give you a flavour of this. But, DAS is not an organisation that rests on its laurels—because, although it has achieved so much, there is yet so much more to do.

In the DAS media release on the occasion of its 25th anniversary, CEO Lee Siang wrote, "From humble beginnings, DAS has spread its wings over the years, growing in stature and significance by keeping our focus on helping people with dyslexia and specific learning differences to achieve their potential. In this 25th year, we want to thank all our partners and our staff for their unstinting dedication and commitment that have made this momentous milestone possible. At the same time, we are forward-focused and will forge ahead to provide even more comprehensive support to individuals with specific learning differences."

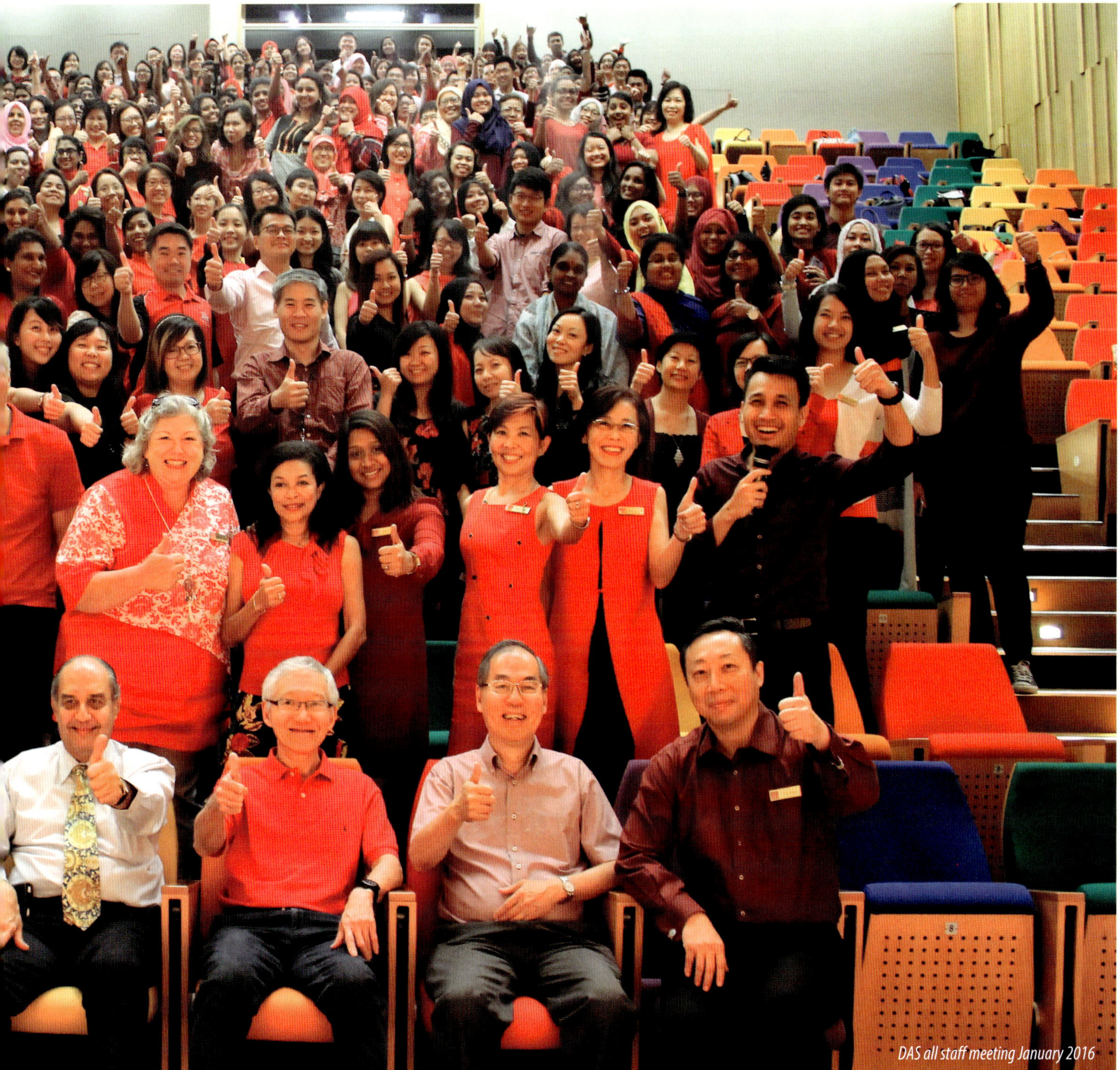

DAS all staff meeting January 2016

BUILDING EXPERTISE FOR THE FUTURE

Positioning itself to be on the cutting age to meet the needs of the future, DAS invests in its educators. In the last two years, DAS has begun to focus on specialist certification for its teaching staff.

While the DAS Academy provides the bulk of the training, there are areas where expertise is lacking. The teaching of Chinese is one area where DAS sends its staff to other local institutions to receive their training. Consultants, like the former Head of the Chinese Curriculum Department in MOE, have been brought in where necessary.

All the teachers of Chinese are now required to obtain the Chinese-teaching diplomas. There are now over 30 people attending math certificate training as DAS strengthens its proficiency in the teaching of maths.

Speech therapy is another important area for DAS to develop further. To that end, DAS set up two scholarships in January 2017 for the NUS speech and language pathology Master degree. The DAS speech and language therapy programme is unique in that it focuses on education. DAS therapists are the only ones working outside the purview of the Ministry of Health.

DAS is encouraging more of its teachers to take up the Masters programme so that they can be equipped to conduct curriculum development and research work. Several teachers are being sponsored by DAS to pursue their Masters degrees,

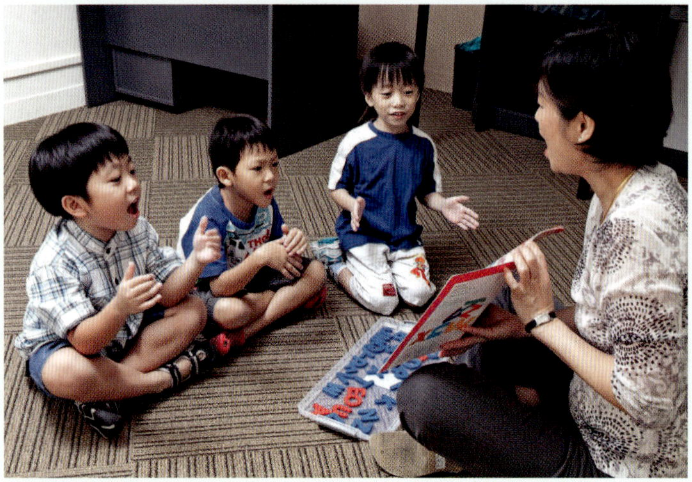

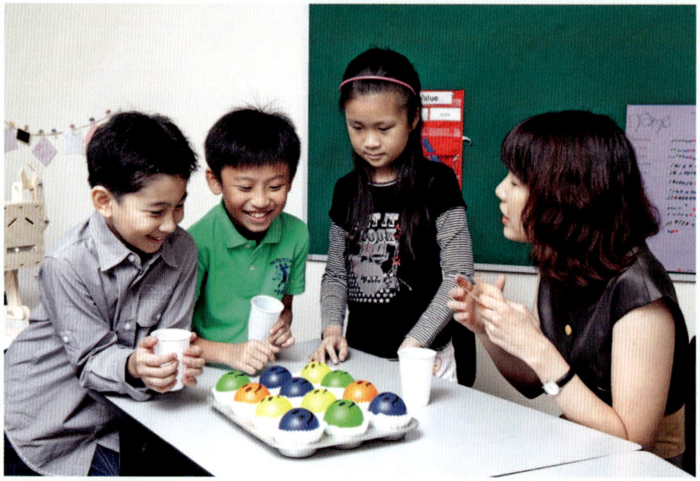

including a candidate for the Masters in Mathematics at NIE and another in Chinese in a joint NUS-Hong Kong University programme.

As there is a constant need for specialist psychologists, DAS has placed five psychologists in the Master in Educational Psychology programme. They will be returning over the next two to three years.

The graduate level of training for psychologists reflects the advances made in the area of assessment service. Previously, graduate specialist psychologists in DAS mainly assessed and diagnosed dyslexia. Since 2016, DAS psychologists have been offering assessment services to clients in a range of learning differences.

These are exciting times, and DAS is on the cusp of exponential growth. Some of its younger managers are in their mid-30s. The fact that they have the opportunity to create something of great significance that is unique in the world is incredible.

Referring to one of the maths teachers in training, DAS CEO Mr Lee Siang said, "If she gets the right qualifications, the right experience, and publishes the right papers, in 10 years' time, she'll be trotting around Asia as the expert in mathematics for dyslexia." That's the kind of opportunity that will be available to her. And many similar opportunities are being given to other DAS staff members.

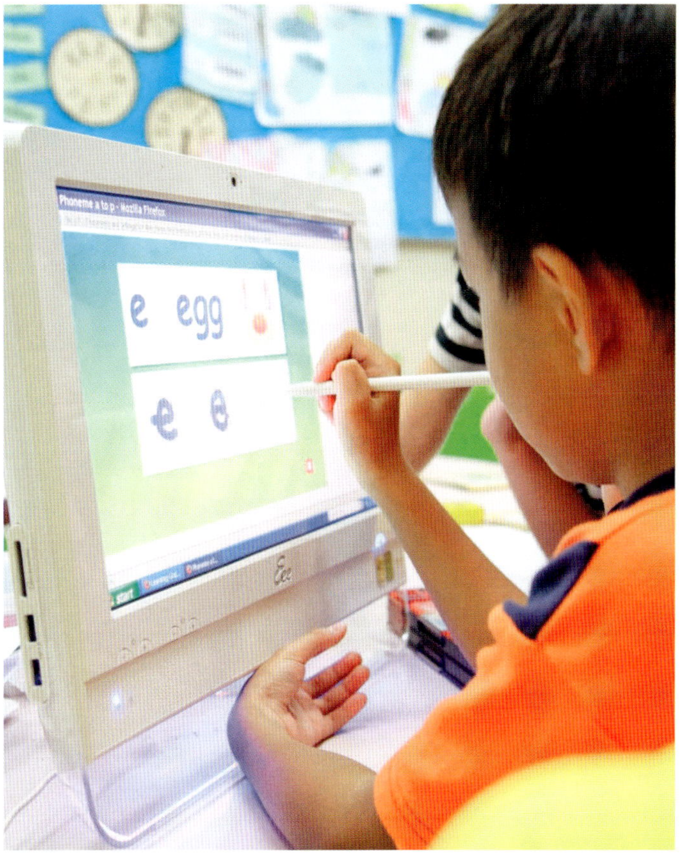

HARNESSING TECHNOLOGY

DAS will also be rolling out a computerised curriculum-based assessment. Developed by an in -house team, the software programme will greatly enhance the monitoring process on the progress of 3,000 DAS students and counting. This is something unique in the world as DAS is the pioneer of this assessment system.

Great excitement is also brewing over developments in the math programme with the launch of the problem sums math curriculum. Previously, DAS only delivered classes in essential math. The new addition of a problem sums math curriculum will help Primary 5 and Primary 6 students to be more successful in PSLE mathematics. That is a huge contribution to the standards of math education in Singapore. As Singapore is highly regarded for its math education by the world, we expect our dyslexic students to enjoy the same regard in time to come.

COMMUNITY OF PRACTICE

Recognising also that many different streams come together to help each dyslexic, DAS CEO Lee Siang highlighted the importance of fostering a community of practice, so that all who are involved in caring for dyslexics can come together from different fields, different expertise, and different experiences to share and to learn. Case conferences are particularly suited for facilitating this and DAS will be looking to organise such activities.

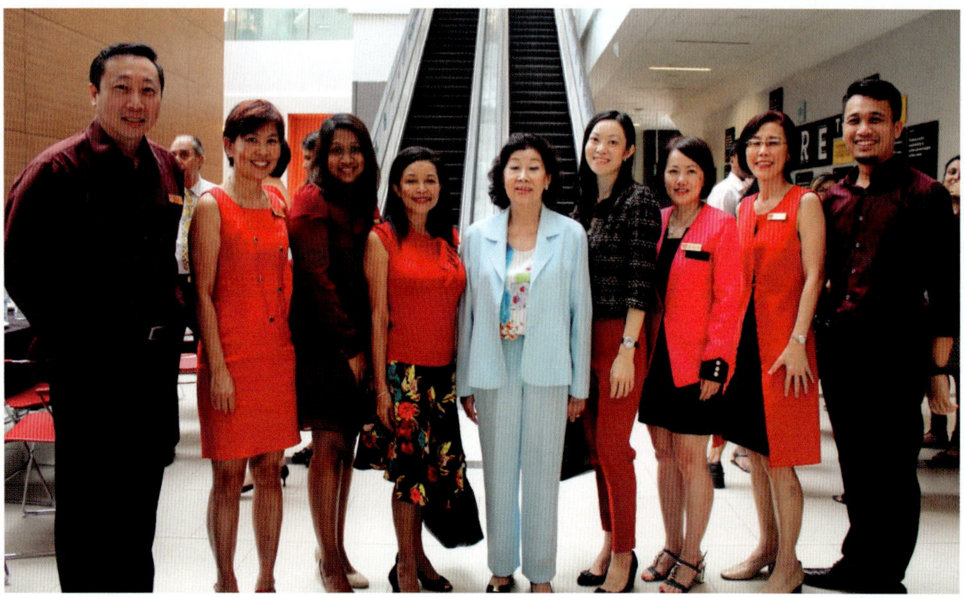

DAS General Management Committee members withMrs Goh Chok Tong in January 2016. (L to R) Mr Lee Siang, DAS CEO; Ms Fanny Foo, Director of Learning Centres and Outreach; Ms Geetha Shantha Ram, Director of MOE-aided DAS Literacy Programme and Staff Professional Development; Ms Anaberta Oehlers-Jaen, Head of DAS International and Programme Director of SES Maths, Specialist Tutoring and Assessments; Mrs Goh Chok Tong, DAS Patron; Ms June Siew, Head of DAS Academy; Ms Chia Soo Chiao, DAS CFO; Ms Quek Gek San, Director of Corporate Services and HR; and Mr Nor Ashraf Bin Samsudin, Director of Specialised Educational Services

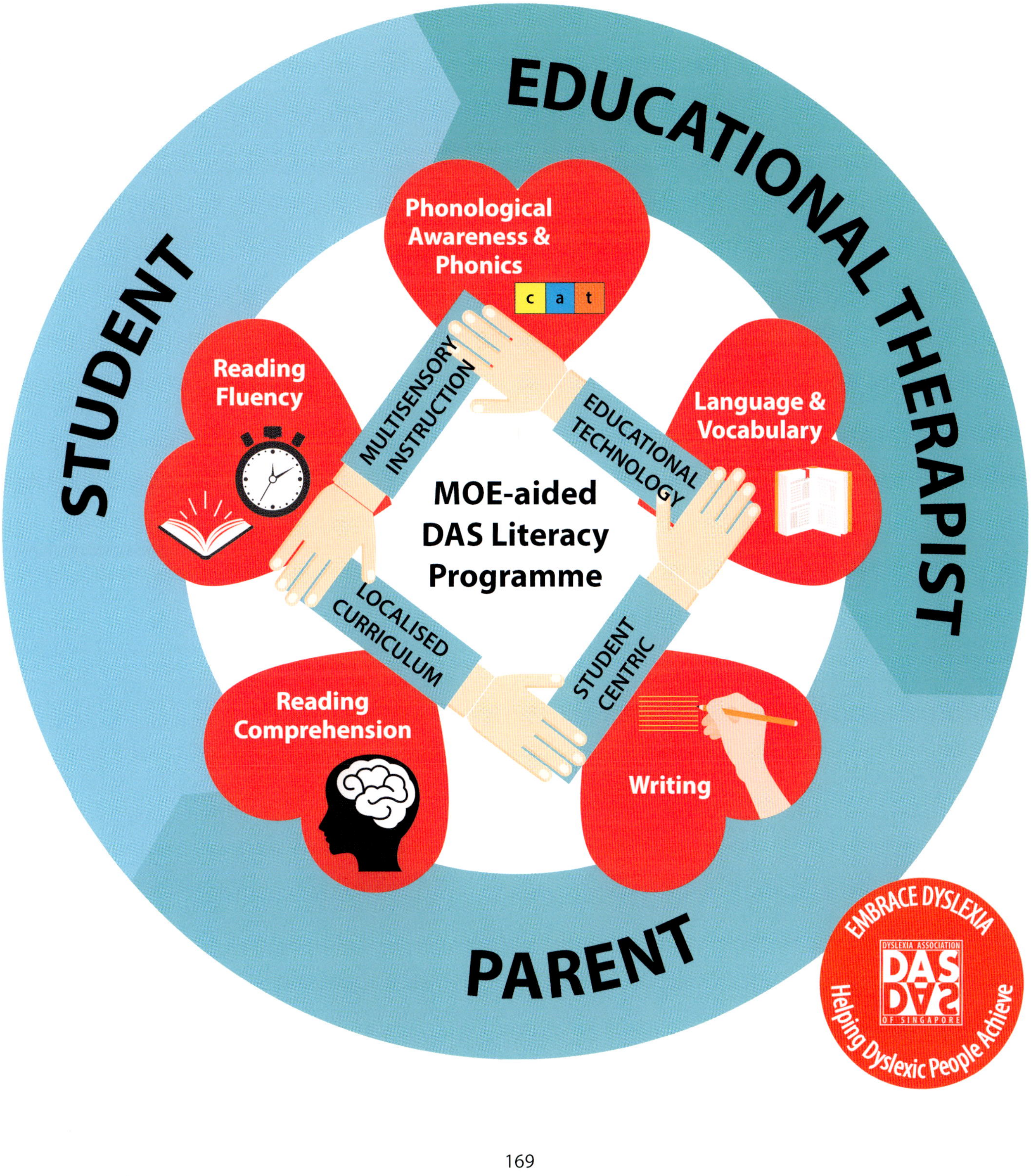
EDUCATIONAL THERAPIST
STUDENT
PARENT
Phonological Awareness & Phonics
c a t
Reading Fluency
Language & Vocabulary
Reading Comprehension
Writing
MULTISENSORY INSTRUCTION
EDUCATIONAL TECHNOLOGY
LOCALISED CURRICULUM
STUDENT CENTRIC
MOE-aided DAS Literacy Programme
EMBRACE DYSLEXIA
DYSLEXIA ASSOCIATION
DAS
OF SINGAPORE
Helping Dyslexic People Achieve

THE NEXT 25 YEARS

As DAS looks toward the next 25 years, DAS CEO Lee Siang expressed his wish for DAS to "go beyond" five areas!

"First of all, we must go beyond support in basic reading and spelling. Children with dyslexia also need support in higher-order skills such as reading comprehension and essay writing. DAS has now added a new writing component and additional reading comprehension content is on its way. This is a natural progression for the DAS's main literacy programme as we expand and improve our curriculum to support dyslexic children in the full range of literacy skills.

Second, DAS must go beyond literacy and the English language. Dyslexics need support in a range of language and academic subjects. We have already initiated Maths, Chinese and Exam Skills programmes designed for dyslexic children. Creating and delivering a wider range of programmes must therefore be a continuing effort of DAS in the coming years.

Third, our support must go beyond academic subjects. We must help our dyslexic clients build on their strengths and talents. Our Speech and Drama Arts programme designed for dyslexic children to boost their confidence and speaking skills is a good example of such a programme. Results have been most encouraging. We are examining how best to provide other non-academic and talent programmes to help dyslexic children develop into productive adults and find employment in industries where they can excel.

Fourth, we must go beyond the current age group we serve. We have always worked with primary and secondary school students. We have started with preschoolers only fairly recently. We are in the process of providing a support programme for post-secondary students and students in institutes of higher learning. It will be a logical next step for us to also provide for those in tertiary education and in the workforce.

Last but not least, we must go beyond just dyslexia. That many dyslexic children have accompanying Specific Learning Differences such as ADHD, Dyspraxia, Dyscalculia, Speech and Language Impairment, etc., is well recognised. DAS must therefore also help our children overcome these issues over and above their dyslexia.

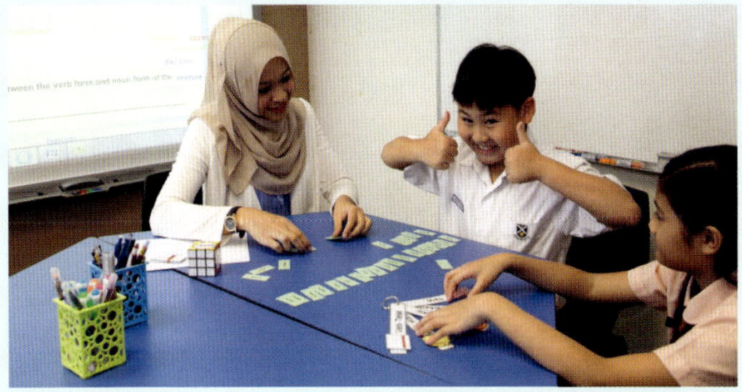

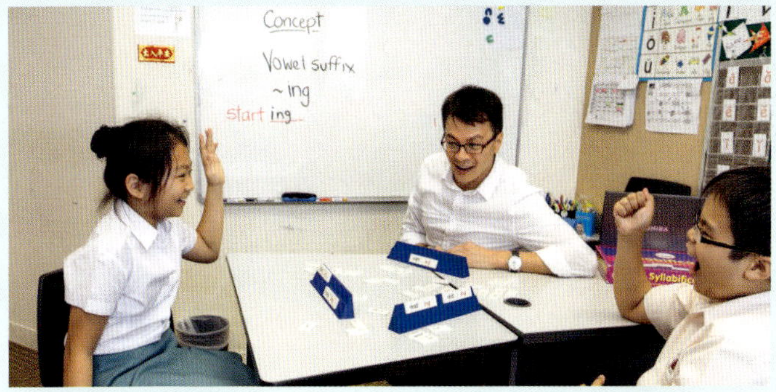

And to help us "go beyond" these five areas, DAS must continue to do two things: We must continue to invest in and develop the professional capability of our staff to deliver high-quality programmes and services. It is also the objective of DAS to build a pool of expertise in dyslexia here in Singapore! The training arm of DAS, DAS Academy, which now delivers programmes up to Masters level, will help us achieve this.

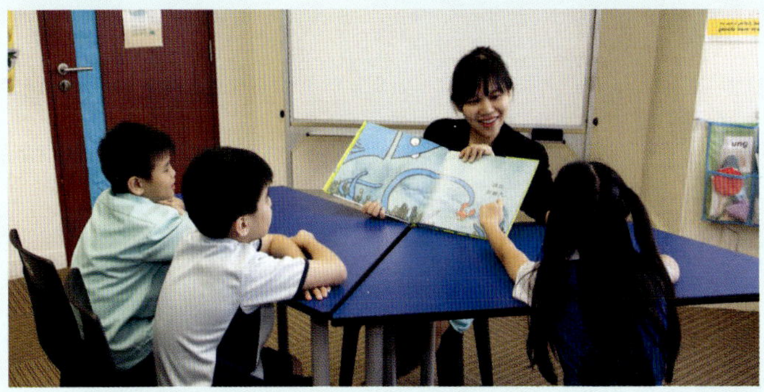

We must also continue to invest in programme evaluation and publish research to ensure that our programmes and services are effective and reliable.

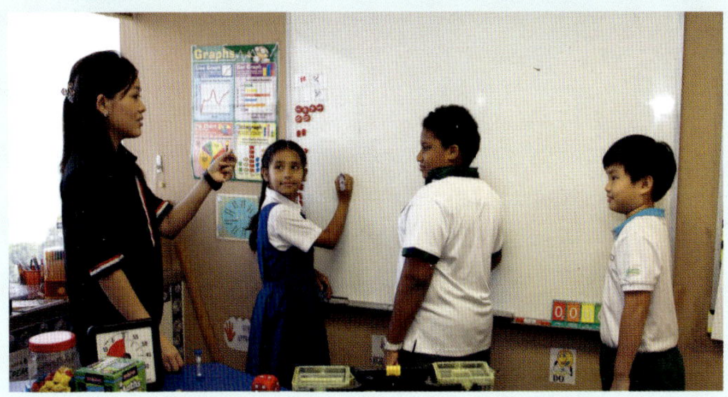

So, as you can see, DAS will continue to be very busy in the next 25 years. We look to the continuing support of the Ministry of Education and all stakeholders to help us achieve our goal of providing a truly comprehensive and holistic range of programmes for our dyslexic clients and bring DAS to a new level."

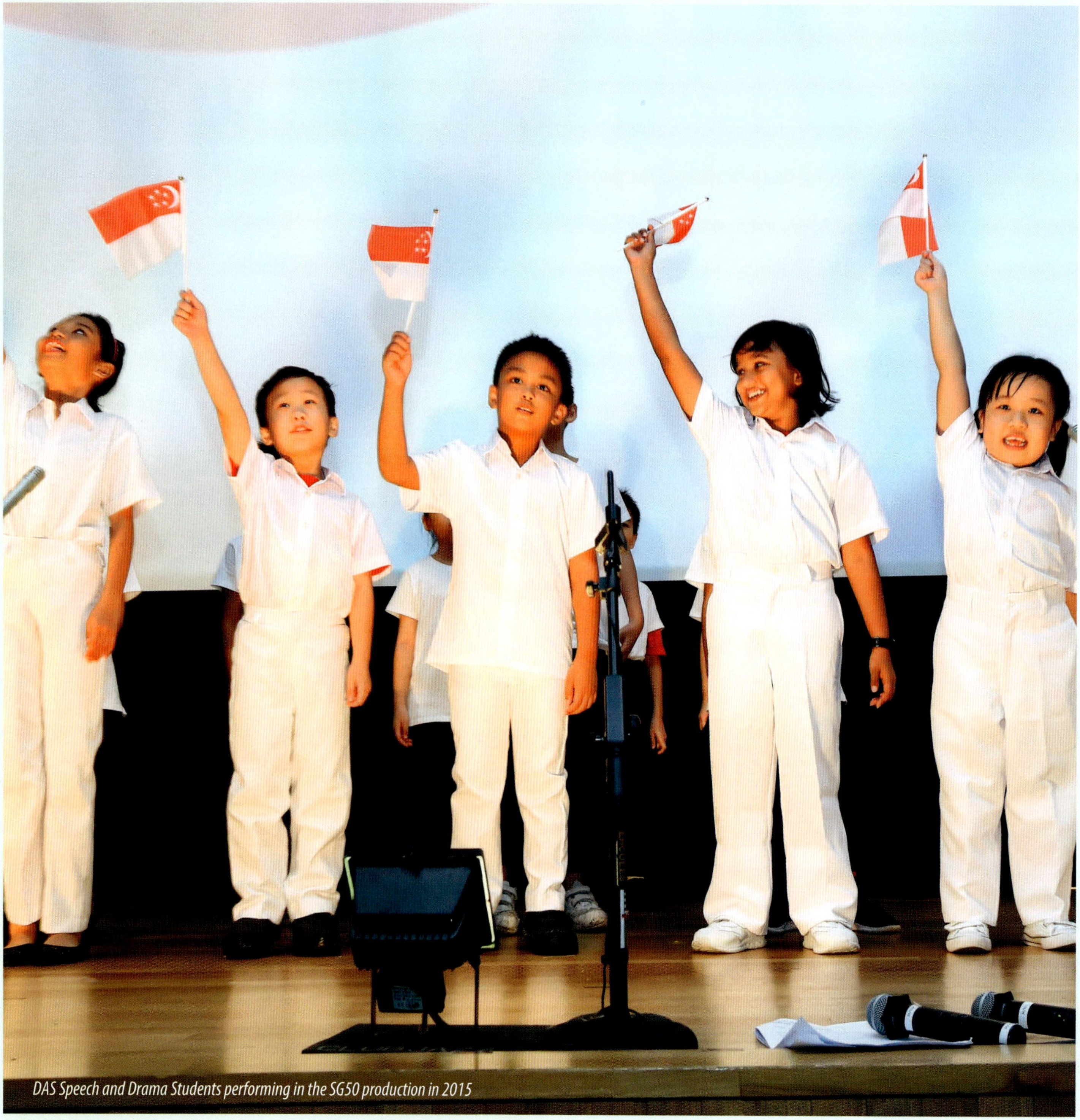

DAS Speech and Drama Students performing in the SG50 production in 2015

CONGRATULATIONS

The reward for work well done is the opportunity to do more.

Jonas Salk

Polio Vaccine creator

CONGRATULATIONS

KOH KOK KHAI

It is with great pleasure that I am writing this message to congratulate the Dyslexia Association of Singapore (DAS) on your 25th Anniversary!

The partnership between the Ministry of Education and DAS, which started in 1995, to provide support for students with dyslexia in our mainstream schools has come a long way. Currently, DAS conducts dyslexia-related training for MOE's Allied Educators (Learning and Behavioural Support), and a dyslexia remediation programme, the MOE-aided DAS Literacy Programme (MAP), for mainstream students. DAS currently runs the MAP in 13 Learning Centres, serving about 3,500 students. This complements MOE's efforts to support students with dyslexia through the School-based Dyslexia Remediation programme that has been made available to all primary schools since 2016. As MOE builds the capacity of our teachers in dyslexia support, we continue to value DAS' partnership in providing additional support for our students.

It has been our pleasure to work with the professional and dedicated staff members of DAS and to witness your significant 25th anniversary milestone. We wish DAS the very best for your future ventures.

With best wishes,

Mr Koh Kok Khai
Director, Psychological Services
Education Services Division
Ministry of Education

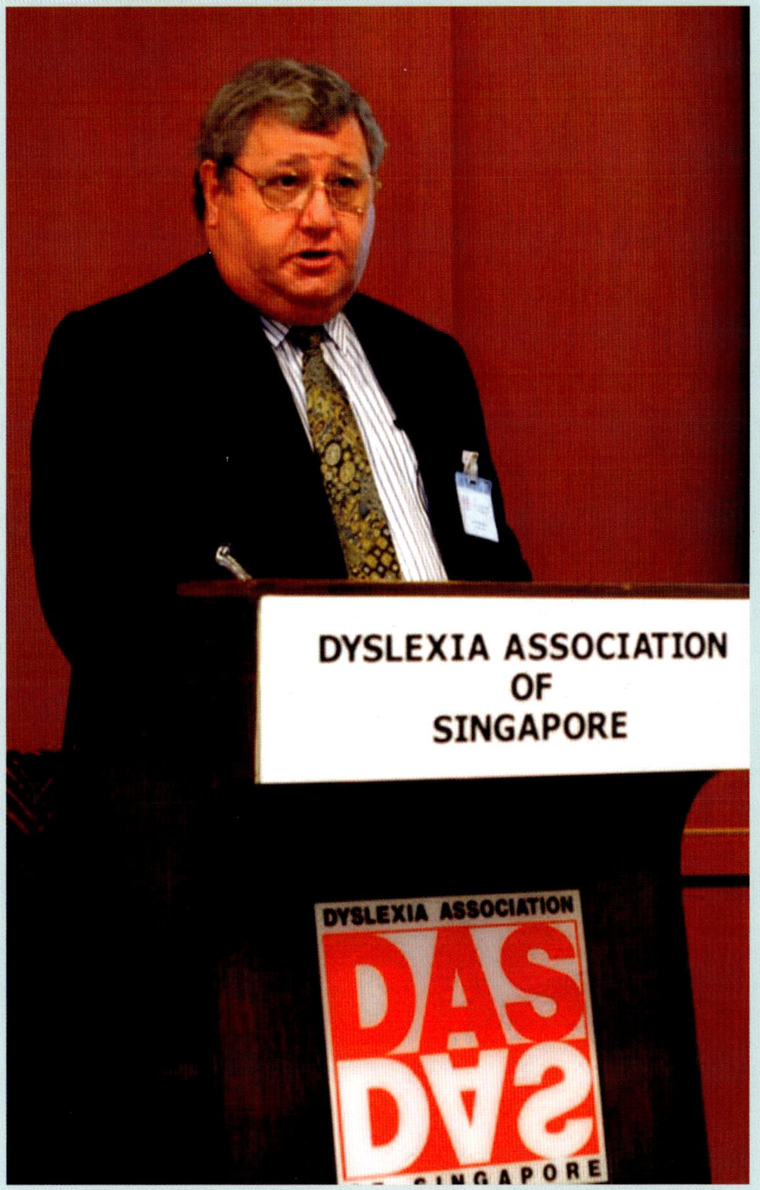

ROBIN MOSELEY

My congratulations to the whole DAS family for making the DAS the success it is today.

I look back on my years with the DAS as EXCO member, part-time Executive Director and finally as full-time CEO some of the most satisfying of my career. It was a privilege to be associated with the DAS for so many years and a huge pleasure to work with so many talented and hard-working individuals.

Now in my retirement, I am very happy in the knowledge that DAS is continuing to thrive and, most importantly, providing the best possible service to the dyslexic population of Singapore.

Congratulations on making it to 25 years of age. I am looking forward to celebrating DAS's 50th birthday!

Best wishes,

Mr Robin Moseley
Former CEO, DAS (2012 – 2014)

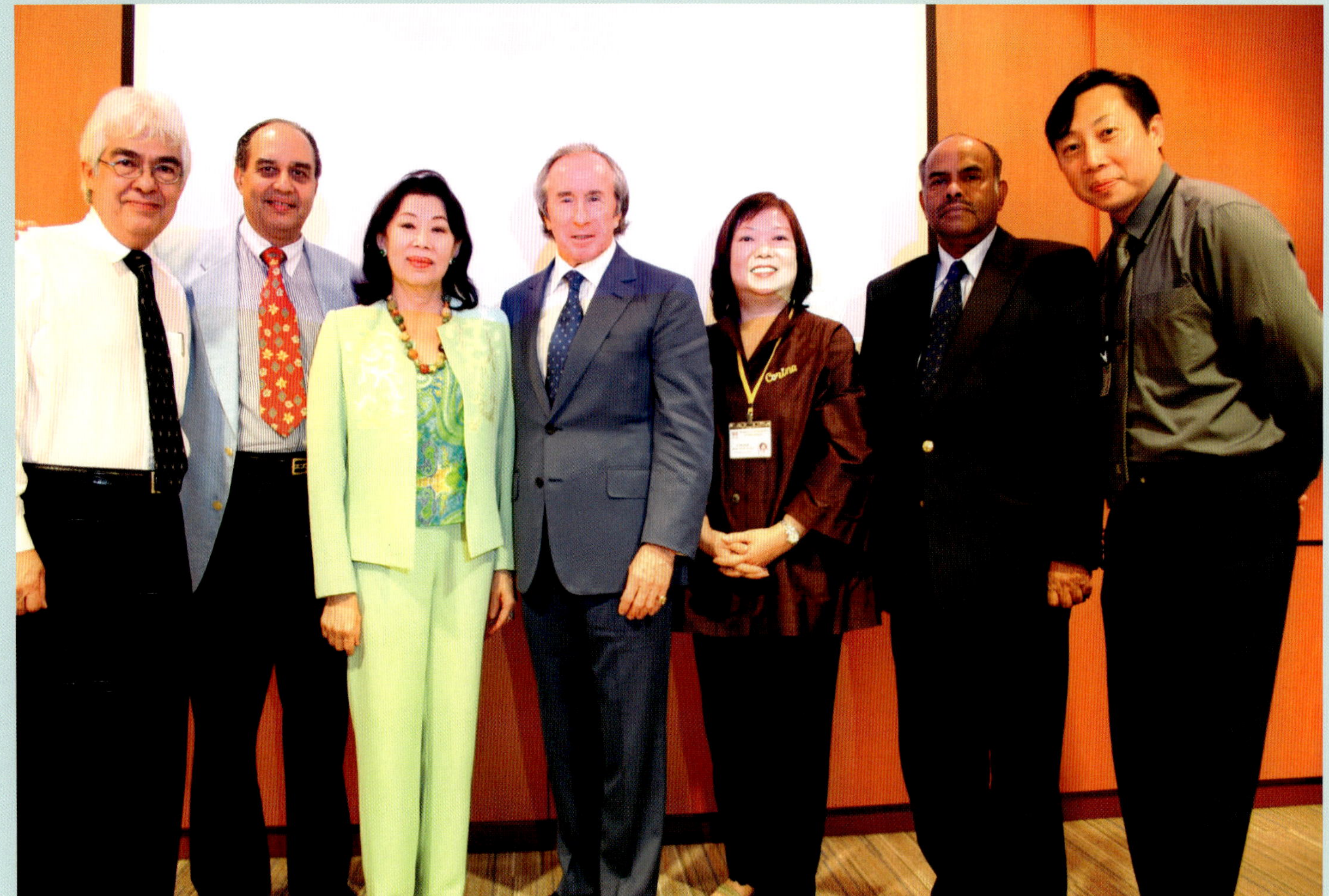

Sir Jackie Stewart visited DAS in 2007, at that time he announced that "DAS could lead the world in this!" (L to R) Mr Derek McCully, DAS Exco; Dr Jimmy Daruwalla, DAS President; Mrs Goh Chok Tong, DAS Patron; Sir Jackie Stewart,; Mrs Corina Lai, DAS CFO; Mr Kesavapany, DAS Exco; and Mr Lee Siang, DAS COO.

Right: Sir Jackie Stewart autographs a model F1 car for a DAS student.

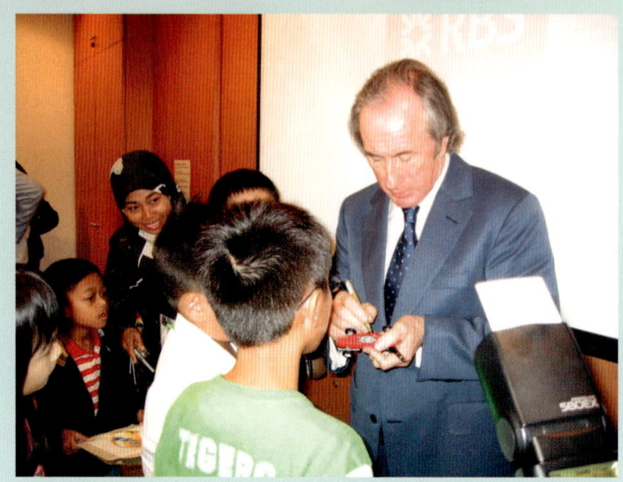

SIR JACKIE STEWART

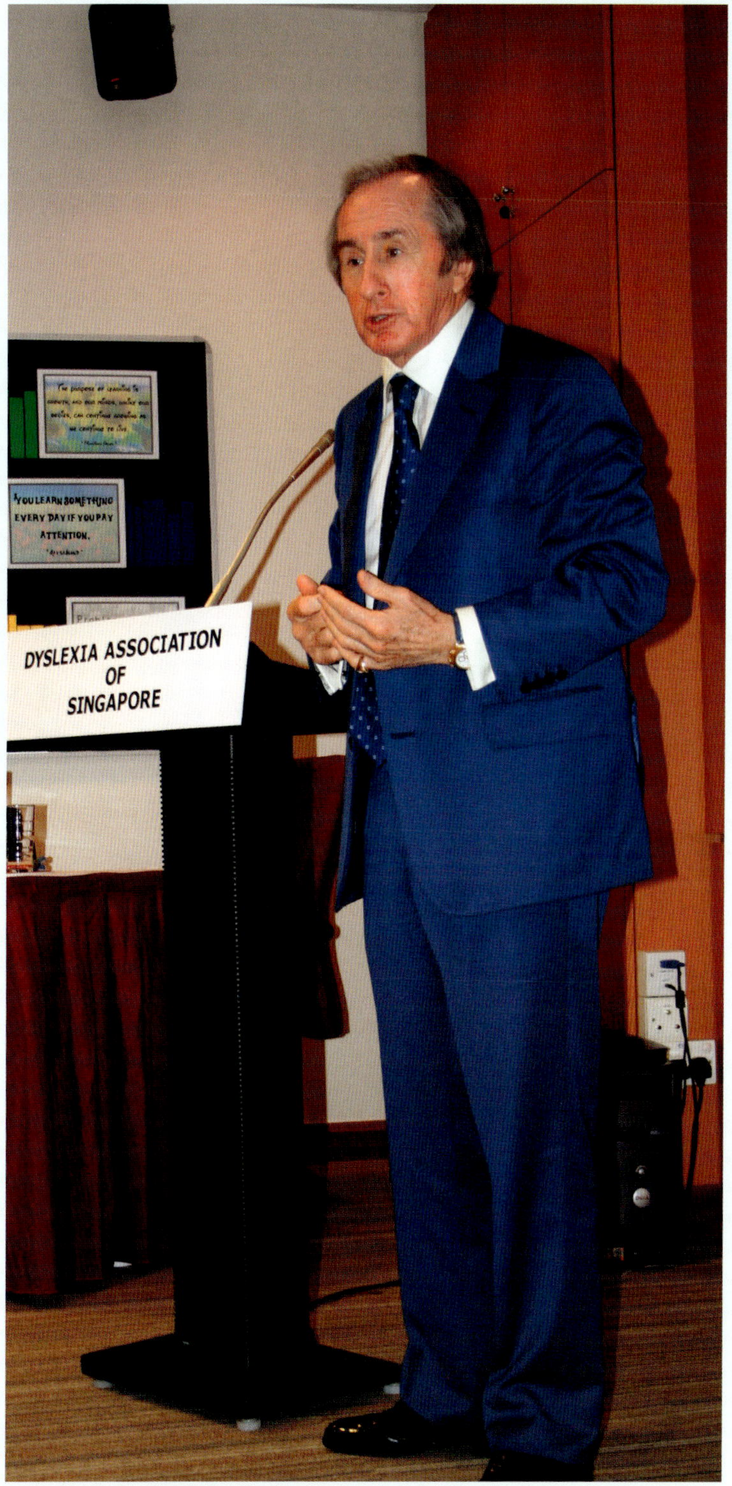
DYSLEXIA ASSOCIATION
OF
SINGAPORE
YOU LEARN SOMETHING EVERY DAY IF YOU PAY ATTENTION.

I visited Singapore quite a few years ago and met up with Dr Vivian Balakrishnan, the then Minister for Community Development, Youth and Sports, who took me to a unit that looked after delinquent boys and almost every one of them had dyslexia or other forms of learning disabilities and they were therefore in custody. There are many young people who have ended up on the wrong side of the road because their schooling did not look after them and educate them correctly.

Singapore can now be very proud of what, with the assistance of the Government, the Dyslexia Association of Singapore has done over these years.

Many congratulations to all of you.

***Sir John Young Jackie Stewart, OBE**, is a British former Formula One racing driver from Scotland. Nicknamed the "Flying Scot", he won three World Driver's Championships between 1965 and 1973. In 2009 he was ranked 5th of the fifty greatest Formula One drivers of all time by journalist Kevin Eason who wrote: "He has not only emerged as a great driver, but one of the greatest figures of motor racing."*

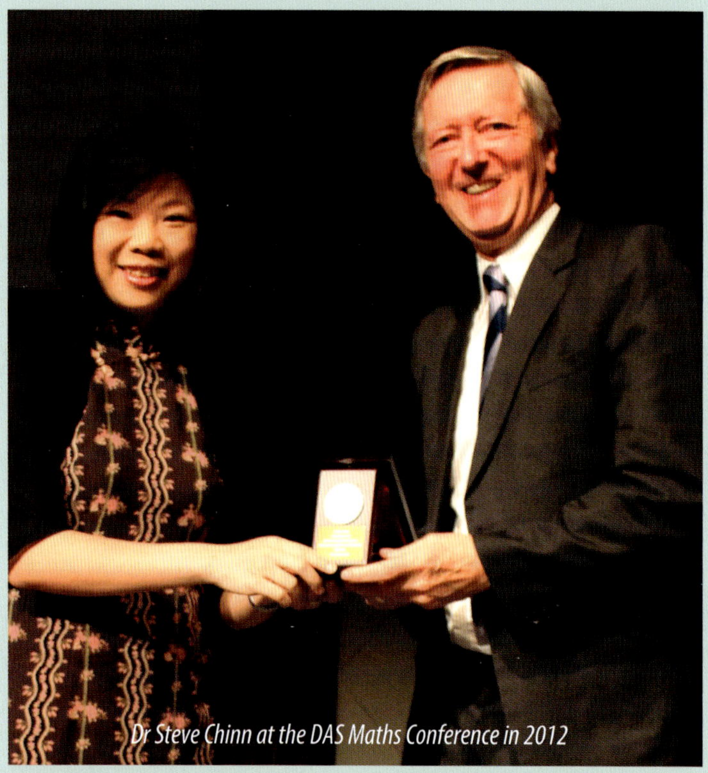

Dr Steve Chinn at the DAS Maths Conference in 2012

DR STEVE CHINN

Many congratulations to DAS. Long may you continue your work in helping so many children and in being such a powerful advocate for all those with dyslexia.

It has been a pleasure and an honour to have been involved with your work, conferences and training and to have met so many of your wonderful team.

Dr Steve Chinn, PhD FRSA
Visiting Professor,
University of Derby, UK

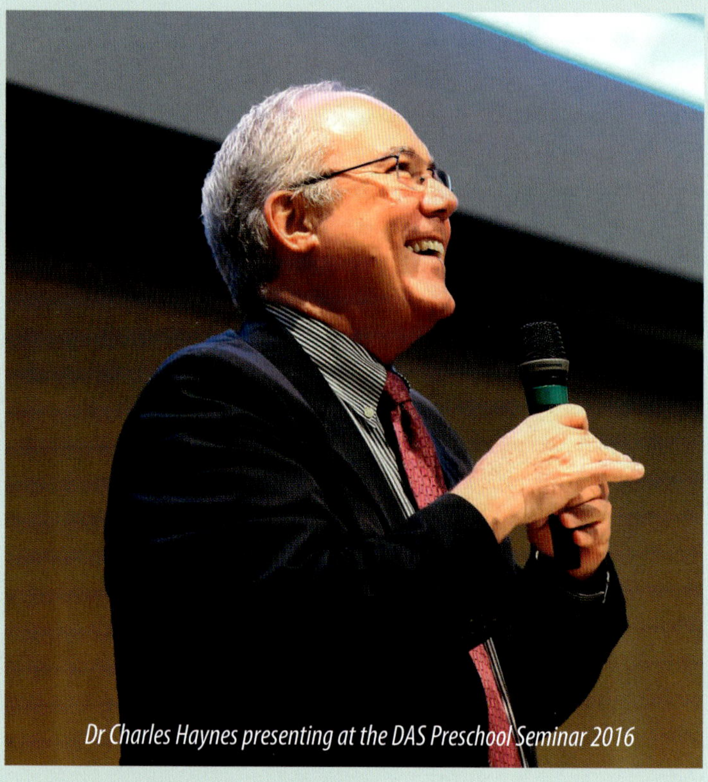

Dr Charles Haynes presenting at the DAS Preschool Seminar 2016

DR CHARLES HAYNES

Happy 25th Anniversary to the Dyslexia Association of Singapore! I am proud to be part of your 'extended family'.

May DAS continue to shine its powerful light of knowledge and caring so that society is transformed and persons with dyslexia and their families may enjoy harmony as well as prosperity.

Dr Charles Haynes, EdD
Professor, MGH Institute of Health Professions
Boston, Massachusetts

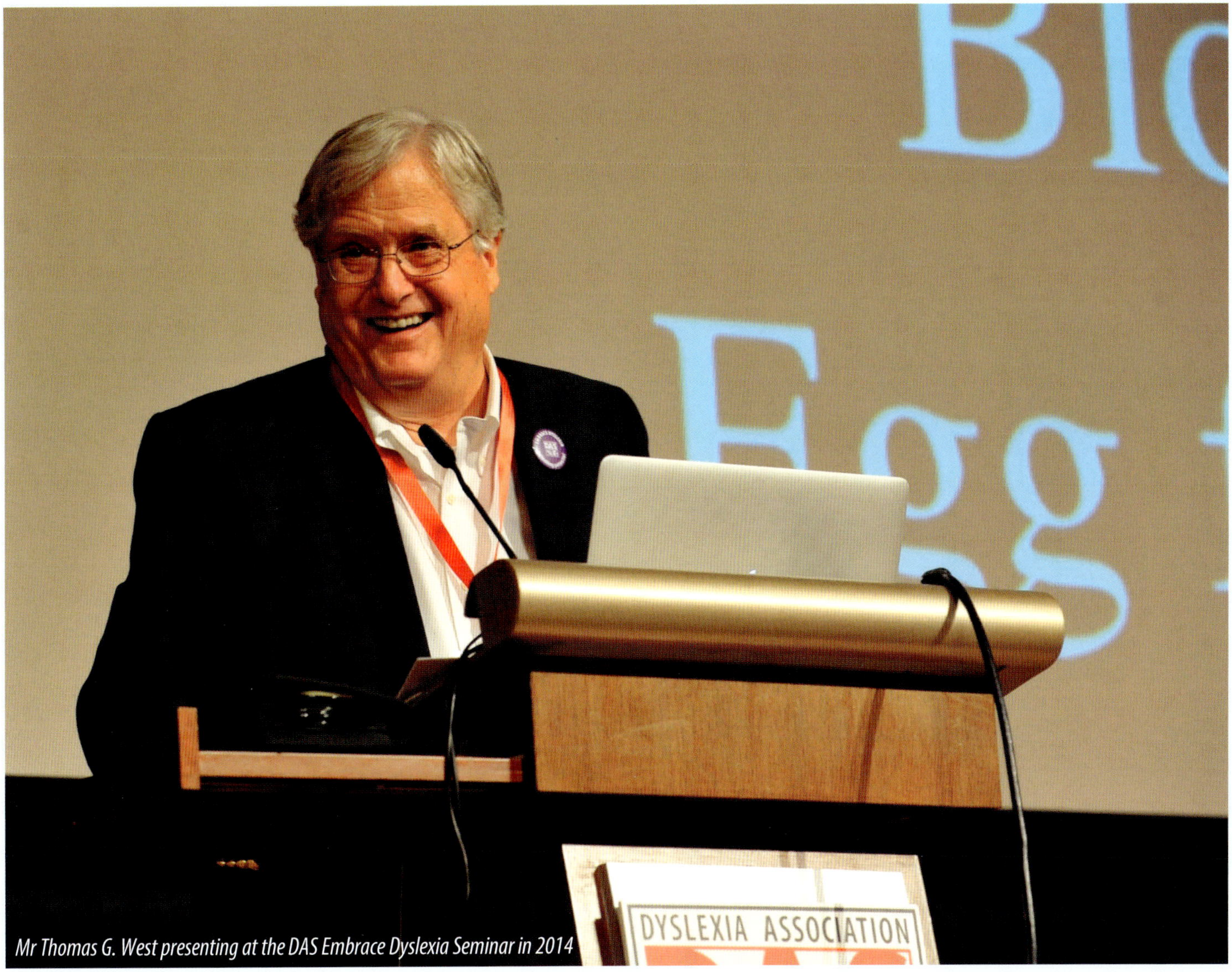

Mr Thomas G. West presenting at the DAS Embrace Dyslexia Seminar in 2014

THOMAS G. WEST

Warm congratulations to DAS at 25! I have been so honoured to be a part of the DAS story. May you long show your light to the world!

Mr Thomas G. West
Author of *Thinking Like Einstein*, *In the Mind's Eye* and *Seeing What Others Cannot See.*

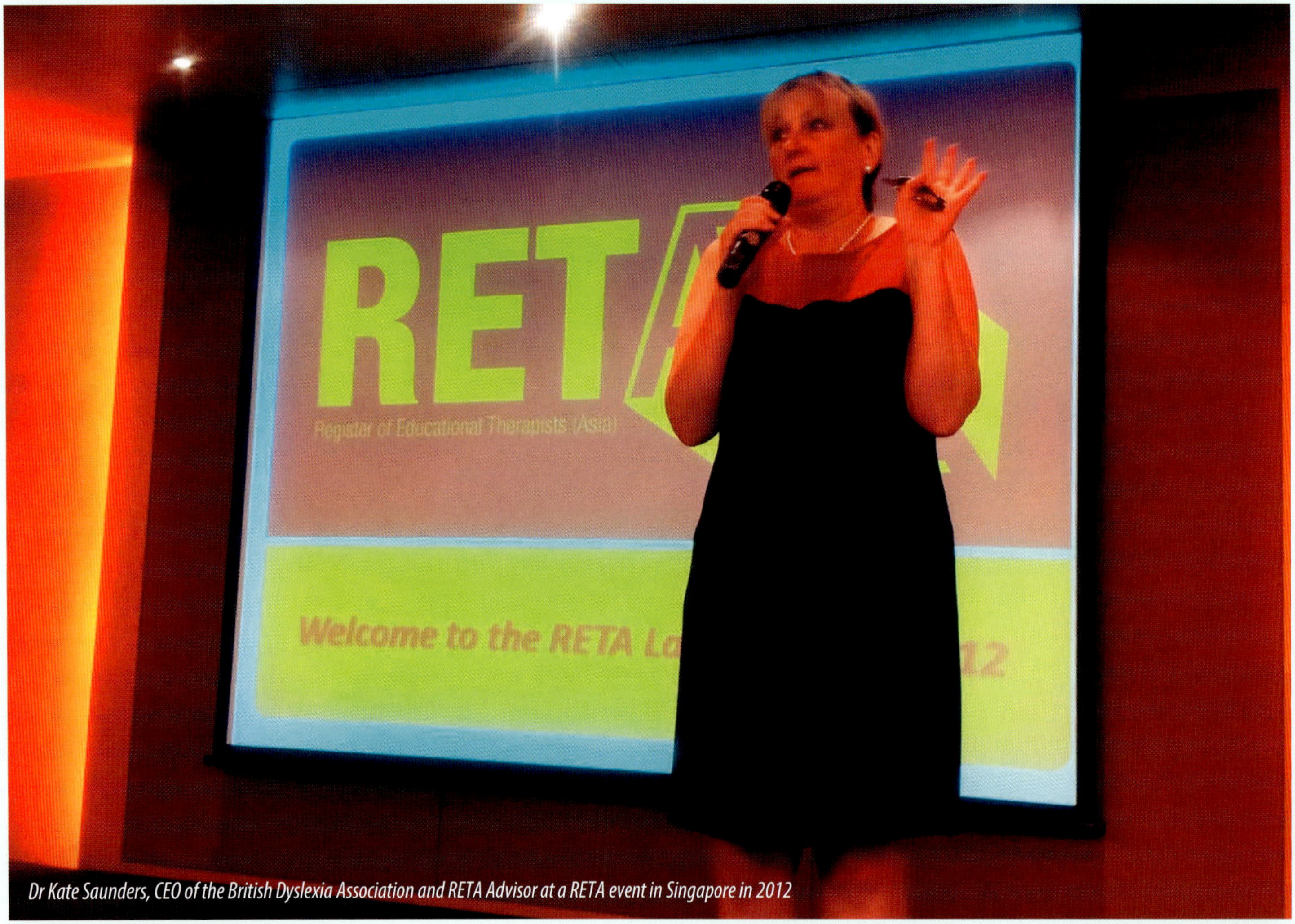

Dr Kate Saunders, CEO of the British Dyslexia Association and RETA Advisor at a RETA event in Singapore in 2012

DR KATE SAUNDERS

Congratulations to DAS on their 25th Anniversary! The British Dyslexia Association congratulates DAS on their work in this field, which goes from strength to strength. We look forward to continued positive collaboration between our organisations, working together to bring about increased awareness and use of Dyslexia Friendly practices, across all age ranges and within all sectors.

Dr Kate Saunders
CEO, British Dyslexia Association

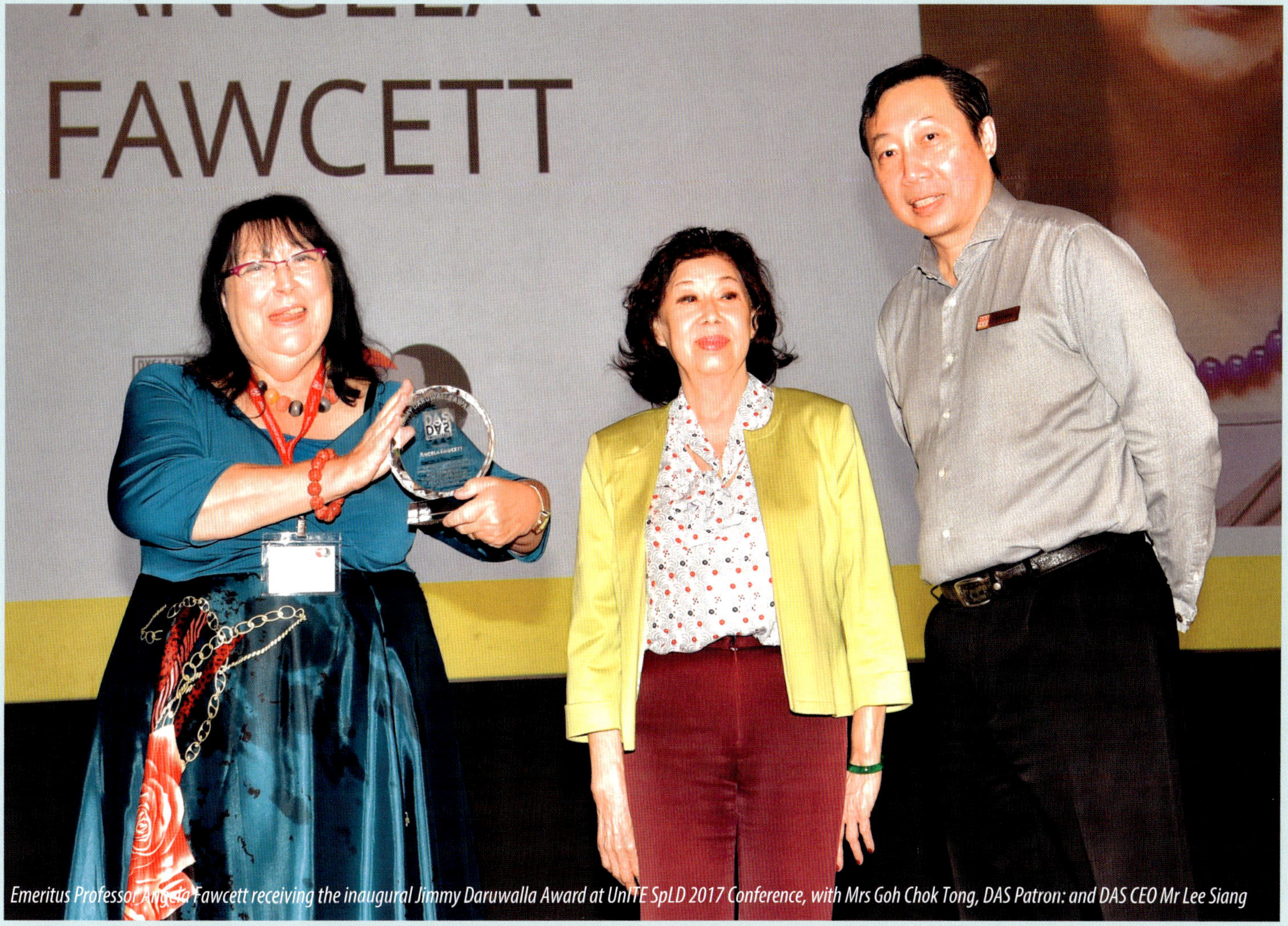

Emeritus Professor Angela Fawcett receiving the inaugural Jimmy Daruwalla Award at UnITE SpLD 2017 Conference, with Mrs Goh Chok Tong, DAS Patron: and DAS CEO Mr Lee Siang

EMERITUS PROFESSOR ANGELA FAWCETT

I would like to wish you all many heartfelt congratulations on the 25th anniversary of DAS! As DAS Research Consultant, I am extremely proud to be associated with such a force for change for dyslexia in Asia and beyond. I wish you joy and even greater success for the next 25 years!

Emeritus Professor Angela Fawcett
Research Consultant, Dyslexia Association of Singapore

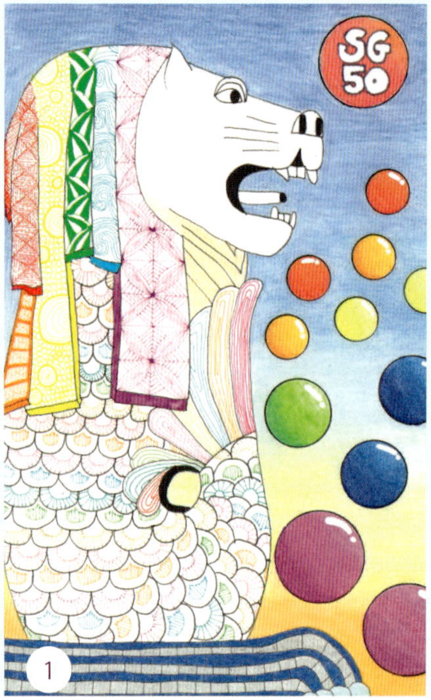

1

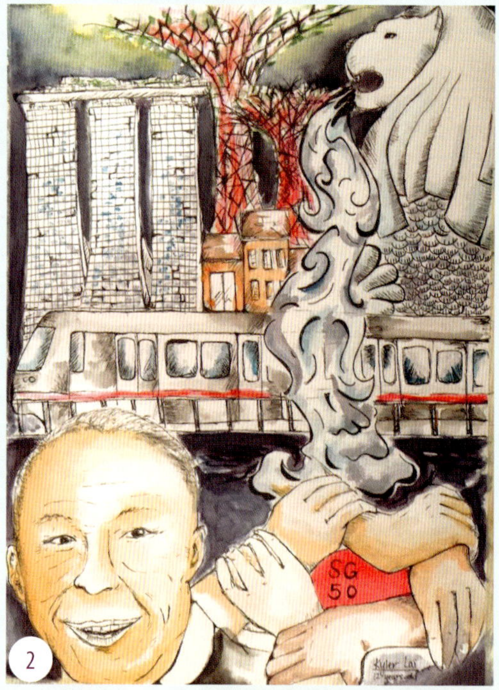

2

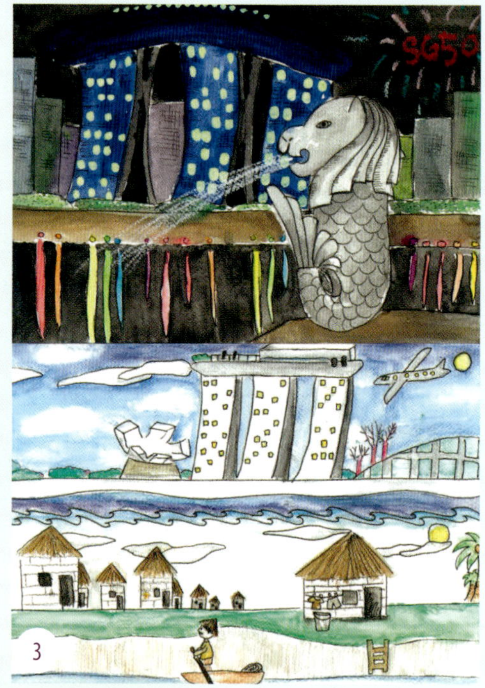

3

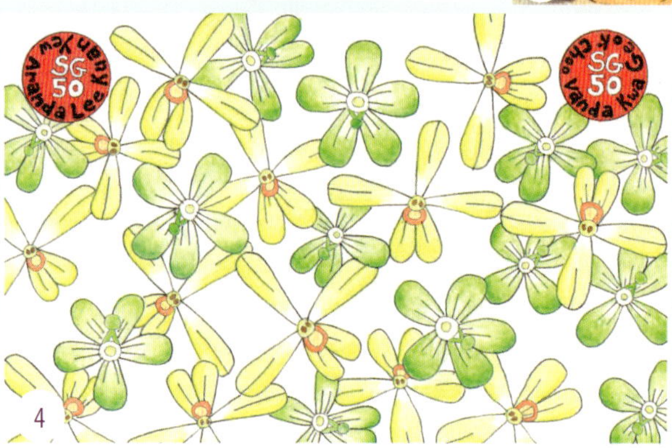

4

5

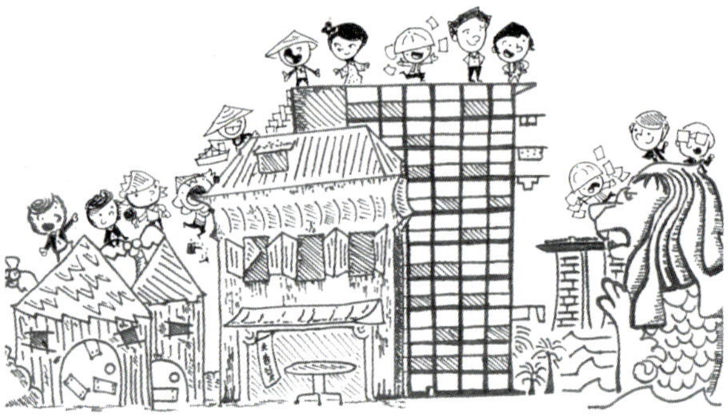

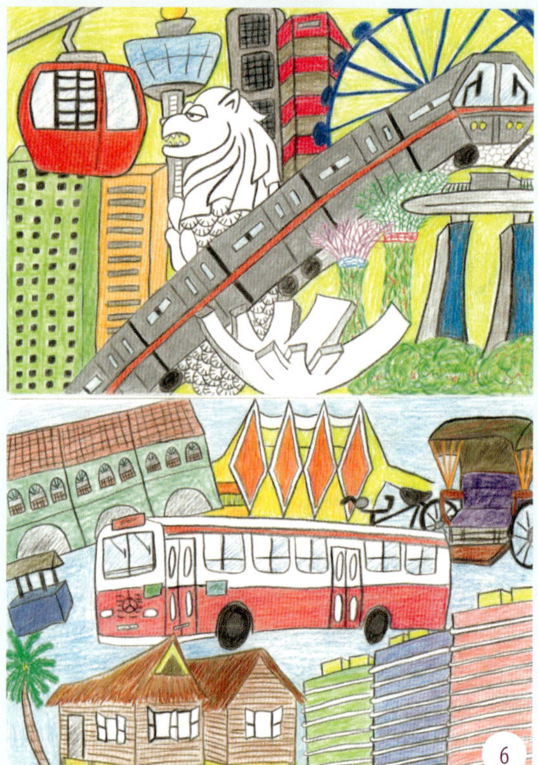

6

EZ-Link—DAS SG50 Card Design Art Competition held in 2015

1. *Yue Jia Xuan, 12*
2. *Kyler Lai, 12*
3. *Casimia Wee Jyen, 12*
4. *Yue Jian Xuan, 12*
5. *William Choo, 15 (Winner—Senior)*
6. *Tang Chun Kit Matthew Hubert, 12 (Winner—Junior)*

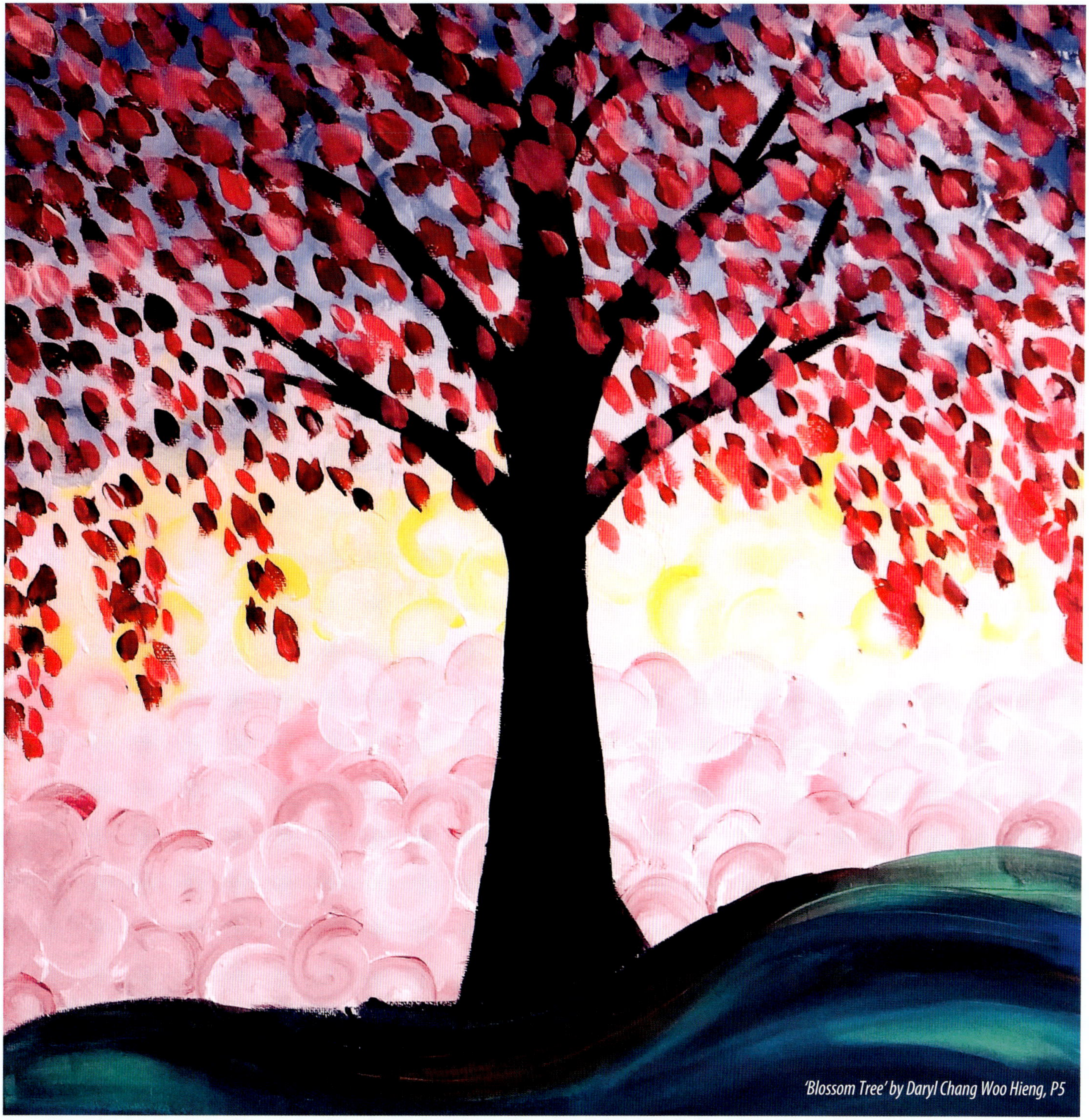

'Blossom Tree' by Daryl Chang Woo Hieng, P5